Ulcerative Colitis: A Complete Study

Ulcerative Colitis:
A Complete Study

Edited by **Eldon Miller**

New Jersey

Published by Foster Academics,
61 Van Reypen Street,
Jersey City, NJ 07306, USA
www.fosteracademics.com

Ulcerative Colitis: A Complete Study
Edited by Eldon Miller

International Standard Book Number: 978-1-63242-413-6 (Hardback)

Printed in the United States of America.

Contents

Preface

In my initial years as a student, I used to run to the library at every possible instance to grab a book and learn something new. Books were my primary source of knowledge and I would not have come such a long way without all that I learnt from them. Thus, when I was approached to edit this book; I became understandably nostalgic. It was an absolute honor to be considered worthy of guiding the current generation as well as those to come. I put all my knowledge and hard work into making this book most beneficial for its readers.

Ulcerative Colitis is a disease in which inflammation develops in the rectum and the colon. This book aims to cater to the needs of readers who hold interest in the field of gastroenterology and specifically, Ulcerative Colitis. It will act as an updated source of reference and knowledge. Reputed experts from distinct specialty fields across the globe have contributed significant amount of information on the disease of Ulcerative Colitis in this extensive book. It is an elaborative source of information comprising of comprehensive data regarding Ulcerative Colitis disease.

I wish to thank my publisher for supporting me at every step. I would also like to thank all the authors who have contributed their researches in this book. I hope this book will be a valuable contribution to the progress of the field.

Editor

Part 1

An Introduction to Ulcerative Colitis

Ulcerative Colitis

Iftikhar Ahmed[1] and Zafar Niaz[2]

[1]*Department of Gastroenterology, University of Bristol / North Bristol NHS Trust, Bristol*
[2]*Mayo Hospital / King Edward Medical University Lahore*
[1]*UK*
[2]*Pakistan*

1. Introduction

Ulcerative colitis (UC) is chronic remitting relapsing disease of gastrointestinal tract which together with Crohn's disease (CD) is often grouped as inflammatory bowel disease (IBD). For a long time, all diarrhoeal diseases were believed to be caused by infectious agents such as bacteria. In 1875 Wilks and Moxon for the first time described UC as a separate entity different from infectious colitis [1]. Later in 1960, formal criteria to differentiate UC from CD were established. UC has an annual incidence of 10-20 per 100,000 compared to 5-10 per 100,000 for CD, however these data are generally considered to be an underestimate [2, 3]. It predominantly affects younger population with a peak incidence between ages 20-40 yrs, however they may affect any age group; and up to 15% of individuals are above 60 yrs of age at the time of diagnosis. Currently IBD is estimated to affect as many as 1.4 million people in the United States and 2.2 millions in Europe [3]. UC usually causes continuous mucosal inflammation and is confined to the large bowel, except in a minority of patients where involvement extends to the terminal ileum, called "backwash ileitis". Bloody diarrhoea, abdominal pain and passage of rectal mucous and blood are the predominant presenting symptoms of UC. In addition, extra-intestinal manifestations are also prevalent in UC although less common than CD; the most common being rheumatological (ankylosing spondylitis, axial arthritis), dermatological (erythema nodosum, pyoderma gangrenosum), and ophthalmological (scleritis, episcleritis) [4]. A small subgroup of patients (approximately 10%) have disease affecting colon with histological features of both CD and UC which is termed as indeterminate colitis [5].

2. Epidemiology

Epidemiological studies have revealed gender-related differences in UC with a slight predominance of males. It is traditionally considered to be most common in Western countries and least common in Asian pacific region, however its low incidence in the later is considered to be due to under-diagnosis and its overlap with infective diarrhoea [6]. The incidence of UC has increased markedly in the West since 1950s. The increase in the incidence of UC precedes that of CD by about 15-20 years [7]. Geographically, the prevalence of the disease has a gradient from North to South and, to a lesser degree, from West to East. The Western-Eastern discrepancy can be attributed to urbanization and a difference in Western lifestyles [8].

The incidence of the disease has been increasing worldwide of late, but the rate of increase has been slowing in highly affected countries [9]. Racial and ethnic observations in different populations reflect genetic, inherited, environmental and behavioural factors. The disease seems to have a characteristic racial-ethnic distribution: blacks are less affected by the UC than whites and the Jewish population is highly susceptible to both UC and CD everywhere, but its prevalence in a particular population nears that of the domestic society in which they live [10]. A study from northern England suggested that the prevalence of UC in 1995 was as high as 243 cases per 100,000 persons [2]. Recent data from Cardiff, UK showed that incidence of CD continue to rise slowly with female preponderance [11], and a similar trend has been seen in juvenile onset CD and UC in Scotland [12].

3. Aetiology

Despite progress in our understanding of its immunopathogenesis, the exact aetiology of UC remains elusive and appears to be polygenic and multifactorial. It is postulated that there is chronic activation of immune and inflammatory cascade in genetically susceptible individual. Environmental factors play a significant role in the disease manifestation, course and prognosis of UC. A rapid increase in its incidence in developed countries, the occurrence of UC in spouses and a lack of complete concordance in monozygotic twins are strong arguments for the role of environmental factors in UC. Observations on temporal trends and geographical distribution point to risk factors associated with a Western lifestyle. Many studies have specifically looked for involvement of factors such as diet, smoking, and several infectious agents but, so far, only smoking cessation can be considered established risk factors for the manifestation of the disease [13]. A strong negative association between appendectomy and UC has been found consistently across many studies; however, the implications of this finding are still obscure [14].

Interaction of these various factors (environmental, microbial and immunological) contributes to the development of chronic intestinal inflammation in a genetically susceptible host. Genetic susceptibility is influenced by the luminal microbiota, which provides antigens and adjuvant that stimulate either pathogenic or protective immune responses.

The gut microbiota has been known to be involved in the induction and perpetuation of immune-mediated bowel inflammation for a long time and the most revealing evidence for its potential involvement came from the study of genetically engineered mice in which colitis did not develop if mice were kept in a germ-free environment [15],[16]. More importantly, UC preferentially occurs in the colon which contains the highest intestinal bacterial concentrations. Moreover, the composition and function of microbiota in UC, and pouchitis are abnormal. Such evidence points towards a strong association between mucosal microbiota and the development of CD. However, few investigators have examined in depth the involvement of disturbed intestinal microbiota composition in the pathogenesis of IBD. This is due to the difficulty in culturing relevant bacteria by conventional means. Over half of the intestinal bacteria are almost impossible to culture; their characterisation requires complex, labour-intensive, and time-consuming methods [17]. Furthermore, identifying bacterial strains can be inaccurate and determining the strain abundance can be difficult.

More recently, the development of advanced molecular techniques has shown a breakdown in the balance between putative "protective" and "harmful" intestinal bacteria [18], [19]. The decreased concentration of protective bacteria that produce short chain fatty acid (SCFA) such as butyrate can enhance mucosal permeability. Conversely, increased concentration of harmful bacteria might increases the production of toxic metabolites such as hydrogen sulfide that increase mucosal permeability and block butyrate metabolism. The increase in mucosal permeability may lead to activation of pathogenic T cell mediated and innate immune response through exposure of bacterial TLR ligands and antigen [20].

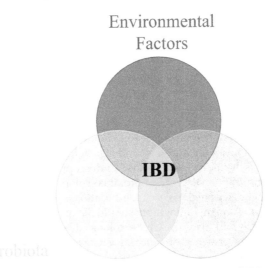

Fig. 1. Possible etiological mechanisms for the development of IBD

Altered composition of gut microbiota has been demonstrated by many studies both in CD and UC and also in pouchitis [21]. There is an increase in gut Enterobacteria mainly *E. Coli* [22], [23] and decrease in the Firmicutes in IBD, although no fundamental difference between CD and UC was found [22],[24] some studies demonstrated microbial difference in active and inactive disease [23], [25].

Other possible mechanisms by which gut microbiota can play a role in immune mediated intestinal injury are; functional alteration in commensal bacteria (such as increased epithelial adherence, mucosal invasion, and resistant to killing) [26], defective containment of commensal bacteria where by defective killing of phagocytosed bacterial and ineffective clearance of bacterial antigen provide a persistent source of mucosal immune stimulation [27] and exaggerated mucosal immune response to commensal bacteria due to discoordinated homeostatic mechanism in intestinal epithelial cells [28] .

4. Diagnosis

Diagnosis of UC is based on clinical assessment followed by a combination of biochemical, endoscopic, radiological, histological, or nuclear medicine based investigations. Endoscopy with histology is considered to be the so called "gold standard" diagnostic modality

History: Important aspects in history of patients with UC are duration and severity of symptoms, recent travel, medication, smoking, family history, stool frequency and consistency, urgency, rectal bleeding, abdominal pain, malaise, fever, weight loss, and symptoms of extra-intestinal manifestations. Majority of patients presents with diarrhoea with or without blood, urgency abdominal pain, rectal bleed and systemic illness. The pattern of symptoms is usually depends on the extent of bowel involvement. For example, patients with pan-colitis are usually systemically ill and present with abdominal pain and bloody diarrhoea compared to those with limited colitis who remains systemically well despite similar symptoms of bloody diarrhoea.

Examination: Examination findings may suggest the severity of disease and extent of involvement. For example, patient with limited colitis and mild disease may have no specific clinical findings on examination and will be systemically well as compared to those with severe disease who may be systemically unwell, hypotensive, tachycardic and may have generalised abdominal tenderness on examination.

Investigation: Initial laboratory workup includes full blood count (FBC), U&Es, liver function tests, and erythrocyte sedimentation rate (ESR) or C reactive protein (CRP), and microbiological testing for infectious diarrhoea including *Clostridium difficile* toxin. Abdominal radiography is also important in patients with suspected severe UC.

Endoscopic investigation: A flexible sigmoidoscopy should be performed to confirm the diagnosis. It enables taking biopsies for histology and also helps excluding other causes for diarrhoea such as infective, ischemic or CMV colitis. Endoscopic changes characteristically extend in continuous fashion from anal verge to proximal colon. Full colonoscopy in acute severe colitis is not recommended as high risks of complications.

Radiological investigations: A plan radiograph should be performed on admission to estimate the extent of disease and also to exclude colonic dilatation. Certain features on abdominal radiograph such as presence of mucosal islands or more than two gas-filled loops of small bowel may suggest severity of the disease and may predict poor response to medical treatment [29].

Generally large bowel radiology is inferior to endoscopy in the diagnosic evaluation of UC but double contrast barium enemas; CT or MRI (with or without contrast) may have a place where endoscopy is contraindicated or unsuitable. Ultrasound scanning is very sensitive for thickened bowel wall in slimmer patients. Capsule endoscopy and white cell scanning lack sensitivity and specificity.

Depending upon the extent of bowel involvement, the disease can be categorized as follows:

- **Proctitis:** Where disease is limited to the rectum only
- **Left sided:** disease involvement limited to the proportion of the colon distal to the splenic flexure
- **Extensive Colitis:** Where bowel involvement extend proximal to the splenic flexure including Pancolitis

Majority of patients have long standing diarrhoea before the diagnosis of UC is eventually made.

The main differential is infective colitis, ischemic colitis, CMV colitis and drug induced colitis.

5. Management

Management is usually depends upon the severity, complexity and extent of disease. No treatment is an option in case of very mild and limited disease. In this section, we discuss in more detail the therapeutic options in sever UC and briefly about mild and moderate disease.

5.1 Management of severe colitis

Acute severe colitis is a serious and life threatening emergency and in about 10% of all newly diagnosed cases, the first presentation is with acute severe colitis. Early recognition and prompt start of treatment is vital to the successful management and prevention of complications. Prior to the discovery of steroids in 1955 the mortality of acute severe UC was described to be as high as 33% in some studies and 75% in other study [30]. Early use of intravenous steroids has reduced the mortality to 7 % and even <1% in specialized centre [31].

Several criteria are in use to define severe colitis. One of the simple and most commonly used criteria is proposed by Truelove and Witts as shown in the table 1.

	Mild UC	Moderate	Severe
Bloody stool / day	< 4	4-6	> 6
Pulse	< 90	90 - 100	> 100
Temp	< 37.5°C	≤ 37.8 °C	>37.8 °C
Hb	>11.5g/dl	> 10.5g/dl	< 10.5 g/dl
ESR	< 20mm /h	< 30 mm/h	> 30 mm/h
CRP	Normal	< 30mg/L	> 30 mg/L
Albumin	Normal	30 - 35	< 30

Table 1. Truelove & Witts criteria for severity of UC [32]

A thorough clinical assessment is important to identify patients at risks and immediate admission to hospital is warranted for all those fulfilling the Truelove and Witts' criteria for severe colitis [32] . Differential diagnosis for these patients will include infective, ischaemic, drug-induced and other inflammatory causes of colitis. Routine lab investigation such as full blood count, electrolyte and liver function tests and inflammatory markers along with plain abdominal radiograph should be carried out and a faecal specimen should be sent to exclude infective causes including C-Difficile. If the mucosa on a plain abdominal radiograph is unremarkable, a sensible approach is to treat decisively with corticosteroids, review the patient within a few days and admit for intensive treatment if there is no improvement. Early sigmoidoscopy and biopsy should be performed as part of the initial assessment of the patient. Biopsies confirm the severity of the inflammation and allow other diagnoses such as cytomegalovirus (CMV), indicated by viral inclusion bodies, to be excluded. CMV colitis can mimic UC and is thought to be responsible for treatment failure in up to 10% of patients labelled as steroid-refractory. Treatment of CMV may obviate colectomy. Care should be taken to monitor and correct electrolytes on a daily basis as almost every patient with severe colitis becomes hypokalaemic during intensive treatment as a result of loss through bowel in the form of diarrhoea and also intensive therapy with steroids contribute to the development of hypokalaemia. Since acute UC is associated with higher risk of venous thromboembolism, unfractionated heparin should be administered for prophylaxis purposes.

5.2 Corticosteroids
Steroids remain the treatment of choice in severe UC and usually given as intravenous Hydrocortisone 100mg four times a day. Early use of IV steroids has shown a significant reduction in mortality and therefore, should not be delayed whilst awaiting microbiological results for possible infective causes. IV treatment is best given for about 5 days while monitoring parameters for response objectively and on satisfactory response to IV steroids; oral Prednisolone can be instituted at 40 mg daily dose and tapered down gradually. It is important to attain a full remission before beginning tapering of steroids or rapid recurrence of symptoms may ensue [33].

Approximately 60% of patients will only show partial response to corticosteroids which can be predicted through objective measures such as lack of clinical improvement and persistent raised inflammatory markers [34]. At presentation, low albumin, high CRP, short duration of illness and prior steroid use all portend an increased risk of medical failure. In an analysis of 189 patients with acute severe UC, a stool frequency >9 in the first 24 h, an albumin <30 g/l or a pulse rate >90 beats per minute after 24 hours of IV steroid was predictive of a 62% failure rate to steroids. Similarly in another prospective study, a stool frequency > 8/day or CRP > 45 mg/l on day 3 of intensive therapy were predictive of the need for colectomy in 85% during that admission [35]. In case of failure of treatment with IV steroids, early use of Ciclosporin or Infliximab is now considered a rescue therapy in order to prevent colectomy.

5.3 Ciclosporin
Ciclosporin is a calcineurin inhibitor and prevents a cascade of downstream events that are necessary for T-cell activation and proliferation.

It is used in an attempt to prevent surgery when intravenous corticosteroids have failed to induce a response [36] or in those with contraindication or intolerance of steroids due to psychoses, severe osteoporosis, uncontrolled diabetes or patient preference . It is usually started after steroid failure preferable on day 3 when little or no response is seen with IV steroids, and is converted to oral cyclosporine 5 mg/kg once a response has occurred. Oral ciclosporin is then generally continued for about 3 months, and azathioprine or mercaptopurine (6-MP) introduced to maintain remission once the steroid dose tapers below 20 mg/day.

5.4 Infliximab
Infliximab is a monoclonal antibody to tumour necrosis factor-α (TNFα) and is established treatment in active CD. In cases of UC, there are only few small trials which have shown its use in case of steroid failure. The recently published Active Ulcerative Colitis Trials (ACTs) 1 and 2 support the use of Infliximab in moderately active UC refractory to aminosalicylates,

steroids or thiopurines [37]. Infliximab has emerged a promising therapeutic option in circumstances where intravenous steroids show signs of failing.

5-aminosalcylic acid (5-ASA) drugs are of little use during severe attacks of colitis and their role is usually reserved for maintenance of remission. Use of opioids and anticholinergic medication should be avoided during the acute attack in order to prevent development of megacolon, and NSAIDs should also be ceased.

5.5 Surgery

Surgical therapy requires a mutual decision by patient, surgeon and physician with consideration of optimum timing and remains a definitive procedure for the treatment of UC. Early involvement of an experienced colorectal surgical team with the gastroenterologist is crucial in decision-making. Close liaison with a stoma therapist is also necessary for continued education, support and postoperative follow-up.

The most commonly performed procedure is a subtotal colectomy and ileostomy initially which later on followed by an elective completion proctectomy and the formation of an ileal-pouch anal anastomosis (IPAA). With timely surgery, a marked improvement in clinical condition is noted within a short span after colectomy. It improves quality of life, provide confidence and control in >90%, allow patients to stop immunomodulators and prevent the long-term risk of cancer. Most follow-up studies of patients undergoing IPAA report an average of six bowel motions per day, but up to 50% experience episodes of faecal leakage at some stage

Surgery is associated with certain complications such as small bowel obstruction, anastomotic stricture, pouch leak and pelvic abscesses, and some late complications such as pouchitis. However, this has to be balanced against the poor outcome of medical therapy in patients who have had an episode of severe colitis.

5.6 Management of Left sided UC

The ECCO guidelines suggest that left sided UC with mild to moderate severity should be initially treated with combined oral and topical mesalazine therapy. Higher doses of mesalazine, usually a daily dose of 4.8gm is more effective than lower doses of 2.4 gm daily. The treatment does of topical mesalazine is usually 1gm daily and various studies have shown no additional benefits with higher topical doses. Treatment with systemic steroids is reserved for cases not responding to combined mesalazine therapy. A usually starting dose of Prednisolone is 40mg daily for 2 weeks which is then tapered down by 5 mg every week. Topical steroids are reserved for patients who are intolerant to topical mesalazine.

5.7 Management of limited UC

The preferred treatment for active proctitis is with topical therapy either with 5ASA based suppository or enema or steroid based enema. The usual daily dose of mesalazine suppositories is 1gm per day and is considered to be better in proctitis than enema. Various studies have shown topical mesalazine to be twice as effective as topical steroids in inducing remission. Therefore, mesalazine suppositories are recommended as first line treatment for active Proctitis while topical steroids are reserved for those who are less responsive or intolerant to topical mesalazine.

A significant proportion of patients with left sided UC or proctitis either remain refractory to treatment with 5ASA medication and steroids or are steroid dependant. Patients refractory to initial treatment would require more intensive treatment such as Infliximab, cyclosporine or Tacrolimus. Those who are steroid dependant would be a candidate for immunosuppressant and Azathioprin has shown better efficacy than mesalazine in inducing and maintaining remission in this groups of patient.

A careful evaluation of patients who remain symptomatic despite initial treatment with mesalazine and or steroids is important and other causes such IBS and CMV colitis with a review of the diagnosis should be considered. Poor compliance with medication is another aspect which should be considered while dealing with treatment refractory patients.

6. References

[1] Wilks S Moxon W *et al.* Lectures on pathological anatomy (Lindsay and Blakiston, Philadelphia) 1875;2nd Edition:408-9.

[2] G. P. Rubin *et al.* Inflammatory bowel disease: epidemiology and management in an English general practice population. *Alimentary Pharmacology & Therapeutics* 2000;14:1553-9.

[3] Loftus EV. Clinical epidemiology of inflammatory bowel disease: incidence, prevalence, and environmental influences. *Gastroenterology* 2004;126:1504-17.

[4] Larsen S, Bendtzen K, Nielsen OH. Extraintestinal manifestations of inflammatory bowel disease: Epidemiology, diagnosis, and management. *Ann Med.* 2010, 422:97-114.

[5] Mitchell P, Rabau M, Haboubi N. Indeterminate colitis. *Techniques in Coloproctology* 2007;11:91-6.

[6] Ahuja V, Tandon RK. Inflammatory bowel disease in the Asia–Pacific area: A comparison with developed countries and regional differences. *Journal of Digestive Diseases*;11:134-47.

[7] Molinie F, Gower-Rousseau C, Yzet T, *et al.* Opposite evolution in incidence of Crohn's disease and ulcerative colitis in Northern France (1988-1999). *Gut* 2004;53:843-8.

[8] Shivananda S, Logan R, EC-IBD Study Group. Incidence of inflammatory disease across Europe: is there a difference between north and south? *Gut* 1996;39:690-7.

[9] Loftus JEV, Silverstein MD, Sandborn WJ, *et al.* Crohn's disease in Olmsted County, Minnesota, 1940-1993: Incidence, prevalence, and survival. *Gastroenterology* 1998;114:1161-8.

[10] Niv Y, Abuksis G, Fraser GM. Epidemiology of Crohn's disease in Israel: a survey of Israeli kibbutz settlements. *The American Journal of Gastroenterology* 1999;94:2961-5.

[11] S. Gunesh *et al.* The incidence of Crohn's disease in Cardiff over the last 75 years: an update for 1996-2005. *Alimentary Pharmacology & Therapeutics* 2008;27:211-9.

[12] Armitage E, Hazel E.; Wilson, David C.; Ghosh, S. Increasing incidence of both juvenile-onset Crohn's disease and ulcerative colitis in Scotland. *European Journal of Gastroenterology & Hepatology* 2001;13:1439-47.

[13] van der Heide F, Dijkstra A, Weersma RK, *et al.* Effects of active and passive smoking on disease course of Crohn's disease and ulcerative colitis. *Inflammatory Bowel Diseases* 2009;15:1199-207.

[14] Koutroubakis IE, Kouroumalis EA. Role of appendicitis and appendectomy in the pathogenesis of ulcerative colitis: a critical review. *Inflamm Bowel Dis* 2002;8:277-86.

[15] Sartor RB, Rath HC, Lichtman SN, *et al.* Animal models of intestinal and joint inflammation. *Baillière's Clinical Rheumatology* 1996;10:55-76.

[16] Sartor RB. Therapeutic manipulation of enteric microflora in IBD: antibiotic, probiotic and prebiotic. *Gastroenterology.* 2004; 126(6): 1620-33.

[17] Suau A, Bonnet R, Sutren M, *et al.* Direct Analysis of Genes Encoding 16S rRNA from Complex Communities Reveals Many Novel Molecular Species within the Human Gut. 1999:4799-807.

[18] Takaishi H, Matsuki T, Nakazawa A, *et al.* Imbalance in intestinal microflora constitution could be involved in the pathogenesis of inflammatory bowel disease. *Int J Med Microbiol* 2008;298:463-72.

[19] Sokol H, Seksik P, Rigottier-Gois L, *et al.* Specificities of the fecal microbiota in inflammatory bowel disease. *Inflamm Bowel Dis* 2006;12:106-11.

[20] Thomas C, Dirk H. Bacteria- and host-derived mechanisms to control intestinal epithelial cell homeostasis: Implications for chronic inflammation. *Inflamm Bowel Dis* 2007, 13(9);1153-1164.

[21] Bibiloni R, Mangold M, Madsen KL, *et al.* The bacteriology of biopsies differs between newly diagnosed, untreated, Crohn's disease and ulcerative colitis patients. *J Med Microbiol.* 2006, 55:1141-9.

[22] Frank DN, St. Amand AL, Feldman RA, *et al.* Molecular-phylogenetic characterization of microbial community imbalances in human inflammatory bowel diseases. *Proc Natl Acad Sci USA.* 2007:13780-5.

[23] Baumgart M, Dogan B, Rishniw M, *et al.* Culture independent analysis of ileal mucosa reveals a selective increase in invasive Escherichia coli of novel phylogeny relative to depletion of Clostridiales in Crohn's disease involving the ileum. *ISME J* 2007;1:403-18.

[24] Kotlowski R, Bernstein CN, Sepehri S, *et al.* High prevalence of Escherichia coli belonging to the B2+D phylogenetic group in inflammatory bowel disease. *Gut* 2007,56(5):669-75.

[25] Darfeuille-Michaud A, Boudeau J, Bulois P, *et al.* High prevalence of adherent-invasive Escherichia coli associated with ileal mucosa in Crohn's disease. *Gastroenterology* 2004;127:412-21.

[26] Korzenik JR. Is Crohn's disease due to defective immunity? *Gut.* 2007,56(1):2-5.

[27] Xavier RJ, Podolsky DK. Unravelling the pathogenesis of inflammatory bowel disease. *Nature* 2007;448:427-34.

[28] Sartor RB. Mechanisms of Disease: pathogenesis of Crohn's disease and ulcerative colitis. *Nat Clin Pract Gastroenterol Hepatol* 2006;3:390-407.

[29] Prantera C LR, Cerro P *et al.* The plain abdominal film accurately estimates the extent of activity in ulcerative colitis. *J Clin Gastroenterol* 1991;13:321-4.

[30] Bulmer T *et al.* Ulcerative Colitis-A survey of ninety five cases. *British Medical Journal* 1933;2:812-5.

[31] Rice-Oxley JM *et al.* Ulcerative colitis: course and prognosis. *Lancet* 1950;1:663-6.

[32] Truelove SC, Witts L. Cortisone in ulcerative colitis: final report on a therapeutic trial. *British Medical Journal* 1955;2:1041-8.

[33] Rosenberg W, Jewell DP. High-dose methylprednisolone in the treatment of active ulcerative colitis. *J Clin Gastroenterol* 1990;12:40-1.

[34 Hawthorne AB *et al.* The BSG IBD Clinical Trials Network. Outcome of inpatient management of severe ulcerative colitis. *Gut* 2002;16:50.

[35] Travis SP, Farrant JM, Ricketts C, *et al.* Predicting outcome in severe ulcerative colitis. Gut. 1996, 38(6):905-10.

[36] Lichtiger S, Present DH, Kornbluth A, *et al.* Cyclosporine in Severe Ulcerative Colitis Refractory to Steroid Therapy. *N Engl J Med* 1994; 330:1841-1845

[37] Rutgeerts P, Sandborn WJ, Feagan BG, *et al.* Infliximab for Induction and Maintenance Therapy for Ulcerative Colitis. 2005:2462-76.

Proteomic Approaches for Biomarker Discovery in Ulcerative Colitis

Manae S. Kurokawa[1], Moriaki Hatsugai[2], Yohei Noguchi[2],
Takuya Yoshioka[1], Hiroyuki Mitsui[3], Hiroshi Yasuda[2] and Tomohiro Kato[1]

[1]*Clinical Proteomics and Molecular Medicine,*
St. Marianna University Graduate School of Medicine,
[2]*Division of Gastroenterology and Hepatology, Department of Internal Medicine,*
St. Marianna University School of Medicine,
[3]*Department of Orthopaedic Surgery, St. Marianna University School of Medicine,*
Kawasaki
Japan

1. Introduction

Ulcerative colitis (UC) as well as Crohn's disease (CD) is one of the major inflammatory bowel diseases (IBD). Although genetic (1), infectious (2), and immunological (3, 4) factors have been reported to be involved in the pathogenesis of UC, the precise etiology remains unclear. UC is now diagnosed based on clinical, radiologic, endoscopic and histopathological findings. Thus, biomarkers for UC have been vigorously explored to diagnose UC accurately and non-invasively. The most clinically useful biomarker for UC at present is perinuclear anti-neutrophil cytoplasmic antibodies (p-ANCA) which is detected in 50-80% of UC patients (5). However, p-ANCA is also detected in 10-40% of CD patients, 30-80% of patients with microscopic polyangiitis, 30-75% of patients with Churg-Strauss syndrome and 50% of patients with rapid progressive glomerulonephritis (5-7). A more sensitive and specific biomarker for UC should be established.

Recently, there have been great advances in proteomics, the science dealing with the comprehensive analysis of protein expression. Proteomics have been applied to search of biomarkers in various diseases (8-10). In this paper, we introduced proteomic studies which explored biomarkers for UC by analyzing proteins in various clinical samples such as sera, peripheral blood mononuclear cells (PBMCs) and colonic mucosa. The comprehensive study can detect unexpected and sometimes novel molecules as a biomarker, which may also lead to elucidation of the pathogenesis of UC.

1.1 Representative methods for proteomics

As an assembly of genes is called as genome (gene + ome), an assembly of proteins is named as proteome (protein + ome). An assembly of low molecular proteins (peptides) is specifically called as peptidome (peptide + ome) (11). Proteomics are the study to comprehensively analyze proteome. There are two major methods for proteomics, 2-dimensional electrophoresis (2DE) and shotgun method (Fig.1).

A. 2-dimensional electrophoresis (2DE)

Extraction of whole proteins from cells or tissue
↓
Isoelectric focusing
↓
Sodium dodecyl sulfate-polyaclylamide gel electrophoresis (SDS-PAGE)
↓
Detection of individual proteins as spots
↓
Comparison of individual protein spot intensity between disease A and disease B
↓
Cut out the gel of the protein spots of interest
↓
In gel digestion of the proteins by a protease
↓
Identification of the proteins by mass spectrometry (MS) and protein database search

B. Shotgun method

Extraction of whole proteins from cells or tissue
↓
Digestion of the mixture of proteins with a protease
↓
Fractionating the obtained peptides by liquid chromatography
↓
Analysis of individual peptides by MS/MS method to identify the original proteins

Fig. 1. Representative methods for proteomics.
The outlines of 2DE and shotgun method are described

2DE is the method to separate cell- or tissue-derived proteins into protein spots by isoelectric focusing and subsequent sodium dodecyl sulfate-polyaclylamide gel electrophoresis (SDS-PAGE) (Fig.2). After the 2DE, protein spots of interest are cut out, and the proteins contained in the spots are identified by mass spectrometry (MS). Both matrix-assisted laser desorption/ionization time-of-flight mass spectrometer (MALDI-TOF/MS) and liquid chromatography-mass spectrometer (LC-MS) are mainly used for the identification. One advantage of 2DE is to visualize the proteome of targeted cells or tissue as protein spots. A representative case is 2-dimensional differential image gel electrophoresis (2D-DIGE) which displays 2 kinds of proteome with different fluoresceines on the same gel (9). 2D-DIGE can visualize and compare proteome of two different samples, for examples, between a patient and a healthy donor, and before and after treatment with a drug. The other advantage of 2DE is to detect at least a part of the difference of post-translational modification, amino acid mutation, and isotypes of one protein as different spots. Disadvantages of 2DE are that it is laborious requiring many manual procedures, and that number of detectable proteins is limited because proteins with low expression levels and with extremely high or low molecular weights/isoelectric points are not visualized and separated, respectively. However, automation of 2DE has been recently developed, and use of a longer isoelectric focusing gel has increased number of detected proteins to achieve more comprehensiveness.

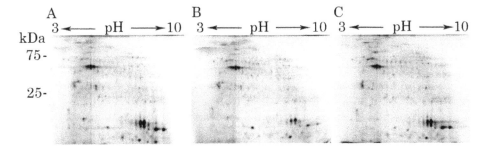

Fig. 2. 2DE analysis of a UC patient.
PBMCs were obtained from patients with UC, CD, and from a healthy subject, and proteins were extracted from the cells to be separated by 2DE. Representative results of a UC patient (A), a CD patient (B), and a healthy subject are shown. pI, isoelectric points; MW, molecular weights

In the shotgun method, mixture of proteins extracted from cells or tissue is digested with a protease. When protein profiles of several disease groups are compared, proteins are sometimes labeled by isotopes such as iTRAQ and ICAT. The obtained peptide mixture was fractionated by liquid chromatography (LC) to be finally analyzed by MS/MS method (LC-MS/MS). To fractionate minutely, 2D-HPLC is useful, for example, using a combination of strong cation exchange column and reverse-phase column. Surface enhanced laser desorption/ionization (SELDI)-TOF/MS is also used, in which proteins/peptides are trapped by radicals and molecules immobilized on protein chips to be directly measured by the MS system. The shotgun method has advantages to detect proteins with low expression levels, to achieve high comprehensiveness because of no limitation of isoelectric points, molecular weights, and hydrophilicity, and to automatize the procedures from fractionation to mass spectrometry. However, the proteome is not visualized, and nature of the original proteins remains unknown in this method.

1.2 Discovery of biomarkers for UC
Proteomic studies using sera, PBMCs, and colonic mucosa have found biomarker candidates for UC by comparison of UC, CD, other colitis, and healthy condition. Comprehensive analysis of a number of proteins makes multivariate analysis possible, which raises not only one protein but a combination of multiple proteins as a biomarker for UC.

2. Serum proteomics

A serum sample is one of the most frequently used clinical samples, which is obtained with low invasiveness. It contains a number of proteins which are physiologically and pathologically important. Serum samples would be an excellent source for the surveillance of biomarker candidates.

As a conventional proteomic study using MALDI-TOF/MS, Nanni et al analyzed serum protein profiles of UC patients, CD patients, and healthy subjects (12). The profiles of 20 peptides extracted based on hydrophobic interaction completely classified all the cases into the original three groups, and UC was predicted with 96.3% prediction ability by cross validation of the classification model. In this study, the 20 peptides were not identified. In contrast, three studies analyzing serum proteins by SELDI-TOF-MS identified the biomarker candidates (Table 1) (13-15). Subramanian et al analyzed sera from UC and CD patients, and detected 12 discriminative peaks with both specificity and sensitivity of approximately 95% (13). Six out of the 12 proteins were identified, including inter alpha trypsin inhibitor 4, apolipoprotein C1, and platelet activated factor 4 variants. Meuwis et al generated classification models by multivariate analysis, whose sensitivity and specificity to discriminate UC from CD were approximately 80% and 90%, respectively (14). Four biomarkers with important diagnostic values were identified as platelet aggregation factor 4 (PF4), myeloid related protein 8 (MRP8), fibrinopeptide A (FIBA), and haptoglobin $\alpha2$ (Hp$\alpha2$). Kanmura et al selected human neutrophil peptides 1-3 (HNP 1-3) from the 27 proteins with significantly different concentration between UC and healthy sera (15). In a larger cohort, concentration of HNP 1-3 were significantly higher in active UC patients compared to that in UC patients in remission, CD patients, patients with infectious colitis, and healthy subjects. Levels of HNP 1-3 decreased after corticosteroid therapy in responders for the drug, whereas the levels were not changed in non-responders. As a new method, Haas et al analyzed serum samples from UC and CD patients by Fourier Transform Near-Infrared Spectroscopy (FT-NIR) (16). The cluster and Artificial Neural Networks (ANN) analyses of the results correctly identified 80% and 69.8% of UC, respectively, suggesting a usefulness of this technology. In addition, a pilot study compared sera between corticosteroid-resistant and -responsive UC patients, and detected 19 proteins with significantly different concentration, which may predict response to the treatment in UC (17).

Proteomics include studies using various kinds of protein arrays. Kader et al used antibody arrays containing 78 cytokines, growth factors and soluble receptors to screen sera from UC and CD patients (18). In UC, only IL-12p40 was significantly upregulated in the remission stage compared to in the active stage (p<0.02). On the other hand, in CD, significantly elevated levels of 4 cytokines including IL-12p40 were found in the remission stage compared to in the active stage (p<0.01). The other 3 cytokines were placenta-derived growth factor, IL-7, and TGF-$\beta1$. In another study using protein arrays, Escherichia coli-derived proteome was served to screen serum antibodies (19). A set of antibodies distinguished UC patients from healthy subjects with 66% accuracy (p<0.05). The other antibody set distinguished UC patients from CD patients with 80% accuracy (p<0.01). The latter set consists of only two kinds of antibodies which recognized YidX and Frv X, suggesting that immune reaction to the 2 proteins from E. coli would be useful for discrimination of UC from CD.

It seems to be difficult to find serum autoantibodies which are more powerful than p-ANCA even using proteomic techniques. Vermeulen et al analyzed serum autoantibodies against commercial human protein arrays (20). 75 proteins reacted more strongly with sera from IBD patients than those from healthy subjects, while 88 proteins showed the opposite pattern. One of the identified proteins as an autoantigen for IBD was pleckstrin homology-like domain, family A, member 1 (Phla1). In a large cohort, 42.8% of the UC patients, 50.0% of the CD patients, (taken together, 46% of the IBD patients), 33.3% of the patients with non-IBD gastrointestinal diseases, and 28.7% of the healthy subjects were positive for the anti-

Phla1 antibodies. Thus, discriminative power between UC and CD, and IBD and controls remained low. The same research group also analyzed serum autoantibodies against α-enolase in IBD by a classic proteomic approach (21). The anti-α-enolase antibodies were detected in 49.0% of the UC patients, 50.0% of the CD patients, 37.8% of the patients with autoimmune hepatitis, 34.0% of the patients with ANCA-positive vasculitis, and 31.0% of the patients with the other gastrointestinal diseases, showing the only limited diagnostic value.

References	Samples	Methods	Identified proteins
Subramanian et al (13)	sera	SELDI-TOF MS	inter alpha trypsin inhibitor 4 apolipoprotein C1 platelet activated factor 4 variants
Meuwis et al (14)	sera	SELDI-TOF MS	platelet aggregation factor 4 (PF4) myeloid related protein 8 (MRP8) fibrinopeptide A (FIBA) haptoglobin α2 (Hpα2)
Kanmura et al (15)	sera	SELDI-TOF MS	Human neutrophil peptide (HNP) 1-3
Kader et al (18)	sera	antibody array	IL-12p40 (upregulated in the remission stage than in the active stage in UC)
Chen et al (19)	sera	E. coli-protein array	YidX Frv X
Vermeulen et al (20)	sera	Human protein arrays	autoantibodies against pleckstrin homology-like domain, family A, member 1 (Phla1)
Vermeulen et al (21)	sera		autoantibodies against α-enolase
Hatsugai et al (9)	PBMCs	2DE, MALDI-TOF MS	cyclophilin A (PPIA) protein S100-A9 (S100A9) peroxiredoxin-2 (PRDX2) carbonic anhydrase 2 (CA2) β-actin (ACTB) annexin A6 (ANXA6) α/β Hydrolase domain-sontaining protein 14B (ABHD14B)

Table 1. Blood biomarker candidates for UC

3. Proteomics of PBMCs

PBMCs, relatively easily prepared from the peripheral blood, contain a number of proteins different from serum proteins. Because UC is considered as an autoimmune disease, analysis of PBMCs which include lymphocytes and monocytes is useful not only for the biomarker surveillance but also for the elucidation of the pathogenesis of UC. However, little has been known about the protein profile of PBMCs in UC.

We comprehensively analyzed proteins in PBMCs from UC, focusing on discrimination of UC from CD (9). PBMC-derived proteins from UC patients, CD patients, and healthy subjects were separated by 2DE, and intensity of individual protein spots was subjected to multivariate analysis to generate differential diagnostic models between UC and CD. As a result, 547 protein spots were detected in the 2DE results. Two diagnostic models were generated using intensity of selected 276 protein spots and further selected 58 protein spots, both of which completely discriminated between UC and CD (sensitivity and specificity were 100% in these models). Eleven out of the 58 protein spots were identified, which were functionally related to inflammation (cyclophilin A, PPIA; protein S100-A9, S100A9), oxidation/reduction (peroxiredoxin-2, PRDX2; carbonic anhydrase 2, CA2), cytoskeleton (β-actin, ACTB), endocytotic trafficking (annexin A6, ANXA6), and transcription (α/β Hydrolase domain-sontaining protein 14B, ABHD14B). Interestingly, the PBMC protein profiles were useful for prediction of disease activity in the UC and the CD patients, and prediction of severity and responses to treatments in the UC patients. Especially, some clinical parameters were predicted by intensity of a few protein spots, for example, intensity of only 2 protein spots for disease activity of the UC. Proteins associated with the activity of UC may be extremely restricted. PBMC protein profile would be a potent biomarker for differential diagnosis of UC from CD, and investigation of the proteins contributing to the discrimination may elucidate the different pathophysiology of UC from CD.

As an antigen-specific model, an IBD model was established using male SD rats by colonic administration of trinitrobenzene sulfonic acid (TNBS) in 50% ethanol (22). Lymphocyte-derived protein profiles from the model rats and the control rats receiving 50% ethanol were compared by 2DE and MALDI-TOF/MS, which revealed different expression of 26 proteins (17, upregulated; and 9, downregulated) included regulators of the cell cycle and cell proliferation, signal transduction factors, apoptosis-related proteins and metabolic enzymes.

4. Proteomic analyses of colonic mucosa from UC

Proteomic analysis of colonic mucosa has demonstrated multiple biomarker candidates. The analyses using clinical samples of the disease-affected sites may highly contribute to elucidation of the pathophysiology of UC, indicating functional difference of various proteins from the other gastrointestinal diseases.

Comparing protein profiles between the UC-affected mucosa and normal mucosa both from UC patients by 2DE and subsequent LC-MS, protein spots showing higher intensity in the UC-affected mucosa than in the normal mucosa were identified (23). They were protocadherin, α-1 antitrypsin, tetratrico-peptide repeat domains, caldesmon, and mutated desmin, associated with inflammation and cell repair (Table 2). Especially, a mutated form of desmin was detected in all the examined UC-affected mucosa, suggesting its potential as a UC biomarker. Another study comparing colonic mucosa from UC patients and healthy subjects by 2DE and MALDI-TOF/MS showed 13 downregulated and 6 upregulated proteins in UC (24), which were involved in mitochondrial function (heat shock protein 70, HSP70; HSP60; H+-transporting two sector ATPase, ATP5B; prohibitin, PHB; malate dehydrogenase, MDH2; voltage-dependent anion-selective channel protein 1, VDAC1; thioredoxin peroxidase 1, PRDX1; PRDX2), energy generation (ATP5B, MDH2, triosephosphate isomerase), cellular antioxidants (PRDX1; PRDX2; selenium binding protein 1, SELENBP1), and stress-response (HSP70, HSP60, PRDX1, PRDX2, PHB, VDAC1). Aberrant activation of nuclear factor of activated T cell (NFAT), and ectopic expression of tumor rejection antigen 1 and poliovirus receptor related protein 1 were detected in the UC-affected colonic mucosa.

References	Samples	Methods	Identified proteins
Fogt et al (23)	colonic mucosa	2DE, LC-MS	protocadherin, α-1 antitrypsin, tetratrico-peptide repeat domains, caldesmon, mutated desmin
Hsieh et al (24)	colonic mucosa	2DE, MALDI-TOF/MS	heat shock protein 70 (HSP70), HSP60, H+-transporting two sector ATPase (ATP5B), *prohibitin (PHB)*, malate dehydrogenase 2 (MDH2), voltage-dependent anion-selective channel protein 1 (VDAC1), thioredoxin peroxidase 1 (PRDX1), *PRDX2*, triosephosphate isomerase, selenium binding protein 1 (SELENBP1), nuclear factor of activated T cell (NFAT), tumor rejection antigen 1, poliovirus receptor related protein 1
Shkoda et al (25)	colonic mucosa	2DE, MALDI-TOF/MS	programmed cell death protein 8, annexin 2A (Both increased in inflamed regions)
Shih et al (26)	colonic mucosa	2DE, IHC	Translocation of NFAT2 into nuclei
Berndt et al (27)	T cells in colon	MELC	Colocalization of NF-kB and poly (ADP-ribose)-polymerase
Naito et al (30)	mouse intesitinal mucosa	2DE, MALDI-TOF/MS	3-Hydroxy-3- methlglutaryl-coenzyme A synthase 2, serpin b1a, protein disulfide-isomerase A3, PRDX6, vimentin

Table 2. Biomarker candidates for UC identified from colonic mucosal cells

Comparison with colonic mucosal proteins between UC and CD revealed their specific characters of UC and common features to IBD (25-27). Intestinal epithelial cells (IECs) from patients with UC, CD, and colon cancer, analyzed by 2DE and MALDI-TOF/MS, showed 21 protein spots with at least 2-fold change between inflamed tissue from the IBD (UC and CD) patients and non-inflamed tissue from the patients with colonic cancer (25). The identified proteins were functionally related to signal transduction, stress response, and energy metabolism. Specifically, Rho-GDP dissociation inhibitor α, which inhibits cell cycle progression, was upregulated in IBD and sigmoid diverticulitis, possibly involving with the destruction of IEC homeostasis under the condition of chromic inflammation. On the other hand, 40 proteins were significantly altered between inflamed and noninflamed regions in the UC patients. The proteins included programmed cell death protein 8 and annexin 2A, both of which were increased in the inflamed regions. In addition, localization of the proteins may indicate the pathophysiological difference of UC and CD (26, 27). NFAT2, increased in the UC-affected colon tissue in the 2DE results, was specifically translocated into nuclei of the UC colonic mucosa, whereas NFAT2 was located exclusively in cytoplasm in the normal and the CD mucosa (26). A modified proteomic method, Multi-Epitope Ligand Cartography (MELC), showed that only CD4+ T cells co-expressing NF-kB were caspase-8+ and poly(ADP-ribose)-polymerase+ in the UC colonic mucosa (27). The colocalization of NF-kB+ and poly(ADP-ribose)-polymerase+ would be the base motif that discriminates UC from CD. Interestingly, the number of CD4+CD25+ T cells was elevated only in the UC mucosa, but not in the CD mucosa and the normal mucosa from patients with colonic cancer, suggesting the specific activation of regulatory T cells in UC.

Other modified methods including cellular or subcellular analyses have brought useful information (28, 29). Effects of inflammatory cytokines of IFNγ, IL-1β, and IL-6 on IBD were investigated human adenocarcinoma cells by 2DE and MALDI-TOF/MS (28). Tryptophanyl tRNA synthetase, indoleamine-2,3-dioxygenase (IDO), heterogenous nuclear ribonucleoprotein JKTBP, IFN-induced p35, proteasome subunit LMP2, and arginosuccinate synthetase were identified as the cytokine-regulated proteins. Overexpression of IDO in IECs was found in the UC and CD mucosa, but not in the diverticulitis and normal mucosa, suggesting that the specific response of IDO to the inflammatory cytokines may be a character of IBD. As a subcellular fractionation analysis, expression levels of 5′ nucleotidase (plasma membrane), malate dehydrogenase (mitochondria), catalase (peroxisomes), LDH (ER), N-acetyl-β-glucosaminidase (lysosomes), and neutral-α-glucosidase (ER) in rectal biopsy homogenates from the UC, CD, and non-rectal CD patients were assayed (29). Reduction of both cytosolic and particulate N-acetyl-β-glucosaminidase was found in the UC patients, whereas a selective reduction in particulate activity was found in the non-rectal CD patients, demonstrating lysosomal alterations in these diseases.

IECs from UC or IBD model mice have been analyzed by proteomics (30-33). Intestinal mucosa from a UC mouse model, made by oral administration of 8.0% dextran sodium sulfate, was analyzed by 2DE and MALDI-TOF/MS (30). Comparison of mucosa from the UC model with that from normal mice revealed 7 altered protein spots. Five proteins were identified from the spots, which were 3-Hydroxy-3-methlglutaryl- coenzyme A synthase 2, serpin b1a, protein disulfide-isomerase A3, PRDX6 and vimentin. To investigate response of IECs against a pathogen, Caco-2 IEC line was co-cultured with Enteropathogenic E. coli (EPEC) to be injected the bacterial proteins through bacterial type III secretion system (TTSS) (31). Among 2,090 host proteins identified by LC-MS, 264 proteins (approximately 13%) were differentially expressed between WT EPEC-cocultured IECs and TTSS-deficient EPEC-cocultured IECs, suggesting that host proteins were potentially involved in EPEC-induced colitis.

Based on an interesting idea that endoplasmic reticulum (ER)-mediated stress responses in IECs may contribute to chronic intestinal inflammation, IECs from Enterococcus faecalis-monoassociated IL-10-deficient mice and WT mice were analyzed by 2DE and MALDI-TOF/MS (32). Increased expression of glucose-regulated ER stress protein (grp)-78 was found in the IL-10-deficient mice. In human, the increased expression of grp-78 was also found in the inflamed colonic tissue from patients with UC, CD and sigmoid diverticulitis. IL-10 was found to inhibit inflammation-induced ER stress response by modulating nuclear recruitment of activating transcriptional factor (ATF)-6 to the grp-78 gene promoter. Another interesting idea is raised from the field of neutrinogenomics, in which environmental factors would contribute to the chronic intestinal inflammation in the genetically susceptible hosts (33, 34). In this respect, TNFDeltaARE/WT mice were prepared, which showed impaired regulation of TNFα synthesis by deletion of an AU-rich motif in the 3′-untranslated region of the TNF gene (35). WT and TNFDeltaARE/WT mice were fed with adequate and low amount of iron, and the adequate iron-fed TNFDeltaARE/WT mice were found to develop severe ileal inflammation. Comparison of IEC-derived proteins between adequate iron-fed WT and TNFDeltaARE/WT mice (inflamed conditions), and that between adequate iron- and low iron-fed

TNFDeltaARE/WT mice (absence of inflammation), by 2DE and MALDI-TOF/MS showed 4 contrarily regulated proteins including aconitase 2, catalase, intelectin 1, and fumarylacetoacetate hydrolase (FAH). These proteins are associated with energy homeostasis, host defense, oxidative, and ER stress responses.

5. Prediction of colorectal cancer associated with UC

UC shows an increased risk of colorectal cancer compared to other inflammatory intestinal diseases. In UC patients, occurrence of colorectal cancer is periodically examined by colonoscopy throughout their lives. To avoid this invasive and expensive examination, a biomarker which predicts occurrence of colorectal cancer in UC will be useful. Further, although UC-associated colon cancer is known to develop from dysplastic lesions caused by chronic inflammation, the molecular mechanism how inflammation leads to carcinogenesis should be elucidated.

Brentnall et al analyzed protein profiles of epithelium from normal colon, nondysplastic colon of UC patients without dysplasia (UC nonprogressors), nondysplastic colon of UC patients with high grade dysplasia or cancer (UC progressors), and high grade dysplastic colon of UC progressors by LC-MS subsequent to strong cation exchange (36). Proteins related to mitochondria, oxidative activity, and calcium-binding proteins were associated with the neoplastic progression in UC. In the early and late stages, Sp1 and c-myc may play roles in UC neoplastic progression, respectively (Table 3). Carbamoyl-phophate synthase 1 (CPS1) and S100P were overexpressed in nondysplastic colon tissue from the UC progressors. The overexpression may be useful for the prediction of dysplasia in UC.

In another study from the same research group, differently expressed proteins between nondysplastic and dysplastic tissue from the UC progressors were detected by LC-MS (37). They were mitochondrial proteins, cytoskeletal proteins, RAS superfamily, proteins related to apoptosis and metabolism, suggesting their importance in the early stages of neoplastic progression in UC. Among such proteins, both TNF receptor-associated protein 1 (TRAP1) and CPS1 were increased in nondysplastic and dysplastic tissue in the UC progressors than in the nonprogressors. Rectal CPS1 staining predicts dysplasia or cancer in the colon with 87% sensitivity and 45% specificity, indicating its feasibility as a biomarker to predict colonic dysplasia or cancer. On the other hand, comparison of UC-associated and sporadic colon cancer cell lines by 2DE and LC-MS showed that the expression of heat shock protein (HSP47) was significantly higher in UC-associated colon cancers, the increase of which was correlated to the progression of neoplastic lesions (38). HSP47 was co-expressed with type I collagen in the cytoplasm, and both of them were released from culture cells into the medium, suggesting the possibility of HSP47 as a biomarker for UC-associated cancer.

Analysis of colonic mucosa by MELC study showed significant increase of NF-kB+ HLA-DR+ cells in CD4+ and CD8+ cell populations in UC patents and patients with colorectal cancer compared to healthy subjects (39). This suggested increase of activated T cells and an altered antigen presentation. In the UC group, NF-kB+ cells were significantly increased in CD45RO+ cell populations, but not in CD45RA+ cell population, suggesting the activation in memory T cells. CD4+CD25+NF-kB+ cells were also specifically increased in the UC group, which indicated the increase of regulatory T cells. The specific activation of such subpopulations of T cells would play protective roles in UC, and loss of the activation may play a role in the progression of colorectal cancer. In an animal model for UC, which was established by repeatedly exposing B6 mice to dextran sodium sulfate (DSS), proteins in colonic mucosa were analyzed by 2DE and MALDI-TOF/MS (40). 38 protein spots were found to be differently expressed in colon tumors compared to normal colon, 27 of which were identified. They included glucose-regulated protein (GRP) 94, HSC70, emolase, PHB and transgelin. Transgelin was found to be significantly reduced in human colon tumors compared with adjacent nontumorous tissues, suggesting that low expression of this protein may be a candidate biomarker of colitis-associated colon cancer.

References	Samples	Methods	Identified proteins
Brentnall et al (36)	colonic mucosa	LC-MS	Sp1, *Carbamoyl-phophate synthase 1 (CPS1)*, S100P
May et al (37)	colonic mucosa	LC-MS	TNF receptor-associated protein 1 (TRAP1), *CPS1*
Araki et al (38)	colon cancer cell lines	2DE, LC-MS	heat shock protein (HSP47)
Berndt et al (39)	T cells in colon	MELC	(Increase of CD45RO+NFkB+ cells and increase of CD4+CD25+NFkB+ cells in UC than in colorectal cancer)
Yeo et al (40)	Mouse colonic mucosa	2DE, MALDI-TOF/MS	transgelin (GRP94, HSC70, enolase, *PHB*, and transgelin were differently expressed in colon tumors in the UC-model mice from those in normal colon)

Table 3. Biomarker candidates to predict complication of colorectal cancer in UC

6. Subproteomic analyses – metabolomics and other studies

As subproteomic analyses, metabolomics which comprehensively analyze metabolites have been performed in IBD patients and also in UC model mice. Because metabolites are easily obtained from urine or fecal samples, use of biomarkers detected by metabolomics may be less-invasive compared to those derived from blood and colonic tissue. In addition to MS analysis, nuclear magnetic resonance (NMR) spectroscopy is frequently used in metabolomics. Metabolomics, which analyze different molecular profiles from proteomics, should also contribute to unraveling the pathophysiology of UC.

Fecal extracts from patients with CD and UC were analyzed by 1H NMR spectroscopy (41). The levels of butyrate, acetate, methylamine, and trimethylamine were found to be lower in both diseases than in healthy subjects. The results may indicate changes of microbial community in gut. In contrast, elevated quantities of amino acids were demonstrated in both diseases, implying malabsorption caused by inflammation. Interestingly, the decreased amounts of amino acids and glycerol, and the increase of butyrate and acetate, in the feces of UC patients contributed to the discrimination of UC from CD (Table 4). A conventional metabolic analysis, in which utilization of n-butyrate, glucose, and glutamine in isolated colonic epithelial cells were evaluated, showed that oxidation of butyrate to CO_2 and ketones was significantly suppressed in UC colonic mucosa compared to normal mucosa (42). The failure of n-butyrate oxidation in UC suggests that UC may be an energy-deficiency disease of the colonic mucosa. To specifically distinguish UC from CD, exoprotease activity was assayed using 2 synthetic peptides as substrates, which were fibrinopeptide A without the N-terminal alanine and complement 3f (43). The two peptides were spiked into serum samples from 3 UC patients, 3 CD patients, and 3 healthy subjects, and the metabolite pattern was analyzed by MALDI-MS and chemometric analysis. Although 100% discrimination of the UC patients from the CD patients and the healthy subjects was achieved, the diagnostic power should be verified with more number of subjects.

References	Samples	Methods	Identified metabolites
Marchesi et al (41)	fecal extracts	NMR	decreased amounts of amino acids and glycerol, and increase of *butyrate* and acetate, compared to those in CD
Roediger et al (42)	IECs of colon	Metabolic analysis	decreased oxidation of *butyrate* to CO2 and ketones

Table 4. Biomarker candidates for UC identified by metabolomics

As an IBD model study, time course of urine metabolites from IL-10-deficient mice were compared with those from control mice by NMR analysis (44). Both groups initially had similar metabolic profiles, then diverged substantially with the onset of IBD. The levels of trimethylamine and fucose changed dramatically in 8wk IL-10-deficient mice, at the timeline of histological injury. In addition, bacterial signaling molecules involved in their communication may serve as potential biomarkers for IBD (45). Profiles of N-acyl homoserine lactones (AHLs), the chemical signaling molecules in Gram-negative bacteria, in saliva from healthy donors and patients with gastrointestinal disorders were analyzed by LC-MS. The levels of AHLs may correlate with the health status of subjects.

7. Conclusion

Novel approaches by proteomics and subproteomics for biomarker discovery of UC, including those of the complication of colorectal cancer, were introduced. Many proteins have been identified and considered to be candidates for UC biomarkers, however, most of them have not established, indicating the broad range of functional abnormality in UC. PRDX2, PHB, CPS1, and butyrate were identified in multiple different studies, suggesting their usefulness as a biomarker for UC or the associated colonic cancer. The candidate biomarkers should be validated with more number of patients with UC, CD, other control diseases, and healthy subjects. Even though simple and less-invasive biomarkers are desirable for clinical examination, if the biomarkers are sensitive and specific enough for the UC diagnosis, examination of colonic mucosa obtained by endoscopy and combination of multiple proteins as the biomarker are also acceptable. Further advances in these approaches would be useful to establish biomarkers for the accurate diagnosis and the disease course prediction, and may be useful to elucidate the complicated disease mechanisms of UC.

8. Acknowledgement

The authors are grateful to Ms Atsuko Nozawa for her technical assistance.

9. References

[1] Thompson AI, Lees CW. Genetics of ulcerative colitis. *Inflamm Bowel Dis* 2011 17:831-48.

[2] Nell S, Suerbaum S, Josenhans C. The impact of the microbiota on the pathogenesis of IBD: lessons from mouse infection models. *Nat Rev Microbiol* 2010 8:564-77.

[3] Koboziev I, Karlsson F, Grisham MB. Gut-associated lymphoid tissue, T cell trafficking, and chronic intestinal inflammation. *Ann N Y Acad Sci* 2010 1207 Suppl 1:E86-93.

[4] Kurokawa MS, Imamura Y, Noguchi Y, Hatsugai M, Tsukisawa S, Matsuda T, Suzuki N, Kato T. Intestinal Behcet's disease. *Curr Trends Immunol* 2009 10:79-91.

[5] Vasiliauskas E. Recent advances in the diagnosis and classification of inflammatory bowel disease. *Curr Gastroenterol Rep* 2003 5:493-500.

[6] Gómez-Puerta JA, Hernández-Rodríguez J, López-Soto A, Bosch X. Antineutrophil cytoplasmic antibody-associated vasculitides and respiratory disease. *Chest* 2009;136:1101-11.

[7] Falk RJ, Jennette JC. Anti-neutrophil cytoplasmic autoantibodies with specificity for myeloperoxidase in patients with systemic vasculitis and idiopathic necrotizing and crescentic glomerulonephritis. *N Engl J Med* 1988 318:1651-7.

[8] Calligaris D, Villard C, Lafitte D. Advances in top-down proteomics for disease biomarker discovery. *J Proteomics* 2011 74:920-34.

[9] Hatsugai M, Kurokawa MS, Kouro T, Nagai K, Arito M, Masuko K, Suematsu N, Okamoto K, Itoh F, Kato T. Protein profiles of peripheral blood mononuclear cells are useful for differential diagnosis of ulcerative colitis and Crohn's disease. *J Gastroenterol* 2010 45:488-500.

[10] Takakuwa Y, Kurokawa MS, Ooka S, Sato T, Nagai K, Arito M, Suematsu N, Okamoto K, Nagafuchi H, Yamada H, Ozaki S, Kato T. AC13, a C-terminal fragment of apolipoprotein A-I, is a candidate biomarker for microscopic polyangiitis. *Arthritis Rheum*, in press.

[11] Xiang Y, Kurokawa MS, Kanke M, Takakuwa Y, Kato T. Peptidomics: identification of pathogenic and marker peptides. *Methods Mol Biol* 2010 615:259-71.

[12] Nanni P, Parisi D, Roda G, Casale M, Belluzzi A, Roda E, Mayer L, Roda A. Serum protein profiling in patients with inflammatory bowel diseases using selective solid-phase bulk extraction, matrix-assisted laser desorption/ionization time-of-flight mass spectrometry and chemometric data analysis. *Rapid Commun Mass Spectrom* 2007 21:4142-8.

[13] Subramanian V, Subramanian D, Pollok RC. Serum protein signatures determined by mass spectrometry (SELDI-TOF) accurately distinguishes Crohn's disease (CD) from ulcerativecolitis (UC). *Gastroenterology* 2008 134:A196.

[14] Meuwis MA, Fillet M, Geurts P, de Seny D, Lutteri L, Chapelle JP, Bours V, Wehenkel L, Belaiche J, Malaise M, Louis E, Merville MP. Biomarker discovery for inflammatory bowel disease, using proteomic serum profiling. *Biochem Pharmacol* 2007 73:1422-33.

[15] Kanmura S, Uto H, Numata M, Hashimoto S, Moriuchi A, Fujita H, Oketani M, Ido A, Kodama M, Ohi H, Tsubouchi H. Human neutrophil peptides 1-3 are useful biomarkers in patients with active ulcerative colitis. *Inflamm Bowel Dis* 2009 15:909-17.

[16] Hass SL, Bocker U, Bugert P, Singer MV, Backhaus JP. Application of Fourier transform near-infrared spectroscopy of serum samples in patients with inflammatory bowel disease-A pilot study. *Gastroenterology* 2008 134:A201.

[17] Din S, lennon AM, Hogarth C, Ho GT, Arnott ID, Hupp T, Satsangi J. Proeomic profiling identifies corticosteroid resistant patients in severe ulcerative colitis. *Gastroenterology* 2005 128:A310.

[18] Kader HA, Tchernev VT, Satyaraj E, Lejnine S, Kotler G, Kingsmore SF, Patel DD. Protein microarray analysis of disease activity in pediatric inflammatory bowel disease demonstrates elevated serum PLGF, IL-7, TGF-beta1, and IL-12p40 levels in Crohn's disease and ulcerative colitis patients in remission versus active disease. *Am J Gastroenterol* 2005 100:414-23.

[19] Chen CS, Sullivan S, Anderson T, Tan AC, Alex PJ, Brant SR, Cuffari C, Bayless TM, Talor MV, Burek CL, Wang H, Li R, Datta LW, Wu Y, Winslow RL, Zhu H, Li X. Identification of novel serological biomarkers for inflammatory bowel disease using Escherichia coli proteome chip. *Mol Cell Proteomics* 2009 8:1765-76.

[20] Vermeulen N, Vermeire S, Michiels G, Joossens M, Rutgeerts PJ, Bosuyt X. Protein microarray experiments for profiling of the autoimmune response in inflammatory bowel disease; identification of PHLA1. *Gastroenterology* 2008 134:A197.

[21] Vermeulen N, Arijs I, Joossens S, Vermeire S, Clerens S, Van den Bergh K, Michiels G, Arckens L, Schuit F, Van Lommel L, Rutgeerts P, Bossuyt X. Anti-alpha-enolase antibodies in patients with inflammatory Bowel disease. *Clin Chem* 2008 54:534-41.

[22] Liu BG, Cao YB, Cao YY, Zhang JD, An MM, Wang Y, Gao PH, Yan L, Xu Y, Jiang YY. Altered protein profile of lymphocytes in an antigen-specific model of colitis: a comparative proteomic study. *Inflamm Res.* 2007 Sep;56(9):377-84.

[23] Fogt F, Jian B, Krieg RC, Wellmann A. Proteomic analysis of mucosal preparations from patients with ulcerative colitis. *Mol Med Report* 2008 1:51-4.

[24] Hsieh SY, Shih TC, Yeh CY, Lin CJ, Chou YY, Lee YS. Comparative proteomic studies on the pathogenesis of human ulcerative colitis. *Proteomics* 2006 6:5322-31.

[25] Shkoda A, Werner T, Daniel H, Gunckel M, Rogler G, Haller D. Differential protein expression profile in the intestinal epithelium from patients with inflammatory bowel disease. *J Proteome Res* 2007 6:1114-25.

[26] Shih TC, Hsieh SY, Hsieh YY, Chen TC, Yeh CY, Lin CJ, Lin DY, Chiu CT. Aberrant activation of nuclear factor of activated T cell 2 in lamina propria mononuclear cells in ulcerative colitis. *World J Gastroenterol* 2008 14:1759-67.

[27] Berndt U, Bartsch S, Philipsen L, Danese S, Wiedenmann B, Dignass AU, Hämmerle M, Sturm A. Proteomic analysis of the inflamed intestinal mucosa reveals distinctive immune response profiles in Crohn's disease and ulcerative colitis. *J Immunol* 2007 179:6255-62.

[28] Barceló-Batllori S, André M, Servis C, Lévy N, Takikawa O, Michetti P, Reymond M, Felley-Bosco E. Proteomic analysis of cytokine induced proteins in human intestinal epithelial cells: implications for inflammatory bowel diseases. *Proteomics* 2002 2:551-60.

[29] O'Morain C, Smethurst P, Levi J, Peters TJ. Subcellular fractionation of rectal biopsy homogenates from patients with inflammatory bowel disease. *Scand J Gastroenterol* 1985 20:209-14.

[30] Naito Y, Takagi T, Okada H, Omatsu T, Mizushima K, Handa O, Kokura S, Ichikawa H, Fujiwake H, Yoshikawa T. Identification of inflammation-related proteins in a murine colitis model by 2D fluorescence difference gel electrophoresis and mass spectrometry. *J Gastroenterol Hepatol* 2010 25:S144-8.

[31] Hardwidge PR, Rodriguez-Escudero I, Goode D, Donohoe S, Eng J, Goodlett DR, Aebersold R, Finlay BB. Proteomic analysis of the intestinal epithelial cell response to enteropathogenic Escherichia coli. *J Biol Chem* 2004 279:20127-36.

[32] Shkoda A, Ruiz PA, Daniel H, Kim SC, Rogler G, Sartor RB, Haller D. Interleukin-10 blocked endoplasmic reticulum stress in intestinal epithelial cells: impact on chronic inflammation. *Gastroenterology* 2007 132:190-207.

[33] Kaput J, Perlina A, Hatipoglu B, Bartholomew A, Nikolsky Y. Nutrigenomics: concepts and applications to pharmacogenomics and clinical medicine. *Pharmacogenomics* 2007 8:369-90.

[34] Haller D. Nutrigenomics and IBD: the intestinal microbiota at the cross-road between inflammation and metabolism. *J Clin Gastroenterol* 2010 44:S6-9.

[35] Werner T, Haller D. Intestinal epithelial cell signalling and chronic inflammation: From the proteome to specific molecular mechanisms. *Mutat Res* 2007 622:42-57.

[36] Brentnall TA, Pan S, Bronner MP, Crispin DA, Mirzaei H, Cooke K, Tamura Y, Nikolskaya T, Jebailey L, Goodlett DR, McIntosh M, Aebersold R, Rabinovitch PS, Chen R. Proteins That Underlie Neoplastic Progression of Ulcerative Colitis. *Proteomics Clin Appl* 2009 3:1326-1337.

[37] May D, Pan S, Crispin DA, Lai K, Bronner MP, Hogan J, Hockenbery DM, McIntosh M, Brentnall TA, Chen R. Investigating neoplastic progression of ulcerative colitis with label-free comparative proteomics. *J Proteome Res* 2011 10:200-9.

[38] Araki K, Mikami T, Yoshida T, Kikuchi M, Sato Y, Oh-ishi M, Kodera Y, Maeda T, Okayasu I. High expression of HSP47 in ulcerative colitis-associated carcinomas: proteomic approach. *Br J Cancer* 2009 101:492-7.

[39] Berndt U, Philipsen L, Bartsch S, Wiedenmann B, Baumgart DC, Hämmerle M, Sturm A. Systematic high-content proteomic analysis reveals substantial immunologic changes in colorectal cancer. *Cancer Res* 2008;68:880-8.

[40] Yeo M, Kim DK, Park HJ, Oh TY, Kim JH, Cho SW, Paik YK, Hahm KB. Loss of transgelin in repeated bouts of ulcerative colitis-induced colon carcinogenesis. *Proteomics* 2006 6:1158-65.

[41] Marchesi JR, Holmes E, Khan F, Kochhar S, Scanlan P, Shanahan F, Wilson ID, Wang Y. Rapid and noninvasive metabonomic characterization of inflammatory bowel disease. *J Proteome Res* 2007 6:546-51.

[42] Roediger WE. The colonic epithelium in ulcerative colitis: an energy-deficiency disease? *Lancet.* 1980 2:712-5.

[43] Nanni P, Levander F, Roda G, Caponi A, James P, Roda A. A label-free nano-liquid chromatography-mass spectrometry approach for quantitative serum peptidomics in Crohn's disease patients. *J Chromatogr B Analyt Technol Biomed Life Sci* 2009 877:3127-36.

[44] Murdoch TB, Fu H, MacFarlane S, Sydora BC, Fedorak RN, Slupsky CM. Urinary metabolic profiles of inflammatory bowel disease in interleukin-10 gene-deficient mice. *Anal Chem* 2008 80:5524-31.

[45] Kumari A, Pasini P, Daunert S. Detection of bacterial quorum sensing N-acyl homoserine lactones in clinical samples. *Anal Bioanal Chem* 2008 391:1619-27.

Part 2

Pathogenesis

3

Protein Kinases and Ulcerative Colitis

Yutao Yan

Emory University, Atlanta, Georgia
USA

1. Introduction

Ulcerative colitis (UC), together with Crohn's disease (CD), collectively called inflammatory bowel disease (IBD), is a chronic, spontaneously remitting, and relapsing disorder of large intestine, characterized by abdominal pain and diarrhea. UC differs dramatically from CD with the respects of disease distribution, morphology, and histopathology; meantime, they share a lot of inflammatory similarities, such as epithelial barrier dysfunction. UC may result in significant morbidity and mortality, with compromised quality of life and life expectancy. While there is no cure for UC, the last two decades have seen tremendous advances in our understanding of the pathophysiology of this intestinal inflammation. Even though the precise etiology of IBD remains elusive, it is accepted that UC arises from abnormal host–microbe interactions, including qualitative and quantitative changes in the composition of the microbiota, host genetic susceptibility, barrier function, as well as innate and adaptive immunity.

Intracellular signaling cascades mediated by protein kinases are the main route of communication between the plasma membrane and regulatory targets in various intracellular compartments. The signaling pathway mediated by protein kinase plays an important role in transducing signals from diverse extra-cellular stimuli (including growth factors, cytokines and environmental stresses) to the nucleus in order to affect a wide range of cellular processes, such as proliferation, differentiation, development and apoptosis, and more importantly, also involved in intestinal inflammation.

In this chapter, we are going to focus on the involvement protein kinases in the pathogenesis of UC, try to shed some light on the clues of intervention of UC.

2. Genetic factor

Population-based studies provided compelling evidence that genetic susceptibility plays an essential role in the pathogenesis of UC, evidence including an 8- to 10-fold greater risk among relatives of UC and greater rates of concordance between twins in UC patients (15.4% in monozygotic vs 3.9% in dizygotic twins) (Cho & Brant, 2011). Some of genes encoding protein kinase like ERK1 (Hugot et al. 1996) and p38α (Hampe et al. 1999) are located in major IBD susceptibility regions on chromosome 16 and 6. Recently, substantial advances have been achieved in defining the genetic architecture of UC since the genome-wide association study (GWAS) analysis heralded a new era of complex disease gene discovery with notable success in CD initially and latterly also in UC. To date, over 60 published IBD susceptibility loci have been discovered and replicated, of which

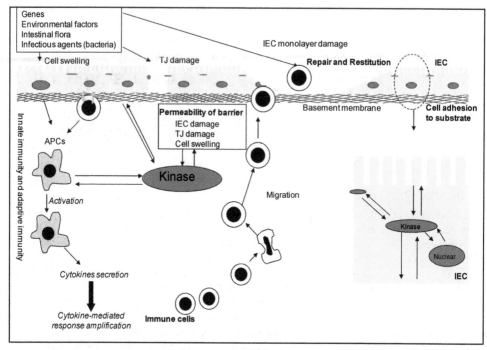

Fig. 1. Pathogenesis of UC. Many different factors, such as genetic factors, environmental factors, and intestinal non-pathogenic or pathogenic bacteria can damage the mucus, epithelium, or the tight junction, to initiate the inappropriate regulation or deregulation of the immune response, leading to the secretion of pro-inflammatory cytokines, decrease in epithelial barrier function and initiation of the inflammation-related signaling pathways. IEC: Intestinal epithelial cell; APC: Antigen presenting cell; TJ: Tightjunction. This model adapted from the model presented previously (Yan 2008)

approximately one third are associated with both UC and CD, although 21 are specific to UC and 23 to CD (Thompson & Lees, 2011). Importantly, most of the genes have been linked to defects in innate and adaptive immunity and epithelial barrier function. Notably, extracellular matrix *gene* 1 (ECM1) (Festen et al. 2010), E-cadherin gene (CDH1), Hepatocyte nuclear factor 4 alpha gene (HNF4a), and laminin B1 (Barrett et al. 2009) are genes implicated in mucosal barrier function, conferring risk of UC; ECM1 interacts with the basement membrane, inhibits matrix metalloproteinase 9 (MMP9), and strongly activate NFκB (Chan et al. 2007; Matsuda et al. 2003). The Wnt/beta-catenin signal transduction pathway has been shown to influence ECM1 expression (Kenny et al. 2005). E-cadherin is the first genetic correlation between colorectal cancer and UC, Chimeric mice with impaired E-cadherin function due to expression of dominant–negative N-cadherin developed colitis despite possessing an intact immune system (Hermiston & Gordon 1995a, 1995b). Notably, all of these 4 genes are regulated or related to protein kinases, for example, HNF4alpha-DNA binding activity is dependent on its phosphorylation by protein kinase A (PKA) (Viollet et al. 1997), while its transcription activity was dependent on AMP-activated protein kinase(AMPK) (Hong et al. 2003).

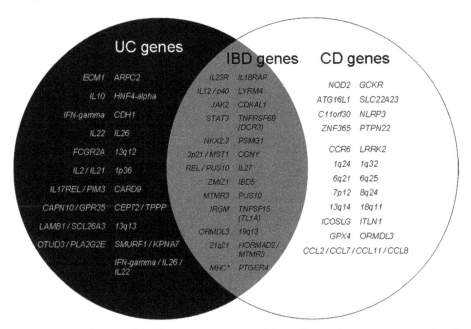

Fig. 2. Susceptible loci for UC. This model is adapted from the model presented previously (Thompson & Lees 2001)

3. Microbiota and immune responses

The human gastrointestinal (GI) tract contains as many as 10^{14} individual bacteria, comprising over 500 different species. These commensal bacteria serves as a primary barrier between the intestinal epithelial cells and the external environment, which is critical to the healthy host, as it modulates intestinal development, maintains a healthy intestinal pH, promotes immune homeostasis, and enhances metabolism of drugs, hormones and carcinogens. Evidence from immunologic, microbiologic, and genetic studies implicates abnormal host-microbial interactions in the pathogenesis of UC. But the mechanisms underlying the involvement of microbiota are elusive, and the effects of microbiota are due to their interaction with other factors, such as immunologic factors, genetic factor or epithelial junction proteins. The postulated mechanisms (Packey & Sartor, 2008) are as followed with little modification: (a) Pathogenic bacteria. A traditional pathogen or functional alterations in commensal bacteria, including enhanced epithelial adherence, invasion, and resistance to killing by phagocytes or acquisition of virulence factors, can result in increased stimulation of innate and adaptive immune responses. (b) Abnormal microbial composition. Decreased concentrations of bacteria that produce butyrate and other short-chain fatty acids (SCFA) compromise epithelial barrier integrity. (c) Defective host containment of commensal bacteria. Increased mucosal permeability can result in overwhelming exposure of bacterial toll like receptor (TLR) ligands and antigens that activate pathogenic innate and T cell immune responses. (d) Defective host immunoregulation. Antigen-presenting cells and epithelial cells overproduce cytokines due to ineffective downregulation, which results in TH1 and TH17 differentiation and inflammation. Dysfunction of regulatory T cells (T-reg) leads to decreased secretion of IL-10 and TGF-β, and loss of immunological tolerance to microbial antigens (an overly aggressive T cell response).

UC is commonly regarded as the consequences of an enhanced inflammatory response or the lack of a down regulatory response to bacteria abnormality. The dysregulated immune response involving the innate (for example, TLR, DC, etc) and the adaptive immune system (e.g. effector T-cells, regulatory T-cells, eosinophils, neutrophils, etc) may follow or precede the macroscopic lesions. Crohn's disease is a predominantly TH1- and TH17-mediated process, while the immunopathogenesis of UC has been a more difficult disease to ascertain, neither IFN-γ (a major Th1 cytokine) nor IL-4 (the major Th2 cytokines) was increased (Fuss et al, 2008). In fact, IL-4 production was found to be decreased in cells extracted from UC tissue and only the fact that an additional Th2 cytokine IL-5 secretion by these cells was somewhat increased hinted that the disease may have a Th2 character. Further, enhanced level of IL-13 was noticed in lamina propria from UC specimens, whereas those from Crohn's disease specimens were producing IFN-γ (Fuss et al, 1996). Fuss (Fuss et al, 2004) found that antigen-presenting cells bearing a CD1d construct (and thus expressing CD1d on its surface, which presents lipid rather than protein antigens to T cells.) could only induce lamina propria mononuclear cells from UC patients but not that of Crohn's disease to produce IL-13. Thereby, the cytokine secretion profile seen in UC was produced from a non-classical CD1 dependent NK T cell whereas the cytokines produced in Crohn's disease were from that of an activated classical Th1 CD4 + T cell. In addition, Lamina propria cells enriched for NK T cells from the patients could be shown to be cytotoxic for epithelial cells and such cytotoxicity was further enhanced by IL-13. Antigens in the mucosal microflora activate NK T cells because of barrier dysfunction that, in turn, cause cytolysis of epithelial cells and the characteristic ulcerations associated with the disease. As suggested, enhancement of cytolytic activity was observed *in vitro* in the presence of IL-13. Further, IL-13 was shown to have direct effects on activation of cytokine transcription. These studies demonstrated that TGF-β transcription was dependent upon IL-13. In short, UC is associated with an atypical TH2 response mediated by a distinct subset of NK T cells that produce IL-13 and are cytotoxic for epithelial cells (Fuss et al. 2008). Further, UC is characterized by the presence of various types of autoantibodies against goblet cells and the isoforms 1 and 5 of human tropomyosin.

The intestinal mucosa must rapidly recognize detrimental pathogenic threats to the lumen to initiate controlled immune responses but maintain hyporesponsiveness to omnipresent harmless commensals. Pattern recognition receptors (PRRs) may play an essential role in allowing innate immune cells to discriminate between "self" and microbial "non-self" based on the recognition of broadly conserved molecular patterns. Toll-like receptors (TLRs), a class of transmembrane PRRs, play a key role in microbial recognition, induction of antimicrobial genes, and the control of adaptive immune responses. Individual TLRs differentially activate distinct signaling events via diverse cofactors and adaptors. To date, at least five different adaptor proteins have been identified in humans: MyD88, Mal/TIRAP, TRIF/TICAM-1, TRAM/Tirp/TICAM-2, and SARM (O'Neill et al. 2003). The first identified so-called "classical" pathway (Cario 2005) involves recruitment of the adaptor molecule MyD88, activation of the serine/threonine kinases of the interleukin 1 receptor associated kinase (IRAK) family, subsequently leading to degradation of inhibitor kB (IkB) and translocation of nuclear factor kB (NFkB) to the nucleus, then result in activation of specific transcription factors, including NFkB, AP-1, Elk-1, CREB, STATs, and the subsequent transcriptional activation of genes encoding pro- and anti-inflammatory cytokines and chemokines as well as induction of costimulatory molecules. All of these various downstream effects are critically involved in the control of pathogen elimination, commensal homeostasis, and linkage to the adaptive immunity. Signaling through different TLRs can result in considerable qualitative differences in TH dependent immune responses by differential modulation of MAPKs and the transcription factor c-FOS (Agrawal et al. 2003). So TLR signalling protects intestinal epithelial barrier and maintains tolerance, but aberrant TLR signalling may stimulate diverse inflammatory responses leading to UC.

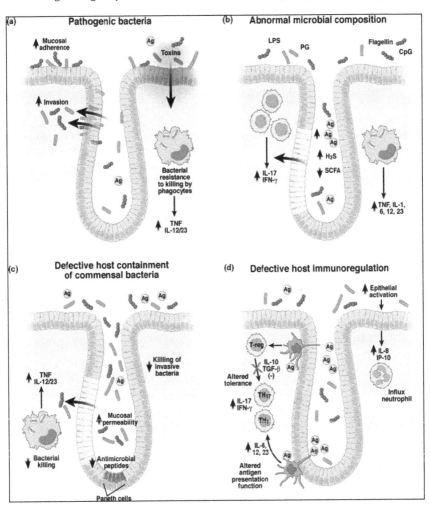

Fig. 3. Proposed mechanisms by which bacteria and fungi induce chronic immune-mediated inflammation and injury of the intestines. This model adapted from the model presented in the work by Dr Sartor (Packey & Sartor 2008) (a) Pathogenic bacteria. (b) Abnormal microbial composition. (c) Defective host containment of commensal bacteria. (d) Defective host immunoregulation

TLR comprise a family of (so far) 11 type-I transmembrane receptors. Different pathogen associated molecular patterns selectively activate different TLRs: (Lipoptroteins) TLR1, 2 and 6; (dsRNA) TLR3; (LPS) TLR4; (Flagellin) TLR5; (ssRNA) TLR7 and 8; (CpG DNA) TLR9. These signals all converge on a single pathway via myeloid differentiation primary response protein MyD88, which activates NFκB. the NFκB pathway was thought to have predominantly pro inflammatory activities and NFκB is activated in the tissues of UC patients and its inhibition can attenuate experimental colitis (Neurath et al 1996).

In intestine, tolerance is an essential mucosal defence mechanism maintaining hyporesponsiveness to harmless lumenal commensals and their products. Several molecular immune mechanisms that ensure tolerance via TLRs in intestinal epithelial cells (IEC) have recently been described, for example, low expression of TLRs at resting conditions in IEC can maintain hyporesponsiveness to microbiota; high expression levels of the downstream signaling suppressor Tollip which inhibits IRAK activation (Otte et al. 2004), ligand induced activation of peroxisome proliferator activated receptor c (PPARc) which uncouples NFkB dependent target genes in a negative feedback loop (Dubuquoy et al. 2003. Kelly et al. 2004), and external regulators which may suppress TLR mediated signalling pathways. Commensal bacteria may assist the host in maintaining mucosal homeostasis by suppressing inflammatory responses and inhibiting specific intracellular signal transduction pathways (Neish et al. 2000), uncoupling NFkB dependent target genes in a negative feedback loop (Dubuquoy et al. 2003) which may lead to attenuation of colonic inflammation (Kelly et al. 2004).

In addition, NF-κB is normally grouped into one of the pro-inflammatory mediators, a protective role for epithelial NF-κB signaling by either bacteria, IL-1, or TNF stimulation of TLRs, or cytokine receptors is demonstrated by conditional ablation of NEMO (IκB kinase) in intestinal epithelial cells causing spontaneous severe colitis (Nenci et al. 2007). Blockade of epithelial NF-κB signaling led to increased bacterial translocation across the injured epithelium, similar to toll like receptor (TLR)4-deficient mice treated with dextran sulphate sodium (DSS) (Fukata et al. 2006).

4. Barrier dysfunction

Generally, intestinal barrier function consists of different level of defense lines, the mucus layer, commensal microbiota, epithelial cells themselves, the junction between lateral epithelial cells, innate and adaptive immune systems and enteric nerve system. Any stresses which interfere with any level of this defense lines could potentially lead to intestinal barrier dysfunction and result in intestinal inflammation.

Epithelial cells form a continuous, polarized monolayer that is linked together by a series of dynamic junctional complexes. Except function as a physical barrier, epithelial cells maintain a mucosal defense system through the expression of a wide range of PRRs, such as TLRs. These PRRs form the backbone of the innate immune system through the rapid response and recognition of the unique and conserved microbial components, (Medzhitov & Janeway. 2002; Akira et al. 2006). Tight junctions are composed of transmembrane proteins (claudins, occludins, and junctional adhesion molecule [JAM]), peripheral membrane or scaffolding proteins (zonula occludens [ZO]), and intracellular regulatory molecules that include kinases and actin. An anatomically and immunologically compromised intestinal epithelial barrier allows direct contact of the intestinal mucosa with the luminal bacteria and plays a crucial role in the development and maintenance of UC by initiating chronic inflammatory responses, although it is unclear whether this is a primary pathogenic process or secondary to inflammation. Since the contribution of genetic factors, microbiota and immune responses to the pathogenesis to UC, we high light the involvement of mucus layer, tight junction itself in the pathogenesis of UC.

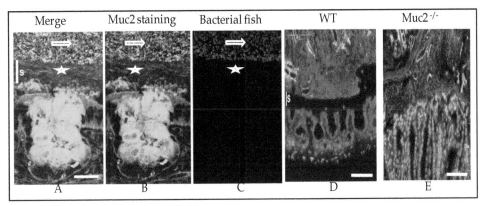

Fig. 4. Merged figure (A) of Muc2immunostaining (green, B) *and FISH analysis using the general bacterial probe EUB338-Alexa Fluor 555* (red, C) of distal colon, it was shown muc2-positive goblet cells and the outer mucus layer (Arrow) and inner mucus layer (Star) on the epithelium. The inner layer (Star) is devoid of bacteria, which can only be detected in the outer mucus layer. The inner mucus generates a spatial separation between the cells and microflora. (Scale bar: 20 μm). (D) FISH using the EUB338-Alexa Fluor 555 probe staining bacteria and DAPIDNA staining in colon show a clear separation of the bacterial DNA and epithelial surface in WT mice, but not in Muc2-/- mice. This separation corresponds to the inner mucus layer (s). (Scale bar: 100m). These models adapted from the models presented previously (Johansson et al. 2008)

4.1 Mucus layer
As mentioned in previous part of this chapter, the digestive tract is home to 10^{14} bacteria and bacteria genome is as many 10 times as human genome, which has evolved to ensure homeostasis. How to manage this enormous bacterial load without overt immune responses from the adaptive and innate systems is not well understood. When the equilibrium is altered, as in the disease ulcerative colitis, inflammatory responses are initiated against the commensal bacteria. An important component, often neglected due to lack of understanding, is the mucus layer that overlies the entire intestinal epithelium as a protective gel-like layer (Johansson et al. 2008). This thick and hyperviscous mucus layer secreted by goblet cells overlies the entire intestinal epithelium as a protective gel-like layer that can extend up to as much as 150 μm thick in mouse colon (and 800 μm thick in rat colon). There exist two different kinds of mucus layer-out layer and inner layer. The majority of microorganisms in the lumen can be found in the outer mucus layer, there is an inner, protected, and unstirred layer that is directly adjacent to the epithelial surface and is relatively sterile. The sterility of this layer contributes to the retention of a high concentration of antimicrobial proteins (such as cathelicidiens, defensins, and cryptidens)

produced by various intestinal epithelial lineages, including enterocytes and Paneth cells. The inner firmly attached mucus layer forms a specialized physical barrier that excludes the resident bacteria from a direct contact with the underlining epithelium. This organization of the colon mucus, as based on the properties of the Muc2 mucin, should be ideal for excluding bacteria from contacting the epithelial cells and thus also the immune system. Alterations or the absence of these protective layers, as in the Muc2$^{-/-}$ mouse colon, allow bacteria to have a direct contact with epithelial cells, to penetrate lower into the crypts and also translocate into epithelial cells. That such a close contact between bacteria and epithelia can trigger an inflammatory response (Johansson et al. 2008; Shen et al. 2009). The surface mucus layer also impacts mucosal permeability, as demonstrated by spontaneous colitis in Muc-2- deficient mice (Bergstrom et al. 2010), and increased DSS-induced colitis in intestinal trefoil factor deficient mice (Mashimo et al. 1996) and in human UC. The importance of the Muc2 mucin in organizing the colon mucus protection is further strengthen by the report that two mouse strains with diarrhea and colon inflammation were shown to have two separate spontaneous mutations in the Muc2 mucin (Heazlewood et al. 2008). Importantly, the production of mucin is regulated by protein kinases, for example, resistin and resistin-like molecule (RELM) beta upregulated mucin expression which dependent on the kinase activities of protein kinase C (PKC), tyrosine kinases, and extracellular-regulated protein kinase (Krimi et al. 2008); Cathelicidin stimulates colonic mucus synthesis by up-regulating MUC1 and MUC2 expression through a mitogen-activated protein kinase pathway (Tai et al. 2008).

4.2 Epithelial cell and its tight junction

The cellular components of the intestinal barrier consist of the complete array of columnar epithelial cell types (enterocyte, paneth cells, enteroendorine cells, and goblet cells) present within the intestine. These cells are polarized with an apical membrane and a basolateral membrane, and apical membrane composition is distinct from the basolateral membrane, for example, the nutrient transporters are located on the apical membrane; they use Na$^+$ ions cotransport to provide the energy and directionality of transport. In contrast, the Na$^+$K$^+$-ATPase, which establishes the Na$^+$ electrochemical gradient, is present on basolateral, but not apical membranes. In addition, the lipid composition of the membrane differs; the apical membrane is enriched in sphingolipids and cholesterol relative to the basolateral membrane. One result of this cellular polarization is that the apical membranes of intestinal epithelial cells are generally impermeable to hydrophilic solutes in the absence of specific transporters. Thus, the presence of epithelial cells, particularly the apical membranes, contributes significantly to the mucosal barrier (Shen et al. 2009). Among the most important structures of the intestinal barrier are the epithelial tight junctions (TJs) that connect adjacent enterocytes together to determine paracellular permeability. The tight junction is composed of multiple proteins including transmembrane proteins such as occludin, tricellulin, claudins and junctional adhesion molecule (JAM). The intracellular portions of these transmembrane proteins interact with cytoplasmic peripheral membrane proteins, including zona occludens (ZO)-1,-2,-3 and cingulin (Mitic & Anderson. 1998). These tight junction and cytoplasmic proteins then interact with F-actin and myosin II, thereby anchoring the tight junction complex to the cytoskeleton. Once thought to be static, the association of these proteins with the tight junction is highly dynamic (Shen et al. 2009) and may play a role in epithelial barrier regulation. Occludin was the first tight junction-associated integral membrane protein identified (Furuse et al. 1993). Although occludin knockout mice exhibit intact intestinal epithelial tight junctions and display no observable barrier defect (Schulzke et al. 2005, Saitou et al. 2000). But *in vitro* studies demonstrate crucial roles in tight junction assembly and maintenance (Yu et al. 2005; Suzuki et al. 2009; Elias et al. 2009). This suggests that further analysis of occludin knockout mice under stressed condition may reveal *in vivo* functions of occludin and provide new insight into mechanisms of tight regulation (Turner 2006). Given the phylogenetic and structural similarities between occludin and tricellulin (Ikenouchi et al. 2005), it may be that the tricellulin accounts for normal intestinal barrier function in occludin knockout mice. This hypothesis could also be applied to inflammatory bowel disease, where intestinal epithelial occludin expression is reduced (Heller et al. 2005). The fact that occludin knockout mice exhibit intact intestinal epithelial barrier function led to the search for additional tight junctional components and ultimately to the discovery of the claudins (Furuse et al. 1998). The claudins are a large family of proteins that also interact with partners on neighboring cells to affect junctional adhesions via extracellular loops. At least 24 different claudin proteins are present in mammals (Van Itallie et al. 2003, 2004, 2006), and these proteins are the primary component of tight junction strands (Furuse et al. 2006). Claudins are expressed in a tissue-specific manner, studies on human intestine confirm the expression of claudins-1, -2, -3, -4, -5, -7, and -8 in the colon, expression of claudins-1, -2, -3, and -4 in the duodenum, and expression of claudins-2 and -4 in the jejunum (Burgel et al 2002; Escaffit et al 2005, Szakal et al. 2010; Wang et al. 2010; Zeissing et al. 2007).

The molecular anatomy of transport through tight junction is not yet clear, at least two routes allow transport across the tight junction, and the relative contributions of different paracellular transport are regulated independently (Fihn et al. 2000; Van Itallie 2008; Watson et al. 2005). One route, the size-dependent pathway, allows paracellular transport of large solutes, including limited flux of proteins and bacterial lipopolysaccharides (Van Itallie 2008; Watson et al. 2005). Although at what size particles are excluded from the leak pathway has not been precisely defined, it is clear that materials as large as whole bacteria cannot pass. Flux across the leak pathway may be increased by cytokines and protein kinases, including IFNγ, TNF (Watson et al. 2005; Wang et al. 2005; Clayburgh et al. 2006), MAPKs, myosin II light chain kinase (MLCK) (Turner 2006) and SPAK (Yan 2011). A second pathway is charge-dependent pathway, characterized by small pores that are defined by tight junction-associated pore-forming claudin proteins (Amasheh et al. 2002; Colegio et al. 2003; Simon et al. 1999). These pores have a radius that excludes molecules larger than 4 A (Van Itallie 2008; Watson et al.2005). Thus, tight junctions show both size selectivity and charge selectivity, and these properties may be regulated individually or jointly by physiological or pathophysiological stimuli. It need to point out that barrier dysfunction may be caused by increased paracellular permeability, but mainly by epithelial damage, including erosion, and ulceration (Zeissig et al. 2004; Schulzke et al.2006). In addition, in epithelial cells, the site of claudin protein polymerization to form strands depends on ZO family protein expression (Furuse & Tsukita 2006), and cells lacking ZO-1 and ZO-2 fail to form tight junctions at all.

Generally, TJ proteins can be subdivided into "tightening" TJ proteins that strengthen epithelial barrier properties (such as occluding and claudin-1 and -4 etc) and "leaky" TJ proteins (like claudin-2) that selectively mediate paracellular permeability. Dysfunctional intestinal barrier is a feature of gut inflammation in humans and has been implicated as a pathogenic factor in IBD for the last 30 years. The factors responsible for barrier dysfunction in UC are similar to those in CD, including an increase in epithelial antigen transcytosis and a change in TJ structure with a reduction in TJ strand count and in the depth of the TJ main meshwork; although, in contrast to CD, strand breaks are not as frequent as in UC (Schmitz et al. 1999; Schurmann et al. 1999). Again, the downregulation of occludin and downregulation of several "tightening" TJ proteins like claudin-1 and -4, together with an upregulation of the pore-forming TJ protein claudin-2 contribute to the barrier defect observed in UC (Heller et al.2005; Oshima et al. 2008). These disruptions of tight junction proteins could lead to a breakdown in the protective barrier and can be used as a portal of entry by the luminal bacteria. This breach in intestinal barrier can result in inflammatory infiltrate and enhanced production of cytokines and other mediators (such as neutrophil) that can further contribute to the altered barrier function.

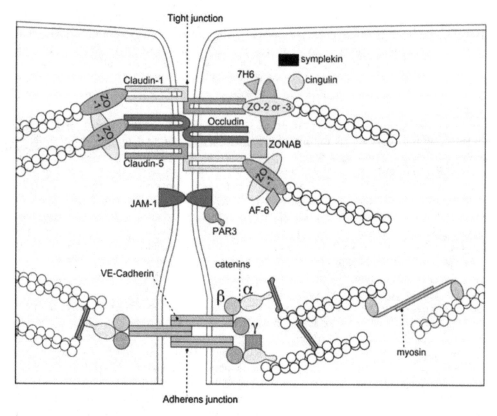

Fig. 5. Molecular composition of tight junctions. This model adapted from the model presented previously:
http://www.ncbi.nlm.nih.gov/pmc/articles/PMC2413111/?tool=pubmed

Mucosal permeability is influenced by several factors. The surface mucus layer also impacts mucosal permeability, as demonstrated by spontaneous colitis in Muc-2- deficient mice (Van der Sluis et al. 2006), and increased DSS-induced colitis in intestinal trefoil factordeficient mice (Mashimo et al. 1996). Luminal microbiota can also compromise the intestinal barrier function (Packey & Sartor, 2008). The third is the integrity of the epithelial cell layer and the basement membrane. Molecularly this can be compromised by downregulating tight junction components Claudins 5 and 6, upregulating pore-forming Claudin 2 (Zessig et al. 2007), which can be accomplished by TNF and IL-13, or increasing epithelial apoptosis, which has been achieved in mice by blocking nuclear factor kappa-B (NFκB) signalling. Genetic factors are involved in the loss of intestinal barrier function (Cho & Brant 2011). Dysregulated innate and adaptive immune system can lead to the enhanced epithelial permeability (Fuss 2008). Finally, autonomic nerve system function affects epithelial permeability, as demonstrated by mice that develop fulminant jejunoileitis following ablation of enteric glial cells (Bush et al. 1998).

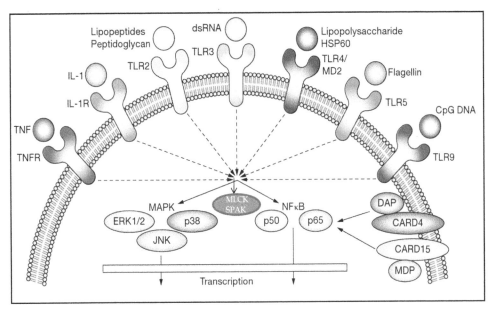

Fig. 6. Binding of microbial adjuvants to extracellular and intracellular pattern-recognition receptors and initiate their function by activating protein kinases. Toll-like receptors on the cell membrane selectively bind to various bacterial, viral or fungal components. This ligation activates conserved signaling pathways that activate NFκB and mitogen-activated protein kinases. These transcription factors stimulate the expression of a number of proinflammatory and antiinflammatory genes. This model adapted and modified from the model presented previously.
http://www.nature.com/nrgastro/journal/v3/n7/full/ncpgasthep0528.html

The increased uptake of antigens and macromolecules from the intestinal lumen mediated through this epithelial barrier dysfunction can further exacerbate the inflammatory process, ending up in a vicious circle. In this manner, barrier dysfunction is a perpetuating principle during gastrointestinal inflammation. Since epithelial TJs are important in the maintenance of barrier function, regulatory changes in their function that are commonly found during intestinal inflammation can have severe consequences. For example, the resulting passive loss of solutes into the intestinal lumen and the subsequent osmotically driven water flow results in "leak flux diarrhea", one of the main consequences of UC. The tight junction is, therefore, the rate-limiting step in transepithelial transport and the principal determinant of mucosal permeability. But it has to be pointed out that barrier dysfunction itself is not sufficient to cause intestinal diseases, such as in MLCK (Turner 2006) and SPAK (Yan 2011) transgenic mice, these two different transgenic mice revealed increased transepithelial permeability, but neither of them demonstrated any UC characterization, for example, these mice develop normal, no significant weight loss, histologically normal crypts were found, no abscesses was noticed.

Recent molecular advances as well as studies of cellular physiology in model epithelia have instead revealed that both the permeability and selectivity of tight junctions can be modulated dynamically by a variety of signals (Mitic et al., 2000). Much of the progress in this field has rested on a significantly enhanced understanding of the proteins that make up the junction itself, as well as those components of the junction on its cytoplasmic face that link the junctional region both to the cellular cytoskeleton and to signal transduction modules (González-Mariscal et al. 2003).

5. Protein kinase and pathogenesis of UC

5.1 Mitogen activated protein kinases (MAPK)

Interestingly, protein kinases are associated with all different level of aspects, demonstrated promising potential as intervention targets against UC. Intracellular signaling cascades are the main route of communication between the plasma membrane and regulatory targets in various intracellular compartments. The evolutionarily conserved mitogen activated protein kinases (MAPK) signaling pathway plays an important role in transducing signals from diverse extra-cellular stimuli (including growth factors, cytokines and environmental stresses) to the nucleus in order to affect a wide range of cellular processes, such as proliferation, differentiation, development, stress responses and apoptosis. MAPK (Coskun et al,2011) signaling cascades, which comprise up to seven levels of protein kinases, are sequentially activated by phosphorylation and also involved in intestinal inflammation. These families can be divided into two groups: the classical MAPKs, consisting of ERK1/2, p38, JNK and ERK5, and the atypical MAPKs, consisting of ERK3, ERK4, ERK7 and NLK (Coulombe & Meloche, 2007). The signalling pathways which the members of these families influence can be independent of each other or overlapping. The classical pathway leading to activation of ERK1/2 is through the upstream activation of the Raf MAPKKKs, which activate sequentially the MAPKKs, MEK1/2, which can specifically bind and phosphorylate ERK1/2. At this stage, and depending upon the signal being propagated, the ERK1/2 proteins commonly then phosphorylate the downstream MAPK activated proteins (MAPKAP) 1/2. However, other proinflammatory proteins such as cytosolic phospholipase A_2 can be activated, as well as several transcription factors including Ets-1, Elk and c-myc. These transcription factors aid the inflammatory process by inducing other related cellular processes such as cell migration and proliferation. Interestingly, a role for ERK1/2, using an ERK1/2 inhibitor, was found in cells of the immune system and colonocytes in the development and progression of IBD, through its mediation in the signalling pathways induced by various cytokines, for example IL-21, and IL-1 (Caruso et al.2007; Kwon et al.2007). Indeed, several studies, cell line cultures and isolated crypts from human biopsies, have shown that it is not only over-expressed in IBD tissue (both colonocytes and cells in the underlying lamina propria), but that its phosphorylation state and therefore activation state is increased significantly during the active stages of IBD (Waetzig et al.2002; Dahan et al.2008). Study also found that Erk activation is involved in claudin-4 protein expression and claudin-4 is involved in the maintenance of the intestinal epithelial cell barrier function (Pinton et al. 2010) as a "tightening" junction protein. Activation of p38/MAPK and Akt signal transduction pathways in the epithelial cells have also been implicated as key mediators of these protective effects (Resta-Lenert and Barrett. 2006). For example, *Lactobacillus GG* (LGG) prevents cytokine-induced apoptosis in both human and mouse intestinal epithelial cells through activating antiapoptotic Akt in a phosphatidylinositol-3-kinase (PI3K)-dependent manner and inhibiting proapoptotic p38/MAPK activation (Yan and Polk. 2002). The p38 family is composed of four members: α, β, γ and δ. Expression of the isoforms varies between tissues. Different ligands, via their respective receptors, are able to activate one or several of p38 targets TAK1, ASK1, MLK3, MEKK1-4 and TAO1-3 (Thalhamer et al.2008). Several studies using the p38 inhibitor, SB203580, have indicated that p38 phosphorylation is increased significantly in IBD tissue (Waetzig et al.2002; Dahan et al.2008). This finding is substantiated further by an *in vitro* study, indicating that inhibition of p38 using the natural IL-1 receptor antagonist, in a colonocyte cell line, leads to reduced IL-6 and -8 production, and an *in vivo* study using a murine model of IBD, where inhibition of p38 reduced significantly cytokine mRNA and NFκB activation (Garat et al.2003; Hollenbach et al.2004). However, Heat-killed *L. brevis* SBC8803 induced Hsps, phosphorylated p38 MAPK, regulated the expression of tumor necrosis factor alpha (TNF-α), interleukin (IL)-1β and IL-12, and improved the barrier function of intestinal epithelia under oxidant stress (Ueno et al. 2011).

There are three JNK isoforms, JNK1, 2 and 3, of which there are 10 splice forms in total. Studies using a specific inhibitor against JNK1/2 in induced IBD in rodent models or with isolated colonic tissue found that proinflammatory cytokine production was reduced in conjunction with reduced inflammatory cell infiltration. Similarly, increased phosphorylation of JNK1/2 was seen in inflamed tissue from IBD patients (Dahan et al.2008; Assi K et al.2006; Mitsuyama et al.2008). RDP58 (Loftberg et al.2002) is a peptide consisting of 9 D-amino acids blocking p38 and JNK, further attenuate UC.

5.2 Serine and threonine kinase
5.2.1 Ste20 related proline/alanine rich kinase (SPAK)

SPAK is defined as a ste20-like proline-/alanine rich kinase that contains an N-terminal series of proline and alanine repeats (PAPA box) followed by a kinase domain, a nuclear localization signal, a consensus caspase cleavage motif, and a C-terminal regulatory region (Johnston et al.2000). Colonic SPAK exists as a unique isoform that lacks the PAPA box and F-α helix loop in the N-terminus (Yan et al.2007). The diversity of domains present in SPAK protein might be associated with a variety of biological roles. For example, SPAK has been shown to play roles in cell differentiation, cell transformation and proliferation, and regulation of chloride transport (Piechotta et al.2002; Gagnon et al.2006). More importantly, a linkage has been established between SPAK and inflammation, SPAK, as an upstream kinase to Na^+-K^+-$2Cl^-$ co-transporter 1 (NKCC1), can phosphorylate Thr203, Thr207, and

Thr212 amino acids on NKCC1, which play an important role in inflammation (Topper et al.1997). Furthermore, we have demonstrated that SPAK can activate p38 pathway (Yan et al. 2007) that is well known involving inflammation. SPAK caused an increase in intestinal permeability, and SPAK transgenic (TG) mice were more susceptible to experimental colitis. Additionally, increased cytokine production and bacterial translocation were associated with the increased colitis susceptibility (Yan Y et al 2011).

5.2.2 Myosin II light chain kinase (MLCK)

MLCK is a specific Serine and threonine kinase which can phosphorylate MLC. It has been found that MLCK activity is required for TNF-induced acute diarrhea. Further, TNF treatment resulted in increased myosin light chain kinase expression (Wang et al. 2005), as a result of transcriptional activation (Graham et al. 2006) in vitro and in vivo. Constitutive MLCK activation accelerates onset and increases severity of experimental UC. MLCK inhibition, either pharmacologically or by genetic knockout, prevented both intestinal epithelial MLC phosphorylation and barrier dysfunction. More remarkably, MLCK inhibition also restored net water absorption, and therefore corrected the TNF-dependent diarrhea (Clayburgh DR).

6. Conclusions

Protein kinase have been implicated in the pathogenesis of a variety of human disorders including UC, continuing progress in the understanding of the roles of protein kinases in intestinal barrier dysfunction, further in IBD pathogeneses offers hope for a new generation of therapeutic strategies targeted at the modulation of protein kinase activity.

7. References

Agrawal, S., Agrawal, A., & Doughty, B.(2003). Cutting edge: different Toll-like receptor agonists instruct dendritic cells to induce distinct Th responses via differential modulation of extracellular signal-regulated kinase-mitogenactivated protein kinase and c-Fos. *J Immunol*. 171: 4984–9.

Akira, S., Uematsu, S., & Takeuchi O.(2006). Pathogen recognition and innate immunity. *Cell*. 124: 783–801.

Amasheh, S., Meiri, N., & Gitter A.(2002). Claudin-2 expression induces cation-selective channels in tight junctions of epithelial cells. *J Cell Sci*. 115: 4969-76.

Assi, K., Pillai, R., & Gomez-Munoz A. (2006). The specific JNK inhibitor SP600125 targets tumour necrosis factor-alpha production and epithelial cell apoptosis in acute murine colitis. *Immunology*. 118: 112–21.

Barrett, J.C., Lee, J.C., & Lees, C.W. (2009). Genome-wide association study of ulcerative colitis identifies three new susceptibility loci, including the HNF4A region. *Nat Genet*. 41:1330–4.

Bergstrom, K.S., Kissoon-Singh, V., & Gibson, L.(2010). Muc2 protects against lethal infectious colitis by disassociating pathogenic and commensal bacteria from the colonic mucosa. *PLoS Pathog*. 6: e1000902.

Burgel, N., Bojarski, C., & Mankertz, J.(2002). Mechanisms of diarrhea in collagenous colitis. *Gastroenterology*. 123: 433-43.

Bush, T.G., Savidge, T.C., & Freeman, T.C. (1998). Fulminant jejuno-ileitis following ablation of enteric glia in a adult transgenic mice. *Cell*. 93: 189–201.

Cario, E. (2005). Bacterial interactions with cells of the intestinal mucosa: Toll-like receptors and NOD2. *Gut*. 54(8):1182-93.

Caruso, R., Fina, D., & Peluso, I.(2007). A functional role for interleukin-21 in promoting the synthesis of the T-cell chemoattractant, MIP-3alpha, by gut epithelial cells. *Gastroenterology*. 132:166–75.

Chan, I., Liu, L., & Hamada, T.(2007). The molecular basis of lipoid proteinosis: mutations in extracellular matrix protein 1. *Exp Dermatol*. 16:881–90.

Cho, J.H., & Brant, S.R. (2011). Recent insights into the genetics of inflammatory bowel disease. *Gastroenterology*. 140:1704–1712.

Clayburgh, D. R., Musch, M.W., & Leitges, M. (2006). Coordinated epithelial NHE3 inhibition and barrier dysfunction are required for TNF-mediated diarrhea *in vivo*. *J Clin Invest*. 116: 2682–2694.

Colegio, O. R., Van Itallie, C., & Rahner, C.(2003). Claudin extracellular domains determine paracellular charge selectivity and resistance but not tight junction fibril architecture. *Am J Physiol Cell Physiol*. 284: C1346–C1354.

Coskun, M., Olsen, J., & Seidelin, J.B.(2011). MAP kinases in inflammatory bowel disease. *Clin Chim Acta*. Mar 18; 412(7-8):513-20-412: 513-20.

Coulombe, P., & Meloche, S. (2007). Atypical mitogen-activated protein kinases: structure, regulation and functions. *Biochim Biophys Acta*. 1773:1376–87.

Dahan, S., Roda, G., & Pinn, D.(2008). Epithelial : lamina propria lymphocyte interactions promote epithelial cell differentiation. *Gastroenterology*.134:192–203.

Dubuquoy, L., Jansson, E.A., & Deeb, S.(2003). Impaired expression of peroxisome proliferator-activated receptor gamma in ulcerative colitis. *Gastroenterology*. 124:1265–76.

Elias, B.C., Suzuki, T., & Seth, A. (2009). Phosphorylation of Tyr-398 and Tyr-402 in occludin prevents its interaction with ZO-1 and destabilizes its assembly at the tight junctions. *J Biol Chem*. 284:1559-69.

Escaffit, F., Boudreau, F., $ Beaulieu, J.F.(2005). Differential expression of claudin-2 along the human intestine: Implication of GATA-4 in the maintenance of claudin-2 in differentiating cells. *J Cell Physiol*. 203: 15–26.

Festen, E.A., Stokkers, P.C., & Van Diemen, C.C. (2010). Genetic analysis in a Dutch study sample identifies more ulcerative colitis susceptibility loci and shows their additive role in disease risk. *Am J Gastroenterol*.105: 395–402.

Fihn, B.M., Sjoqvist, A., & Jodal, M. (2000). Permeability of the rat small intestinal epithelium along the villus– crypt axis: effects of glucose transport. *Gastroenterology*. 119: 1029–36.

Fukata, M., Chen, A., & Klepper, A. (2006). Cox-2 is regulated by Toll-like receptor-4 (TLR4) signaling: role in proliferation and apoptosis in the intestine. *Gastroenterology*. 131:862–77.

Furuse, M., Hirase, T., & Itoh, M. (1993). Occludin: a novel integral membrane protein localizing at tight junctions. *J Cell Biol*. 123:1777-88.

Furuse, M., Sasaki, H., & Fujimoto, K.(1998). A single gene product, claudin-1 or -2, reconstitutes tight junction strands and recruits occludin in fibroblasts. *J Cell Biol.* 143:391-401.

Furuse, M., & Tsukita, S.(2006). Claudins in occluding junctions of humans and flies. *Trends Cell Biol.* 16:181-8.

Fuss, I.J., Neurath, M., & Boirivant, M.(1996) Disparate CD4+ lamina propria (LP) lymphokine secretion profiles in inflammatory bowel disease. Crohn's disease LP cells manifest increased secretion of IFN-γ, whereas ulcerative colitis LP cells manifest increased secretion of IL-5. *J Immunol.* 157: 1261-70.

Fuss, I.J., Heller, F., & Boirivant, M.(2004). Nonclassical CD1d-restricted NK T cells that produce IL-13 characterize an atypical Th2 response in ulcerative colitis. *J Clin Invest.* 113:1490-7.

Fuss, I.J.(2008). Is the Th1/Th2 paradigm of immune regulation applicable to IBD? *Inflamm Bowel Dis.* Suppl 2:S110-2.

Gagnon, K.B., England, R., & Delpire, E.(2006). Characterization of SPAK and OSR1, regulatory kinases of the Na-K-2Cl cotransporter. *Mol Cell Biol.* 26:689-698.

Garat, C., & Arend, W.P.(2003). Intracellular IL-1Ra type 1 inhibits IL-1-induced IL-6 and IL-8 production in Caco-2 intestinal epithelial cells through inhibition of p38 mitogen-activated protein kinase and NF-kappaB pathways. *Cytokine.* 23:31-40.

González-Mariscal, L., Betanzos, A., & Nava, P.(2003). Tight junction proteins. *Prog Biophys Mol Biol.* 81:1-44.

Graham, W.V., Wang, F., & Clayburgh, D.R. (2006). Tumor necrosis factor-induced long myosin light chain kinase transcription is regulated by differentiation-dependent signaling events. Characterization of the human long myosin light chain kinase promoter. *J Biol Chem.* 281: 26205-15.

Hampe, J., Shaw, S.H., & Saiz, R. (1999). Linkage of inflammatory bowel disease to human chromosome 6p. *Am J Hum Genet.* 65:1647-55.

Heazlewood, C. K., Cook, M.C., & Eri, R.(2008). Aberrant mucin assembly in mice causes endoplasmic reticulum stress and spontaneous inflammation resembling ulcerative colitis. *PLoS Med.* 5: e54.

Heller, F., Florian, P., & Bojarski, C., (2005). Interleukin-13 is the key effector Th2 cytokine in ulcerative colitis that affects epithelial tight junctions, apoptosis, and cell restitution. *Gastroenterology.* 129:550-64.

Hermiston, M.L., Gordon, J.I. (1995). Inflammatory bowel disease and adenomas in mice expressing a dominant negative N-cadherin. *Science.* 270:1203-1207.

Hermiston, M.L., Gordon, J.I. (1995). In vivo analysis of cadherin function in the mouse intestinal epithelium: essential roles in adhesion, maintenance of differentiation, and regulation of programmed cell death. *J Cell Biol.*129:489-506.

Hong, Y.H., Varanasi, U.S., & Yang, W. (2003). AMP-activated protein kinase regulates HNF4alpha transcriptional activity by inhibiting dimer formation and decreasing protein stability. *J Biol Chem.* 278:27495-501.

Hugot, J.P., Laurent-Puig, P., & Gower-Rousseau, C. (1996). Mapping of a susceptibility locus for Crohn's disease on chromosome 16. *Nature.* 379:821-23.

Ikenouchi, J., Furuse, M., & Furuse, K.(2005) Tricellulin constitutes a novel barrier at tricellular contacts of epithelial cells. *J Cell Biol.* 171:939-45.

Johansson, M. E., Phillipson, M., & Petersson, J.*(2008)*. The inner of the two Muc2 mucin-dependent mucus layers in colon is devoid of bacteria. *Proc Natl Acad Sci USA* 105: 15064–9.

Johnston, A.M., Naselli, G., & Gonez, L.J. (2000). SPAK, a STE20/SPS1-related kinase that activates the p38 pathway. *Oncogene*. 19:4290–4297.

Kelly, D., Campbell, J.I., & King, T.P. (2004). Commensal anaerobic gut bacteria attenuate inflammation by regulating nuclear-cytoplasmic shuttling of PPARgamma and RelA. *Nat Immunol*. 5:104–12.

Kenny, P.A., Enver, T., & Ashworth, A. (2005). Receptor and secreted targets of Wnt-1/beta-catenin signaling in mouse mammary epithelial cells. *BMC Cancer*.5:3.

Krimi, R.B., Kotelevets, L., & Dubuquoy, L.(2008). Resistin-like molecule beta regulates intestinal mucous secretion and curtails TNBS-induced colitis in mice. *Inflamm Bowel Dis*. 14:931-41.

Kwon, K.H., Ohigashi, H., & Murakami, A.(2007). Dextran sulfate sodium enhances interleukin-1 beta release via activation of p38 MAPK and ERK1/2 pathways in murine peritoneal macrophages. *Life Sci*. 81:362–71

Loftberg, R., Neurath, M., & Ost, A.(2002). Topical NFkB antisense oligonucleotides in patients with active distal colonic IBD. A randomised controlled pilot trial. *Gastroenterology*. 122: A60.

Mashimo, H., Wu, D.C., & Podolsky, D.K. *(1996)*. Impaired defense of intestinal mucosa in mice lacking intestinal trefoil factor. *Science*. 274: 262–5.

Matsuda, A., Suzuki, Y., & Honda, G.(2003). Large-scale identification and characterization of human genes that activate NF-kappaB and MAPK signaling pathways. *Oncogene*. 22:3307–18.

Medzhitov, R., & Janeway, C.A. Jr.(2002). Decoding the patterns of self and nonself by the innate immune system. *Science*. 296:298–300.

Mitic, L.L., & Anderson, J.M. (1998). Molecular architecture of tight junctions. *Annu Rev Physiol*. 60:121-42.

Mitsuyama, K., Suzuki, A., & Tomiyasu, N.(2006). Pro-inflammatory signaling by Jun-N-terminal kinase in inflammatory bowel disease. *Int J Mol Med*. 17:449–55.

Neurath, M.F., Pettersson, S., & Meyer zum Büschenfelde, K.H.(1996) Local administration of antisense phosphorothioate oligonucleotides to the p65 subunit of NF-κB abrogates established experimental colitis in mice. *Nat Med*. 2: 998–1004.

Nenci, A., Becker, C., & Wullaert, A.(2007). Epithelial NEMO links innate immunity to chronic intestinal inflammation. *Nature*. 446: 557–561.

Neish, A.S., Gewirtz, A.T., & Zeng, H.(2000). Prokaryotic regulation of epithelial responses by inhibition of IkappaB-alpha ubiquitination. *Science*. 289:1560–3.

O'Neill, L.A., Fitzgerald, K.A., & Bowie, A.G.(2003). The Toll-IL-1 receptor adaptor family grows to five members. *Trends Immunol*. 24:286–90.

Oshima T, Miwa H, Joh T (2008). Changes in the expression of claudins in active ulcerative colitis. *J Gastroenterol Hepatol*.23(suppl 2): S146–150.

Otte, J-M., Cario, E., & Podolsky, D.K.(2004). Mechanisms of cross hyporesponsiveness to Toll-like receptor bacterial ligands in intestinal epithelial cells. *Gastroenterology*. 126:1054-70.

Packey, C.D., & Sartor, R.B. (2008). Interplay of commensal and pathogenic bacteria, genetic mutations, and immunoregulatory defects in the pathogenesis of inflammatory bowel diseases. *J Intern Med.* 263:597-606.

Piechotta, K., Lu. J., & Delpire, E. (2002). Cation chloride cotransporters interact with the stress-related kinases Ste20-related proline-alanine-rich kinase (SPAK) and oxidative stress response 1 (OSR1). *J Biol Chem.* 277:50812-50819.

Pinton, P., Braicu, C., & Nougayrede, J.P.(2010). Deoxynivalenol impairs porcine intestinal barrier function and decreases the protein expression of claudin-4 through a mitogen-activated protein kinase-dependent mechanism. *J Nutr.* 140:1956-62.

Resta-Lenert, S., & Barrett, K.E. (2006). Probiotics and commensals reverse TNFalpha-and IFN-gamma-induced dysfunction in human intestinal epithelial cells. *Gastroenterology.* 130:731-746.

Saitou, M., Furuse, M., & Sasaki, H.(2000). Complex phenotype of mice lacking occludin, a component of tight junction strands. *Mol Biol Cell.* 11:4131-4142.

Schulzke, J.D., Gitter, A.H., & Mankertz, J. (2005). Epithelial transport and barrier function in occludin-deficient mice. *Biochim Biophys Acta.* 1669:34-42.

Schulzke, J.D., Bojarski, C., & Zeissig, S.(2006). Disrupted barrier function through epithelial cell apoptosis. *Ann NY Acad Sci.* 1072:288-299.

Schmitz, H., Barmeyer, C., & Fromm, M.(1999). Altered tight junction structure contributes to the impaired epithelial barrier function in ulcerative colitis. *Gastroenterology.* 116: 301-9.

Schurmann, G., Bruwer, M., & Klotz, A. (1999). Transepithelial transport processes at the intestinal mucosa in inflammatory bowel disease. *Int J Colorectal Dis.* 14: 41-6.

Shen, L., Su, L., & Turner, J.R.(2009). Mechanisms and functional implications of intestinal barrier defects. *Dig Dis.* 27:443-9.

Simon, D.B., Lu, Y., & Choate, K.A. (1999). Paracellin-1, a renal tight junction protein required for paracellular Mg2+ resorption. *Science.* 285:103-106.

Suzuki, T., Elias, B.C., & Seth, A. (2009). PKC eta regulates occluding phosphorylation and epithelial tight junction integrity. *Proc Natl Acad Sci U S A.* 106:61-66.

Szakal, D.N., Gyorffy, H., & Arato, A. (2010). Mucosal expression of claudins 2, 3, and 4 in proximal and distal part of duodenum in children with coeliac disease. *Virchows Arch.* 456: 245-250.

Tai, E.K., Wong, H.P., & Lam, E.K.(2008). Cathelicidin stimulates colonic mucus synthesis by up-regulating MUC1 and MUC2 expression through a mitogen-activated protein kinase pathway. *J Cell Biochem.* 104:251-8.

Thalhamer, T., McGrath, M.A., & Harnett, M.M.(2008). MAPKs and their relevance to arthritis and inflammation. *Rheumatology (Oxf).* 47:409-14.

Thompson, A.I., & Lees, C.W.(2011). Genetics of ulcerative colitis. *Inflamm Bowel Dis.* 17:831-48.

Topper, J.N., Wasserman, S.M., & Anderson, K.R. (1997). Expression of the bumetanide-sensitive Na-K-Cl cotransporter BSC2 is differentially regulated by fluid mechanical and inflammatory cytokine stimuli in vascular endothelium. *J Clin Invest.* 99:2941-49.

Turner, J.R.(2006). Molecular basis of epithelial barrier regulation: from basic mechanisms to clinical application. *Am J Pathol*. 169:1901-9.

Ueno, N., Fujiya, M., & Segawa, S. (2011). Heat-killed body of lactobacillus brevis SBC8803 ameliorates intestinal injury in a murine model of colitis by enhancing the intestinal barrier function. *Inflamm Bowel Dis*. Jan 6. [Epub ahead of print]

Van der Sluis, M., De Koning, B.A., & De Bruijn, A.C. (2006). Muc 2-deficient mice spontaneously develop colitis, indicating thatMuc 2 is critical for colonic protection. *Gastroenterology*. 131: 117–29.

Van Itallie, C.M., Fanning, A.S., & Anderson, J.M.(2003). Reversal of charge selectivity in cation or anion-selective epithelial lines by expression of different claudins. *Am J Physiol Renal Physiol*. 285:F1078-1084.

Van Itallie, C.M., & Anderson, J.M. (2004). The molecular physiology of tight junction pores. *Physiology(Bethesda)*. 19:331-338.

Van Itallie, C.M., & Anderson, J.M.(2006). Claudins and epithelial paracellular transport. *Annu Rev Physiol*. 68:403-429.

Van Itallie C.M., Holmes, J., & Bridges, A., (2008). The density of small tight junction pores varies among cell types and is increased by expression of claudin-2. *J Cell Sci*. 121:298-305.

Viollet, B., Kahn, A., & Raymondjean, M.(1997). Protein kinase A-dependent phosphorylation modulates DNA-binding activity of hepatocyte nuclear factor 4. *Mol Cell Biol*. 17: 4208-4219.

Wang, F., Graham, W.V., & Wang, Y.(2005). Interferon-γ and tumor necrosis factor-α synergize to induce intestinal epithelial barrier dysfunction by up-regulating myosin light chain kinase expression. *Am J Pathol*. 166: 409–419.

Wang, N., Yu, H., & Ma, J.(2010). Evidence for tight junction protein disruption in intestinal mucosa of malignant obstructive jaundice patients. *Scand J Gastroenterol*. 45: 191–9.

Watson, C.J., Hoare, C.J., & Garrod, D.R. (2005). Interferon-γ selectively increases epithelial permeability to large molecules by activating different populations of paracellular pores. *J Cell Sci*. 118: 5221–30.

Waetzig, G.H., Seegert, D., & Rosenstiel, P., (2002). p38 Mitogen-activated protein kinase is activated and linked to TNF-alpha signaling in inflammatory bowel disease. *J Immunol*. 168:5342–51.

Yan, F., & Polk, D.B. (2002). Probiotic bacterium prevents cytokine-induced apoptosis in intestinal epithelial cells. *J Biol Chem*. 277:50959 –50965.

Yan, Y., Nguyen, H., & Dalmasso, G.(2007). Cloning and characterization of a new intestinal inflammation-associated colonic epithelial Ste20-related protein kinase isoform. *Biochim Biophys Acta*. 1769:106–116.

Yan, Y., Laroui, H., & Ingersoll, S.A. (2011). Overexpression of Ste20-Related Proline/Alanine-Rich Kinase Exacerbates Experimental Colitis in Mice. *J Immunol*. 187:1496-505.

Yu, A.S., McCarthy, K.M., & Francis, S.A.(2005). McCormack JM, Lai J, Rogers RA, Lynch RD, Schneeberger EE: Knockdown of occludin expression leads to diverse phenotypic alterations in epithelial cells. *Am J Physiol Cell Physiol*. 288:C1231-1241.

Zeissig, S., Bojarski, C., & Buergel, N. (2004). Downregulation of epithelial apoptosis and barrier repair in active Crohn's disease by tumour necrosis factor alpha antibody treatment. *Gut.* 53:1295-1302.

Zeissig, S., Burgel, N., & Gunzel, D.(2007). Changes in expression and distribution of claudin 2, 5 and 8 lead to discontinuous tight junctions and barrier dysfunction in active Crohn's disease. *Gut.* 56: 61–72.

4

Defensins in Ulcerative Colitis

Zhanju Liu[1] and Yurong Yang[2]
*[1]Department of Gastroenterology, The Shanghai Tenth People's Hospital,
Tongji University, Shanghai,
[2]College of Animal and Veterinary Engineering,
Henan Agricultural University, Zhengzhou
China*

1. Introduction

Defensins and cathelicidins are the two major endogenous antimicrobial peptide families in mammals, which are abundant components of phagocytic leukocytes and are released by epithelial cells at mucosal surfaces. Defensins are antimicrobial peptides produced at a variety of epithelial surfaces. In the small intestine Paneth cells secrete α-defensins and additional antimicrobial peptides at high levels in response to cholinergic stimulation and when exposed to bacterial antigens. In the intestinal tract α- and β-defensins contribute to host immunity and assist in maintaining the balance between protection from pathogens and tolerance to normal flora. However, attenuated expression of these defensins compromises host immunity and hence may alter the balance toward inflammation. Altered defensins production is suggested to be an integral element in the pathogenesis of ulcerative colitis (UC). Recent years, the defensins have attracted great attention because of their roles in the organism defense system. This review highlights the current knowledge of defensins, distribution, structures, the diverse functions in the immune response and the changes of defensins expression in UC and the potential role in the pathogenesis of UC.

2. Structures of defensins

Antimicrobial peptides are gene-encoded natural antibiotics produced by virtually every life form studied (Boman, 1995; Zasloff, 2002). In mammals, defensins are a major (if not predominant) group of antimicrobial peptides. In the 1980s, Lehrer et al. first found a series of small molecules cationic peptides with similar structures to rabbit and human neutrophil cytoplasmic granules, which were first named "defensins" (Lehrer et al., 1980). A fundamental characteristic of defensins peptides is the presence of three intramolecular disulfide bonds (Ganz, 2003). The defensins are thus subdivided into three subgroups (designated α-, β-, and θ-defensins). The subgroups are based largely on the connectivity of three cystine linkages (Table 1), but structural features of the gene and precursor are also further distinguishing characteristics.

The three-dimensional structures of several α- and β-defensins have been determined by both nuclear magnetic resonance (NMR) and X-ray crystallography techniques (Hill et al., 1991; Zhang et al., 1992; Pardi et al., 1992; Skalicky et al., 1994; Zimmermann et al., 1995;

Sawai et al., 2001). Although crystal structures of some defensins are made up of dimers or multimers, it has not been yet clear whether these multimers are the biologically relevant to different forms of defensins.

Defensins	Peptide size	Cysteine Linkages	Size	Expression Sites	Expression Patterns	Species Distribution
α-defensins	30~34 aa	1-6, 2-4, 3-5	90-105 aa	Neutrophils, Macrophage, Paneth cells, Reproductive epithelia	Mostly constitutive	Primates Rodents Rabbits
β-defensins	36~44 aa	1-5, 2-4, 3-6	60-70 aa	Mucosal epithelia and Skin, Ruminant, Heterophils, Epididymis	Mostly inducible	Primates Rodents Ruminants Birds Crustaceans
θ-defensins	18 aa (two connected hemi-peptides of 9 aa each)	1-1', 2-3, 2'-3'	90 aa	Neutrophils	Constitutive	Non-human primates

Table 1. Comparison of α-defensins, β-defensins and θ-defensins

The 3D structures of α- and β-defensins contain a canonical triple-stranded antiparallel β-sheet motif. Solution and crystallographic analyses of β-defensins have revealed that the α- and β-defensins folds are similar as the amphipathicity is produced by the distribution of polar and hydrophobic side chains on the peptide surfaces. However, both β-defensins possess short α-helical segments that α-defensins lack. There is no evident relationship between β-sheet content and antimicrobial activity, and knowledge of the general structural factors that modulate the antimicrobial spectrum and activity of defensins is for the most part lacking.

The solution structures of closed circular rhesus θ-defensin-1 (RTD-1) and its open chain analog (oRTD-1) have been determined by two-dimensional NMR. RTD-1 and oRTD-1 adopt very similar structures in water, containing an extended β-hairpin, structure with turns at one end in oRTD-1 or in both ends in circular RTD-1. The double stranded β-sheet region of the two molecules is flexible, and, because the structures and flexibilities of RTD-1 and oRTD-1 are similar, the reduced antimicrobial activity of oRTD-1 relative to circular RTD-1 is attributable to the charged N- and C-termini of the oRTD-1 molecule (Trabi et al., 2001; Ouellette, 2006). In contrast to many antimicrobial peptides, RTD-1 has no amphiphilic character, even though surface models of RTD-1 exhibit a certain clustering of positive charges.

3. Characteristics of defensins distribution

Defensins are abundant in cells and tissues that are involved in host defense against microbial infections. Notably, the specific tissue distribution of defensins diverged rapidly during vertebrate evolution (Table 2). To date, 12 different human α-defensins and 48 human β-defensins, 22 mouse α-defensins and 26 mouse β-defensins have been identified and isolated (http://defensins.bii.a-star.edu.sg). In the alimentary tract of mammals, α-defensins are highly expressed and largely confined to the small intestine, whereas β-defensins are found to be inducible expression at sites of infection or inflammation.

Species	Neutrophil defensins	Paneth cell defensins	Epithelial cell defensins
Human	α	α	α and β
Rhesus monkey	α and θ	Not determined	β
Mouse	none	α	α and β
Rat	α	α	β
Pig	Not detected in granule extracts	Not determined	β
Cow	β	none	β
Chicken	β	Not determined	β

Table 2. Diverse patterns of defensins expression in vertebrates

In human, α-defensins are expressed primarily in neutrophils, NK cells, certain T cell subsets, and in Paneth cells of the small intestine, where they may regulate and maintain microbial balance in the intestinal lumen. Moreover, low levels of α-defensins expression have been observed in epithelial cells of digestive tract, urogenital tract of mammalian and the kidney of rabbit. Human α-defensin-1, -2, -3, and -4, also known as neutrophil polypeptide (HNP), are located primarily in neutrophils, while human α-defensin-5 and -6 (HD-5, HD-6) are secreted by the small intestinal Paneth cells. Mature α-defensins consist of 29-36 amino acids including six conserved cysteine residues.

β-defensins are the most widely distributed, being secreted by leukocytes and epithelial cells of many kinds. For example, they can be found on the tongue, skin, cornea, salivary glands, kidneys, esophagus, and respiratory tract. It has been suggested that some of the pathology of cystic fibrosis arises from the inhibition of β-defensins activity on the epithelial surfaces of the lungs and trachea due to higher salt content. β-defensins were first found from tracheal epithelium cells of cattle and in granulocytes of cattle (Diamond et al., 1991). The first human β-defensin (HBD-1) was discovered in 1995, which is mainly expressed in kidney, urogenital tract and other epithelial cells (Bensch et al., 1995). In 1997 Harder et al. first isolated and purified HBD-2 from the skin of psoriasis patients (Harder et al., 1997), and it is mainly expressed in damaged skin, oral mucosa and epithelium of infected lungs. HBD-3 is observed to be mainly expressed in human keratinocytes and airway epithelial cells. HBD-4 is mainly expressed in testis, uterus, neutrophils, thyroid, lung and kidney. In addition, HBD-5 and HBD-6 are only present in testicular cells (Harder et al., 2001; Garcia et al., 2001). β-defensins are composed of 36-42 amino acid residues, containing 6 conserved cysteine residues.

θ-defensins are rare and thus far have been found only in the leukocytes of the rhesus macaque (Tran et al., 2008), and the olive baboon, Papio anubis, being vestigial in humans and other primates (Angie & Michael 2008; Garcia et al., 2008). Interestingly, θ-defensins are negative in humans and New World monkeys (Garcia et al., 2008; Nguyen et al., 2003). θ-defensins are macrocyclic octadecapeptides expressed only in old world monkeys and orangutans, and produced by the pair-wise, head-to-tail splicing of nonapeptides derived from their respective precursors. Rhesus θ-defensin-1 (RTD-1) is a unique cyclic antimicrobial peptide first identified in rhesus macaque leukocytes (Tang et al., 1999), and produced by a novel post-translational processing pathway involving the excision of two 9-amino-acid oligopeptides from a pair of propeptides that is further stabilized by three disulfide bonds. θ-defensins possess broad antimicrobial properties *in vitro* against bacteria, fungi, and viruses (Owen et al., 2004; Tran et al., 2008; Wang et al., 2004). Nevertheless, they exhibit very low levels of toxicity *in vitro* (Tran et al., 2008) and *in vivo*, indicating that they may have utilities as therapeutic agents.

4. Biosynthesis of defensins

4.1 Regulation of α-defensins biosynthesis

α-defensins genes map to 8p21–8pter through 8p23 in human and are syntenic in mice (Ouellette, 2006; Ouellette et al., 1989b; Patil et al., 2004; Sparkes et al., 1989), which are expressed predominantly in myeloid cells or in Paneth cells (Selsted & Ouellette, 1995).

4.1.1 Transcriptional regulation

Myeloid α-defensins mRNA are expressed almost exclusively in the bone marrow, where they are found at the highest levels in promyelocytes and at lower levels in myeloblasts and myelocytes (Yount et al., 1995). Enteric α-defensins occur exclusively in Paneth cells in normal small bowel (Cunliffe et al., 2001; Ouellette et al., 1999; Ouellette et al., 2000; Porter et al., 1997b; Selsted et al., 1992). Myeloid and Paneth cell α-defensins genes differ in that genes expressed in cells of myeloid origin consist of three exons, whereas those expressed in Paneth cells have only two exons (Bevins et al., 1996; Huttner et al., 1994; Jones & Bevins, 1992; Jones & Bevins, 1993; Lala et al., 2003). In Paneth cell α-defensins genes, the 5′-untranslated region and the preprosegment are coded by exon 1, but an additional intron interrupts the 5′-untranslated region of myeloid α-defensins gene transcripts (Ouellette & Selsted, 1996).

The differentiation of Paneth cells is determined by continuous Wnt signaling via the frizzled-5 receptor, and transcription of α-defensins genes in Paneth cell is mediated by β-catenin/TCF-4 recognition sites in the 5′-upstream regions of the gene transcription start sites as well as upstream of the gene coding for matrix metalloproteinase-7 (MMP-7), the mouse α-defensins convertase (Andreu et al., 2005; He et al., 2004; Pinto & Clevers, 2005; Van et al., 2005). Monocytes and NK cells also contain α-defensins mRNAs and peptides, but regulatory elements equivalent to β-catenin/TCF-4 sites in Paneth cell α-defensins genes remain to be found in myeloid α-defensins gene promoters.

4.1.2 Posttranslational activation of α-defensins

Both α- and β-defensins are initially synthesized as preprodefensins, consisting of a characteristic amino terminal signal sequence, a propiece, and the mature peptide at the carboxy terminal end of the prepropeptide. The processing and release of α-defensins seem to be peptide- and host species-specific. α-defensins have been isolated from primate leukocytes and neutrophils of several rodents including rats, rabbits, guinea pigs, and hamsters. Myeloid α-defensins RNAs are expressed almost exclusively in the bone marrow, where they occur at the highest levels in promyelocytes and at lower levels in myeloblasts and myelocytes. Although neutrophils contain high levels of α-defensins peptides, defensins mRNAs are degraded during neutrophil differentiation. In contrast, circulating monocytes contain both α-defensins mRNAs and peptides. The proteolytic pathway required to produce mature HNPs from their proforms is active only in myeloid cells (Valore & Ganz,

1992). Newly synthesized proHNPs are processed to mature defensins and then the mature peptides are stored in cytoplasmic granules. The propiece of proHNPs is important for the normal cellular trafficking during defensins biosynthesis and functions as an intramolecular inhibitor of defensins cytotoxicity (Liu & Ganz, et al., 1995; Valore et al., 1996).

Unlike human neutrophil defensins, Paneth cell defensins HD-5 and HD-6 are stored as precursor in the secretory granules of Paneth cells (Ghosh et al., 2002). The biosynthesis of Paneth cell pro-α-defensins involves post-translational proteolytic activation. Although the enzymes that mediate pro-α-defensins processing in myeloid and epithelial cells are likely to differ, the overall processing schemes are similar in that all are processed from precursor by specific proteolytic cleavage steps.

Evidences have been shown that α-defensins are present in murine Paneth cells under germ-free conditions (Salzman et al., 2007; Ouellette & Lualdi, 1990; Putsep et al., 2000), and in human Paneth cells prenatally (Mallow et al., 1996). These findings indicate that α-defensins expression is independent on bacterial stimulation. In contrast, expression of Reg3γ and angiogenin in Paneth cells is closely associated with the presence of microbes in the intestinal lumen.

Transcription levels of α-defensins in Paneth cells are directed, in part, through factors intimately linked to cellular differentiation (Batlle et al., 2002). Clevers and colleagues have shown that Tcf7-L2 (also known as Tcf-4) is a key transcription factor for α-defensins expression in Paneth cells. Activity of this transcription factor is linked to Wnt/β-Catenin signaling gradients in the crypt and appears to represent a master regulator for Paneth cell differentiation (Van et al., 2005). Defensins expression is found to be low in human neonates (Mallow et al., 1996), unweaned mice (Ouellette & Cordell, 1988; Ouellette et al., 1989a) and rats, but increases dramatically with maturation. Aside from this developmental pattern, α-defensin expression is relatively constitutive under most conditions. However, levels vary significantly in association with some disease states (Kelly et al., 2004; Wehkamp et al., 2004, 2005).

Additional regulatory mechanisms of α-defensins activity are granule secretion and proteolytic processing of precursor peptides (Bevins, 2004). Paneth cells secrete their dense secretory granules into the crypt lumen in response to bacterial products (including muramyl dipeptide, a component of bacterial peptidoglycan), but not to fungal or protozoal stimuli (Qu et al., 1996; Ayabe et al., 2000). These findings suggest that *in vivo* control of α-defensins secretion in Paneth cells may be linked to microbial sensors. Interestingly, recent studies have identified that Paneth cells could express nucleotide oligomerization domain (NOD)2 (a critical intracellular pattern recognition receptor for muramyl dipeptide), whose precise functions in Paneth cells are yet to be clearly determined (Lala et al., 2003; Rumio et al., 2004; Kobayashi et al., 2005). Cholinergic agonists can also stimulate α-defensins secretion by a mechanism that appears to involve both increased cytosolic Ca^{2+} and mIKCa1 potassium channels (Satoh et al., 1995; Ayabe et al., 2002).

Proteolytic processing is an important step in regulating expression of active Paneth cell-derived defensins. Paneth cell-derived α-defensins, like myeloid-derived α-defensins, are initially expressed as amino acid prepropeptides. After removal of the N-terminal signal sequence, the Paneth cell-derived α-defensins propeptides require processing by an endopeptidase to produce a mature active peptide. However, there are differences in this general theme when comparing with rodents and primates. MMP-7 (also known as matrilysin), an endoprotease expressed in mouse Paneth cells, is essential for processing of the α-defensins propeptide to active mature peptides in mice (Wilson et al., 1999; Ouellette,

2005; Selsted & Ouellette, 2005). MMP-7 processes the α-defensins propeptides to their active mature peptide counterparts at precisely the same cleavage site *in vitro* as identified *in vivo* (Selsted et al., 1992; Shirafuji et al., 2003). Polymorphic isoforms of α-defensins containing mutations at MMP-7 cleavage site exist in some mouse strains, which influence post-translational processing and yield differences in mature peptides. Characterization of Paneth cell-derived α-defensins suggests that MMP-7 is also the endoprotease responsible for processing in rats (Qu et al., 1996). In rhesus macaques, characterization of Paneth cell-derived α-defensins indicates that trypsin is likely the endoprotease responsible for processing in these primates as well (Tanabe et al., 2004a, 2004b). In contrast, MMP-7 is not detected in human Paneth cells, and trypsin is the endoprotease expressed in Paneth cells, which is responsible for processing of α-defensins propeptides (Ghosh et al., 2002).

In humans Paneth cell-derived α-defensins are stored in secretory granules as propeptides (Ghosh et al., 2002; Cunliffe, et al., 2001). The propeptide trypsinogen is also stored in these same Paneth cell granules. Current hypotheses point that trypsinogen is activated to trypsin after secretion, which then converts proHD5 into mature HD5 in either the crypt or intestinal lumen. In contrast, some of the α-defensins pool in mouse Paneth cells is processed intracellularly and stored as mature MMP-7-cleaved peptides (Ouellette, 2005; Selsted & Ouellette, 2005). Since proteolytic processing is central to the biology of Paneth cell α-defensins, it will be interesting to determine how and why rodents and primates diverged in their mechanisms for achieving this important post-translational modification.

Evidence for the key role of Paneth cell α-defensins in host defense against orally ingested pathogens comes from murine models. Targeted disruption of the MMP-7 gene, which encodes the processing endoprotease of murine Paneth cell α-defensins precursors, has shown to impair the ability of mice to produce active cryptdin. Compared to their wild-type littermates, the MMP-7 null mice cannot effectively clear orally administered noninvasive *Escherichia coli*, and they succumb more rapidly to lower doses of virulent Salmonella enterica serovar Typhimurium. However, MMP-7 may have other biological functions that could have altered the susceptibility to these bacterial challenges. Therefore, Salzman et al. utilized a complementary approach to analyze Paneth cell α-defensins function (Salzman et al., 2003). Mice were genetically engineered to express the human Paneth cell α-defensins HD5. Under transcriptional control of HD5's own endogenous promoter, these transgenic mice expressed HD5 in Paneth cells. Expression levels of the transgene were similar to those of the endogenous α-defensins (cryptdins), pointing that this murine model can assess the biological effects of physiologically relevant levels of HD5. The transgenic mice were more resistant to orally administered Salmonella. Thus, these two models point to a central role for Paneth cell α-defensins in innate immunity of the small intestine against orally ingested pathogens.

4.2 Regulation of β-defensins biosynthesis

It is likely that β-defensins gene products are produced and stored as mature peptides because pro-β-defensins have not been recovered from natural producing cells and insect cells, in which transfected with β-defensins cDNA always release bioactive mature β-defensins (Aono et al., 2006; Shi, 2007). HBD-1 is constitutively expressed in the epithelial cells in the small intestine and colon and its expression is not influenced by inflammation or bacterial infection. Despite normally absent, HBD-2 and HBD-3 can be induced in normal colon epithelial cells (O'Neil et al., 1999; Fahlgren et al., 2004). Induction of HBD-2 is an NFκB-dependent process in the intestinal epithelium because blocking NF-κB activation could inhibit the upregulation of HBD-2 in response to IL-1 stimulation or bacterial infection (O'Neil et al., 1999; Voss et al., 2006). Unlike professional phagocytes and Paneth cells, epithelial cells expressing β-defensins do not have visible granules. How β-defensins are stored and released from intestinal epithelial cells remains obscure.

4.3 Regulation of θ-defensins biosynthesis

Rhesus θ-defensins peptides assemble from two distinct precursor molecules with each hemi-precursor contributing a nine-amino acid moiety to the final RTD-1 peptide, although the molecular mechanisms that catalyze or facilitate θ-defensins assembly in primates are not understood (Tang et al., 1999). Rhesus pro-RTDs are products of different genes that resemble the three-exon myeloid α-defensins genes, except that they are truncated by stop codons in exon 3. In addition to heterodimeric RTD-1, homodimeric θ-defensins RTD-2 and -3 have also been isolated from monkey neutrophils (Tran et al., 2002; Leonova et al., 2001). α-defensins gene mutations that give rise to the θ-defensins genes (DEFT) apparently arise in Old World monkeys, because rhesus DEFT homologs have not been found in prosimians or in New World monkeys (Lehrer, 2004). Humans, chimpanzees, and gorillas lack θ-defensins, because the DEFT genes of those species harbor mutations that create premature stop codons in the prepro regions of the precursors. However, at least one mutant human DEFT gene still is actively transcribed, and its nonfunctional mRNA accumulates to high abundance at several sites of expression (Cole et al., 2002).

5. Role of defensins in immune response

In the gastrointestinal tract, these peptides have bactericidal activity by forming micropores in the phospholipid bilayer of bacterial membranes, causing loss of structural integrity and collapse of the bacterial cells. This antimicrobial quality allows defensins to protect the host epithelium and stem cells from virulent pathogens and also help to regulate the number and composition of commensal microbiota (Ramasundara et al., 2009).

5.1 Defensins in innate immunity

The innate immunity is the most primitive defense system against pathogens, which has not only the generalized mechanical barriers and antibacterial action, but also includes functional defense barrier built by phagocytosis and inflammatory response.

5.1.1 Antibacterial activity

Defensins have a broad antibacterial spectrum, which can effectively kill Gram-negative and -positive bacteria, fungi, spirochetes, and some parasites. Importantly, α-defensins have stronger activity against Gram-positive bacteria, while the β-defensins have stronger activity against Gram-negative and -positive bacteria. HBD-3 has stronger bactericidal activity against *Staphylococcus aureus*, *Streptococcus pyogenes*, *Pseudomonas aeruginosa*, *Escherichia coli* and *Actinomycetes in vitro* (Maisetta et al., 2005).

The α- and β-defensins expressed in the alimentary tract of human and mice have activity profiles and expression patterns that overlap with other mammalian peptides (Table 3). Intestinal α-defensins have microbicidal activities against many Gram-positive (*L. monocytogenes*, *S. aureus*) and Gram-negative bacteria (*E. coli*, *S. typhimurium*). Similarly, HD5 is active against many bacterial species and the fungus *C. albicans* (Porter et al., 1997a; Ghosh et al., 2002; Ericksen et al., 2005). Surprisingly, initial reports indicate that HD6 has very poor antibacterial activity *in vitro*, despite similar ionic charge properties as HD5 (Ericksen et al., 2005). The most abundant β-defensins, expressed chiefly in the stomach and colon, also have bactericidal activity *in vitro*. HBD-2 is microbicidal against *P. aeruginosa*, *E. coli* and *C. albicans*, but less activity against Gram-positive *S. aureus* (Harder et al., 1997). In contrast, the more cationic HBD-3 has activity against *S. aureus* (Harder et al., 2001) and is less sensitive to the ionic composition of the assay medium. HBD-1 has antibacterial activity (Valore et al., 1998), but it is not potent *in vitro* like HD6.

Defensins	Mr (kDa)	Tissue distribution	Stimuli
HNP 1-4	3.5-4.5	Sparse lamina propria neutrophils in active inflammation seen in scattered intestinal epithelial cells	Increased in active inflammation but possibly a result of increased neutrophilic influx
HD-5, HD-6	3.5-4.5	Paneth cells and some villous epithelial cells in normal duodenum, jejunum and ileum Paneth cell metaplasia	Constitutively expressed, however processing is required for biological activity
HBD-1	3.5-4.5	Colonic epithelia (and some other mucosal epithelia)	Constitutively expressed
HBD-2, -3, -4	3.5-4.5	Colonic epithelia (and some other mucosal epithelia) Colonic plasma cells	IL-1α and entero-invasive bacteria
Cryp-4	5.1	Paneth cells	Uncertain

Table 3. Defensins in the gut of human and mouse

5.1.2 Chemotactic activity

Various defensins have been reported to have chemotactic activity for monocytes, T cells and dendritic cells. In the case of HBD-1 and HBD-2, which attract memory T cells and immature dendritic cells, the chemoattractant activity might be due to defensins binding to the chemokine receptor CCR6. Although the physiological importance of this interaction has not yet been shown, the high concentrations of HBD-2 in inflamed skin make it probable that this defensins could compete effectively with the natural CCL20, despite the higher affinity of the latter for the CCR6. Recent structural analysis of CCL20 has indicated marked similarities to HBD-2 in the putative receptor binding region of CCL20. The role of this region in the chemotactic activity of HBD-2 needs to be confirmed by mutating the amino-acid residues that are suspected to be involved in its interaction with CCR6. Human neutrophil defensins HNP1-3 have been reported to be chemotactic for monocytes, naive T cells and immature dendritic cells (Territo et al., 1989; Chertov et al., 1996; Yang et al., 1999; 2000), but a specific receptor has not been identified. Mouse β-defensin-2 acted as a peptide adjuvant when it was linked to a non-immunogenic tumour antigen (Biragyn et al., 2002). This immunostimulatory activity was shown to depend on TLR-4 and its ability to induce dendritic-cell maturation. It is not yet certain how this receptor can bind with mouse β-defensin-2 as well as the many other ligands attributed to it, or whether some of these molecules function as efficient carriers for lipopolysaccharide, the main ligand of TLR-4.

5.1.3 Paneth cell defensins regulate innate immune responses by NOD2 or TLRs

TLRs which are the major pattern recognition receptors of innate immunity, by recognizing pathogen associated molecular patterns, activating the innate immune system to produce proinflammatory cytokines and defensins resist damage caused by pathogens (Elphick & Mahida, 2005). NOD2 is a new pattern recognition molecule, participating in the anti-bacterial and anti-invasion effect of host cell by the identification of intracellular bacterial components. The absence of NOD2 leads to the disorder of NF-κB, resulting in imbalance of cytokine production and defensins secretion disorders. Kobayashi et al. found that the levels of two cryptdins expression were significantly reduced when NOD2 gene mutated in mice (Kobayashi et al., 2005). NOD2 mutations have impact on Paneth cell α-defensins expression, whereas α-defensins are the main effector molecule which Paneth cells play a major role in innate immunity. Therefore, intestinal epithelium could regulate the expression of defensins secretion to activate and regulate innate immune responses by NOD or TLRs through pattern recognition receptors.

5.1.4 Blocking ACTH activity

Evidences have demonstrated that some defensins have a role in inhibiting the effects of adrenocorticotropic hormone (ACTH) by binding to ACTH receptor (Zhu et al., 1987, 1989; Solomon et al., 1991; Tominaga et al., 1990). Although such activity could inhibit the production of the immunosuppressive hormone cortisol, and could therefore be useful in responding to infections, the physiological role of this *in vitro* interaction has not yet been shown.

5.1.5 Other activities of defensins

It has been reported that defensins have the ability to activate nifedipine-sensitive calcium channels in mammalian cells (MacLeod et al., 1991; Bateman et al., 1996). The structural basis of this effect is not understood. Certain mouse Paneth cell defensins could promote chloride secretion, probably by forming channels in the apical membrane of epithelial cells (Lencer, et al., 1997; Merlin et al., 2001). This activity is limited to a subset of mouse Paneth cell defensins, and its structural basis is not yet known.

5.2 Defensins in acquired Immunity

Evidences have demonstrated that α- and β-defensins have chemotactic activities, indicating that defensins are involved in attracting T cells recycling and promoting immature dendritic cells and monocytes homing to the site of infection. HNP-1 and HNP-2 could enhance severe immune deficiency (SCID) mice T cell recycling (Lillard et al., 1999). Intraperitoneal administration of human neutrophil peptide (HNP) significantly increased the production of keyhole limpet henocyanin (KLH)-specific IgG1, IgG2a and IgG2b antibodies 14 days after immunization. These results indicate that defensins function as potent immune adjuvants by inducing the production of lymphokines, which promote T cell-dependent cellular immunity and antigen-specific Ig production, and that defensins appear to act as neutrophil-derived signals that promote adaptive immune responses (Tani et al., 2000).

Increasing data have shown that β-defensins participate in acquired immunization mainly by chemotactic induction or direct activation of antigen presenting cells, such as dendritic cells, to activate the T cells, resulting in enhanced specific immune response (O'Neil et al., 1999). Previous study has confirmed that defensins contribute to host defense by disrupting the cytoplasmic membrane of microorganisms (Yang et al., 1999, 2000). Human α-defensins are also chemotactic for immature dendritic cells and memory T cells. Human α-defensins was selectively chemotactic for cells stably transfected to express human CCR6, a chemokine receptor preferentially expressed by immature dendritic cells and memory T cells. The α-defensin-induced chemotaxis is sensitive to pertussis toxin and inhibited by antibodies to CCR6. The binding of iodinated LARC, the chemokine ligand for CCR6, to CCR6-transfected cells was competitively displaced by α-defensins. Thus, α-defensins may promote adaptive immune responses by recruiting dendritic and T cells to the site of microbial invasion through interaction with CCR6. In addition, defensins are also able to activate macrophages via TLR signaling and trigger acquired immune system. Evidence has shown that in cooperation with the IL-1 related protein kinase (IRAK), β-defensin-2 as TLR-4 endogenous ligand could combine with TLR4, leading to NK-κB activation and migration to the nucleus to activate cytokine gene transcription, upregulation of costimulatory molecules expression and dendritic cells maturation, thereby activate T cells, trigger a strong specific immune response (Biragyn et a1., 2002; Means et a1., 2000).

6. Role of defenins in the pathogenesis of UC

Inflammatory bowel disease (IBD) is chronic, relapsing and debilitating conditions that have significant impact on quality of life. IBD includes two main conditions, UC and Crohn's disease (CD), which are defined based on characteristic endoscopic and histological findings. UC is characterised by superficial inflammation limited to the mucosa of the colon. In contrast, CD is characterised by discontinuous skip lesions that can occur anywhere in the gastro-intestinal tract with transmural inflammation and non-caseating granulomas.

The pathogenesis of IBD is not clearly understood, and its presentation regarding disease localization, progression and response to therapies is unpredictable. In the intestinal tract, defensins contribute to host immunity and assist in maintaining the balance between protection from pathogens and tolerance to normal flora. However, attenuated expression of defensins compromises host immunity and hence may alter the balance toward inflammation. Altered defensins production is suggested to be an integral element in the pathogenesis of IBD (Table 4).

Defensins	Ulcerative colitis	Ileal Crohn's disease	Colonic Crohn's disease
HNP 1-4	upregulate (infection)	Unknown	Unknown
HD-5, HD-6	Upregulate, Paneth cell metaplasia	Downregulate, especially NOD2 mutation paitent	Upregulate, Paneth cell metaplasia
HBD-1	Downregulate	Downregulate	Downregulate
HBD-2, -3	Upregulate (infection)	No obvious change	No obvious change
HBD-4	Upregulate	No obvious change	No obvious change
Cryp-2	Upregulate	Unknown	Unknown
Cryp-4	Unknown	Unknown	Downregulate

Table 4. Defensins expression in ulcerative colitis, and colonic and ileal Crohn's disease

6.1 α-defensins in UC
6.1.1 Paneth cell-derived α-defensins in UC

α-defensins are highly expressed by Paneth cells (Fig. 1). These cells are located at the base of the crypts of Lieberkühn and are distributed from the duodenum to the ileum. Their location in the crypts suggests an essential role of protecting the epithelial stem cells, located in close proximity. Paneth cells are filled with large apically located granules (Fig. 1A) and have ultrastructural hallmarks (an extensive endoplasmic reticulum and well-developed Golgi) of prototypical secretory cells. The development of small intestine gland is imperfect in newborn BALB/c mice, and no Paneth cells were seen 4 days before. However, Paneth cells could be detected in small intestine gland 6 days after birth (Fig. 1C). In addition to α-defensins, human Paneth cells also secrete lysozyme, Reg 3γ, and phospholipase A2 (Ouellette & Bevins, 2001). Of these antimicrobials, the α-defensins are the most abundant. In addition, mouse Paneth cells also express numerous cryptdin-related peptides (Fig. 1B) and angiogenin (Ouellette & Bevins, 2001; Hornef et al., 2004).

Numerous data have proven that intestinal luminal microbes play an important role in the pathogenesis of IBD (Janowitz et al., 1998; Sartor, 2001; Marteau et al., 2004; Strober et al., 2007). NOD2, the aforementioned intracellular peptidoglycan receptor for muramyl dipeptide is the first susceptibility gene identified for IBD (Hugot et al., 2001; Ogura et al., 2001). Mutations in NOD2 are likely responsible for the genetic predisposition to disease in approximate one third of patients with CD, especially for ileal disease (Bonen & Cho, 2003; Hugot 2004). NOD2 is expressed in macrophages and Paneth cells. Since Paneth cell antimicrobials may affect the microbial composition of the small intestine, deleterious changes in the bacterial microbiota that result from altered Paneth cell function might contribute to the pathogenesis of IBD (Ouellette & Bevins, 2001; Fellermann et al., 2003).

Wehkamp et al. have reported that low levels of Paneth cell α-defensins mRNA and protein are present in inflamed ileum of CD patients as compared to non-IBD controls (Wehkamp et al., 2004, 2005). Interestingly, the specific decrease in α-defensins is more pronounced in CD patients with NOD2 gene mutation. Consistent with this, Kobayashi et al. reported a decrease expression of Paneth cell α-defensins (cryptdin) and cryptdin related sequences in NOD2-knockout mice (Kobayashi et al., 2005). As compared to wild-type controls, the NOD2-knockout mice are more susceptible to gastric, but not systemic, challenges with the Gram-positive bacterium *Listeria monocytogenes*. The decreased expression of Paneth cell antimicrobials in the NOD2-knockout mice is proposed to underlie the increased susceptibility.

6.1.2 α-defensins by colonic Paneth cells

Evidences have shown that HD-5 and HD-6 are not present in normal colonic mucosa. However, Cunliffe et al. detected HD5 in the colonic crypt region of IBD samples (Cunliffe et al., 2001). The appearance of these defensins is due to the phenomenon of Paneth cell metaplasia during colonic inflammation. HD-5 mRNA expression is enhanced in both idiopathic and nonidiopathic inflammatory states of the large bowel, whereas HD-6 is specifically related to CD and UC. Immunohistochemical staining has confirmed that the presence of HD-5 in colonic epithelium may be of importance in maintaining the mucosal barrier and controlling microbial invasion in IBD (Yamaguchi et al., 2009).

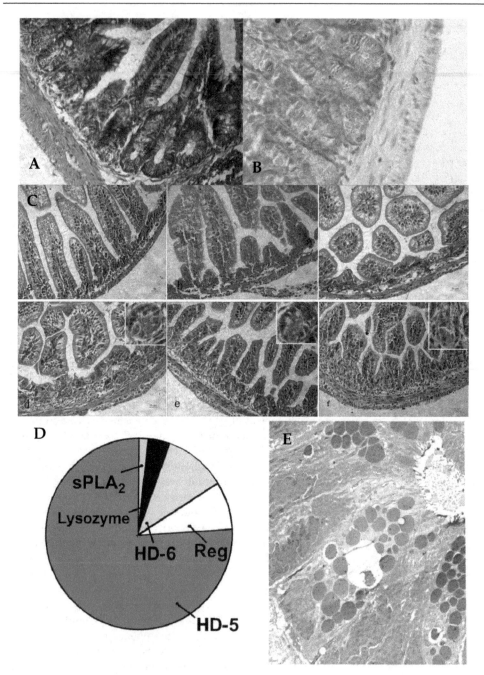

Fig. 1. Paneth cell granules contain α-defensins
A: Hematoxylin-eosin stain of small intestinal crypt shows Paneth cell granules (Bright Red) containing α-defensins in ileum of BALB/c mice. Abundant large secretory vesicles of

Paneth cells are adjacent to the crypt lumen. Scale bar = 20 μm.

B: Immunohistochemical staining demonstrates Cryptdins-4 in the granules of Paneth cell in the ileum crypts of BALB/c mice. Scale bar = 10 μm.

C: The Paneth cells in intestine of newborn BALB/c mice. The development of small intestine gland is imperfect in newborn BALB/c mice, and no Paneth cells were seen 4 days before. However, Paneth cells could be detected in small intestine gland 6 days after birth. a: duodenum, 4 days; b: jejunum, 4 days; c: ileum, 4 days; d: duodenum,10 days; e: jejunum, 10 days; f: ileum, 10 days. Scale bar = 20 μm

D: Real-time PCR analysis of mRNA encoding Paneth cell α-defensins (HD-5 and HD-6) antimicrobial peptides in human ileum.

E: Immunogold electron microscopy localizes HD5 to Paneth cell secretory granules. Transmission electron micrograph of human ileum crypt with immunogold staining for HD5. Defensin-rich granules were found exclusively in Paneth cells

6.1.3 Other α-defensins in the gut

Human HNP-1, -2, -3, and -4 have been found to be present in the granules of polymorphonuclear cells and intestinal epithelial cells, where they participate in systemic innate immunity (Cunliffe, 2003). Cunliffe and colleagues have observed that the mRNA levels of HNP-1, -2, and -3 are significantly increased in inflamed mucosa of IBD patients compared with controls (Cunliffe, 2003), indicating that a-defensins are also involved in the pathogenesis of IBD.

Evidences have shown that expression of HNP-1, -2 and -3 mRNA is highly increased in inflamed colon of UC patients than in healthy controls. Further research also proved that the expression levels of HNP1-3 mRNA, NO and MDA is significantly higher in colonic mucosa of UC patients than in that of normal controls. The expression of HNP-1, -2, and -3 mRNA is correlated with the levels of NO and MDA in the inflamed mucosa in UC patients, the induction of HNP-1, -2, and -3 is involved in the process of inflammation and damage of UC. HNP-1, -2, and -3, NO and MDA might have synergistic effects on colonic inflammation (Cunliffe et al., 2002, 2003). These HNPs are also significantly increased in sera of IBD patients compared with controls, and being significantly correlated with CD activity index, peripheral white blood cell counts, serum CRP values and TNF-α levels (Yamaguchi et al., 2009).

6.2 β-defensins in UC
6.2.1 Inducible β-defensins in UC

Evidences have shown that expression of the inducible β-defensins is significantly increased in inflamed mucosal of UC patients compared with controls. Moreover, HBD-2 expression has also been found to be significantly increased in inflamed colon of UC patients compared with that in controls and CD patients (Wehkamp et al., 2002). In mucosal biopsies, HBD-1 expression is marginally decreased in both CD and UC patients, while HBD-2 is increased exclusively in UC but not in CD. Interestingly, expression of HBD-3 is found to be strongly correlated with HBD-2 in UC (Wehkamp et al., 2003).

6.2.2 Colonic β-defensins

It has been reported that epithelial cells and plasma cells in the lamina propria of colon express HBD. Importantly, expression of HBD-1 is constitutively, while expression of HBD-

2, -3, and -4 is induced by various inflammatory and bacterial stimuli. The pathway responsible for induction of HBD is not completely understood, however it has been presumed that NOD2 signaling is involving in triggering transcription expression of HBD genes (Voss et al., 2006). Colonic plasma cells also express HBD-2, -3 and -4, but it is unclear whether this expression is constitutive or inducible (Rahman et al., 2007).

Previous studies have found that colonic mucosa HBD-1 expression is decreased in UC, and this reduction may result in the decrease of antibacterial activity of mucosal immune system, leading to bacterial invasion secondary inflammatory response. Further studies suggest that defensins deficiency is due to mucosal surface destruction as a result of inflammatory changes, indicating that reduced defensins expression is a symptom of the disease and not the cause (Ramasundara et al., 2009).

Relative low level of HBD-2 expression is found in epithelial cells of normal colon, but significantly increased in inflamed colon (O'Neil et al., 1999). In feces from healthy control individuals, low levels of HBD-2 were detectable, which are also markedly increased under inflammatory conditions (Kapel et al., 2009). In a study by Wehkamp and associates, HBD-2 mRNA was detectable in only 18% of control biopsies compared to 34% in CD and 53% in UC (Wehkamp et al., 2002). In addition, there was increased HBD-2 expression in inflamed compared to non-inflamed areas of CD patients and similarly in UC (Wehkamp et al., 2003). O'Neil and colleagues also demonstrated that HBD-2 mRNA was expressed by colonic epithelial cells in response to stimulation by proinflammatory mediators IL-1α and entero-invasive bacteria (O'Neil et al, 1999; Fahlgren et al, 2003). In addition, HBD-3 and HBD-4 are expressed minimally in normal intestinal epithelium, and that there was no difference in expression for patients with colonic CD. In contrast, there was a significant increase of HBD-3 and HBD-4 in UC (Fellermann et al., 2006; 2007).

Overall, HBD-1 is constitutively expressed in normal intestinal epithelial cells and play foundational defense roles in the mucosal immune, while HBD-2, -3 and -4 could be inducted to express in inflamed mucosa of UC patients and play a defense role in inflammation response.

7. Defensins therapy in UC

Imbalance of intestinal mucosal immunity is an important condition for the pathogenesis of UC, and the defensins is an important factor to maintain the immune response in intestinal mucosa. Defensins play an important role in the prevention and treatment of mucosal inflammation. Consistent with this, evidences have proven that defensins could inhibit the development of neonatal colitis in mice caused by *Escherichia coli* (Sherman et al., 2005). Moreover, defensins also have certain effects on the inhibition of bacterial translocation and control of intestinal infection, which may substitute for antibiotics in the prevention of bacterial infection and some inflammatory diseases. Therefore, monitoring of defensins will help us to evaluate the severity of inflammation (Hiratsuka et al., 1998). A new approach using defensins therapy may shed some light on management of infectious and inflammatory conditions such as UC. HBD-1-expressing *Escherichia coli* clone has been generated, and defensins protein with biological activity is purified (Cipakova et al., 2004, 2005). HBD-2 gene was also cloned from the lesions of human condyloma acuminatum, and an expression vector was constructed and transformed into *Escherichia coli* (Fang et al., 2002). These approaches may allow us to have a clinical trial in the treatment of UC in the future.

8. Outlook

Since innate immune responses in the gut are directed against luminal bacteria, a defect in the expression and/or function of defensins could give rise to an increase in frequency and severity of intestinal infections. Such a deficiency could lead to gradual bacterial invasion, inflammation and a loss of tolerance to gut bacteria. Although this presumes that a defensins deficiency is a primary event in the pathogenesis of IBD, it also possible that the deficiency is a secondary event, occurring as a consequence of the disease. The pathogenesis of UC is not clear, but increasing data have suggested that the abnormalities of intestinal mucosal immune system play a decisive role in the occurrence and development, while the intestinal defenses play an important role in maintaining the balance of mucosal immune. Defensins function as the effective and regulatory molecules of the immune system in the gut. Further study on relationship between defenses and UC will be conducive to understand the pathogenesis of UC, but also provide new approaches for the treatment.

9. References

Andreu P, Colnot S, Godard C, Gad S, Chafey P, Niwa-Kawakita M, Laurent-Puig P, Kahn A, Robine S, Perret C, Romagnolo B. (2005). Crypt-restricted proliferation and commitment to the Paneth cell lineage following Apc loss in the mouse intestine. *Development*, Vol.132, No.6, (March 2005), pp. 1443–1451, ISSN 09501-1991

Aono S, Li C, Zhang G, Kemppainen RJ, Gard J, Lu W, Hu X, Schwartz DD, Morrison EE, Dykstra C, Shi J. (2006). Molecular and functional characterization of bovine beta-defensin-1. *Veterinary Immunoologyl Immunopathoologyl*, Vol.113, No.1-2, (September 2006), pp. 181-190, ISSN 0165-2427

Ayabe T, Satchell DP, Pesendorfer P, Tanabe H, Wilson CL, Haqen SJ, Ouellette AJ. (2002). Activation of Paneth cell alpha-defensins in mouse small intestine. *Journal of Biological Chemestry*, Vol.277, No.7, (February 2002), pp. 5219-5228, ISSN 0021-9258

Ayabe T, Satchell DP, Wilson CL, Parks WC, Selsted ME, Ouellette AJ. (2000). Secretion of microbicidal alpha-defensins by intestinal Paneth cells in response to bacteria. *Nature Immunology*, Vol.1, No.2, (Auguest 2000), pp. 113-118, ISSN 1529-2908

Bateman A, MacLeod RJ, Lembessis P, Hu J, Esch F, Solomon S. (1996). The isolation and characterization of a novel corticostatin/defensin-like peptide from the kidney. *Journal of Biological Chemestry*, Vol.271, No.18, (May 1996), pp. 10654-10659, ISSN 0021-9258

Batlle E, Henderson JT, Beghtel H, van den Born MM, Sancho E, Huls G, Meeldijk J, Robertson J, van de Wetering M, Pawson T, Clevers H. (2002). Beta-catenin and TCF mediate cell positioning in the intestinal epithelium by controlling the expression of EphB/ephrinB. *Cell*, Vol.111, No.2, (Octomber 2002), pp.251-263, ISSN 0092-8674

Bensch KW, Raida M, Mägert HJ, Schulz-Knappe P, Forssmann WG. (1995). hBD-1: a novel beta-defensin from human plasma. *FEBS Letters*, Vol.368, No.2, (July 1995), pp. 331-335, ISSN 0014-5793

Bevins CL, Jones DE, Dutra A, Schaffzin J, Muenke M. (1996). Human enteric defensin genes: chromosomal map position and a model for possible evolutionary relationships. *Genomics*, Vol.31, No.1, (January 1996), pp. 95-106, ISSN 0888-7543

Bevins CL. The Paneth cell and the innate immune response. (2004). *Current Opinion in Gastroenterology*, Vol.20, No.6, (November 2004), pp. 572-580, ISSN 0267-1379

Biragyn A, Ruffini PA, Leifer CA, Klyushnenkova E, Shakhov A, Chertov O, Shirakawa AK, Farber JM, Segal DM, Oppenheim JJ, Kwak LW. (2002). Toll-like receptor 4-dependent activation of dendritic cells by beta-defensin 2. *Science*, Vol.298, No.5595, (November 2002), pp. 1025-1029, ISSN 0036-8075

Boman HG. Peptide antibiotics and their role in innate immunity. (1995). *Annual Review of Immunology*, Vol.13, (no date), pp. 61-92, ISSN 0732-0582

Bonen DK, Cho JH.(2003). The genetics of inflammatory bowel disease. *Gastroenterology*, Vol.124, No.2, (Feburary 2003), pp. 521-536, ISSN 0016-5085

Chertov O, Michiel DF, Xu L, Wang JM, Tani K, Murphy WJ, Longo DL, Taub DD, Oppenheim JJ. (1996). Identification of defensin-1, defensin-2, and CAP37/azurocidin as T-cell chemoattractant proteins released from interleukin-8-stimulated neutrophils. *Journal of Biological Chemestry*, Vol.271, No.6, (February 1996), pp. 2935-2940, ISSN 0021-9258

Cipakova I, Hostinová E, Gasperík J, Velebný V. (2004). High-level expression and purification of a recombinant hBD-1 fused to LMM protein in Escherichia coli. *Protein Expression and Purification*, Vol.37, No.1, (September 2004), pp. 207-212, ISSN1046-5928

Cipakova I, Hostinová E. (2005). Production of the human-beta-defensin using Saccharomyces cerevisiae as a host. *Protein Peptide Letters*, Vol.12, No.6, (Auguest 2005), pp. 551-554, ISSN 0929-8665

Cole AM, Hong T, Boo LM, Nguyen T, Zhao C, Bristol G, Zack JA, Waring AJ, Yang OO, Lehrer RI. (2002). Retrocyclin: a primate peptide that protects cells from infection by T- and M-tropic strains of HIV-1. *Proceedings of the National Academy of Sciences USA*, Vol.99, No.4, (Feburary 2002), pp. 1813-1818, ISSN 1091-6490

Cunliffe RN, Kamal M, Rose FR, James PD, Mahida YR. (2002). Expression of antimicrobial neutrophil defensins in epithelial cells of active inflammatory bowel disease mucosa. *Journal of Clinical Pathology*, Vol.55, No.4, (Aprial 2002), pp. 298-304, ISSN 2153-3539

Cunliffe RN, Rose FR, Keyte J, Abberley L, Chan WC, Mahida YR. (2001). Human defensin 5 is stored in precursor form in normal Paneth cells and is expressed by some villous epithelial cells and by metaplastic Paneth cells in the colon in inflammatory bowel disease. *Gut*, Vol.48, No.2, (Feburary 2001), pp. 176-185, ISSN 00017-5749

Cunliffe RN. (2003). Alpha-defensins in the gastrointestinal tract. *Molecular Immunology*, Vol.40, No.7, (November 2003), pp. 463-467,ISSN 0161-5890

Diamond G, Zasloff M, Eck H, Brasseur M, Maloy WL, Bevins CL. (1991). Tracheal antimicrobial peptide, a cysteine-rich peptide from mammalian tracheal mucosa: peptide isolation and cloning of a cDNA. *Proceedings of the National Academy of Sciences USA*, Vol.88, No.1, (May 1991), pp. 3952-3956, ISSN 1091-6490

Elphick DA, Mahida YR. (2005). Paneth cells: their role in innate immunity and inflammatory disease. *Gut*, Vol.54, No.12, (July 2005), pp. 1802-1809, ISSN 00017-5749

Ericksen B, Wu Z, Lu W, Lehrer RI. (2005). Antibacterial activity and specificity of the six human (alpha)-defensins. *Antimicrobial Agents Chemotherapy*, Vol.49, No.1, (January 2005), pp. 269-275, ISSN 0066-4804

Fahlgren A, Hammarstrom S, Danielsson A, Hammarstrom ML. (2003). Increased expression of antimicrobial peptides and lysozyme in colonic epithelial cells of patients with ulcerative colitis. *Clinical Experimenal Immunology*, Vol.131, No.1, (January 2003), pp. 90-101, ISSN 0009-9104

Fahlgren A, Hammarstrom S, Danielsson A, Hammarstrom ML. (2004). beta-Defensin-3 and -4 in intestinal epithelial cells display increased mRNA expression in ulcerative colitis. *Clinical Experimenal Immunology*, Vol.137, No.2, (Auguest 2004), pp. 379-385, ISSN 0009-9104

Fang X, Peng L, Xu Z, Wu J, Cen P. (2002). Cloning and expression of human beta-defensin-2 gene in Escherichia coli. *Protein Peptide Letters*, Vol.9, No.1, (Feburary 2002), pp. 31-37, ISSN 0929-8665

Fellermann K, Stange DE, Schaeffeler E, Schmalzl H, Wehkamp J, Bevins CL, Reinisch W, Teml A, Schwab M, Lichter P, Radlwimmer B, Stange EF. (2006). A chromosome 8 gene-cluster polymorphism with low human beta-defensin 2 gene copy number predisposes to Crohn disease of the colon. *American Journal of Human Genetics*, Vol.79, No.3, (Semptember 2006), pp. 439-448, ISSN 0002-9297

Fellermann K, Wehkamp J, Herrlinger KR, Stange EF. (2003). Crohn's disease: a defensin deficiency syndrome? *European Joournal of Gastroenterology and Hepatology*, Vol.15, No.6, (June 2003), pp. 627-634, ISSN 0954-691X

Ganz T. Defensins: antimicrobial peptides of innate immunity. (2003). *Nature Review of Immunology*, Vol.3, No.9, (September 2003), pp. 710-720, ISSN 1474-1733

Garcia AE, Osapay G, Tran PA, Yuan J, Selsted ME. (2008). Isolation, synthesis, and antimicrobial activities of naturally occurring theta-defensin isoforms from baboon leukocytes. *Infection and Immunity*, Vol.76, No.12, (December 2008), pp. 5883-5891, ISSN 0019-9567

Garcia AE, Selsted ME. (2008). Olive baboon theta-defensins. *FASEB Journal*, Vol.22, (April 2008), Meeting Abstracts, pp. 673.11, ISSN 0892-6638

Garcia JR, Krause A, Schulz S, Rodríguez-Jiménez FJ, Klüver E, Adermann K, Forssmann U, Frimpong-Boateng A, Bals R, Forssmann WG. (2001). Human beta-defensin 4: a novel inducible peptide with a specific salt-sensitive spectrum of antimicrobial activity. *FASEB Journal*, Vol.15, No.10, (Auguest 2001), pp. 1819-1821, ISSN 0892-6638

Ghosh D, Porter E, Shen B, Lee SK, Wilk D, Drazba J, Yadav SP, Crabb JW, Ganz T, Bevins CL. (2002). Paneth cell trypsin is the processing enzyme for human defensin-5. *Nature Immunology*, Vol.3, No.6, (June 2002), pp. 583-590, ISSN 1529-2908

Harder J, Bartels J, Christophers E, Schröder JM. (1997). A peptide antibiotic from human skin. *Nature*, Vol.387, No.6636, (June 1997), pp. 861, ISSN 0028-0836

Harder J, Bartels J, Christophers E, Schroder JM. (2001). Isolation and characterization of human beta-defensin-3, a novel human inducible peptide antibiotic. *Journal of Biological Chemistry*, Vol.276, No.8, (Feburary 2001), pp. 5707-5713, ISSN 0021-9258

Harder J, Siebert R, Zhang Y, Matthiesen P, Christophers E, Schlegelberger B, Schröder JM. (1997). Mapping of the gene encoding human beta-defensin-2 (DEFB2) to chromosome region 8p22-p23.1. *Genomics*, Vol.46, No.3, (December 1997), pp. 472-475, ISSN 0888-7543

He XC, Zhang J, Tong WG, Tawfik O, Ross J, Scoville DH, Tian Q, Zeng X, He X, Wiedemann LM, Mishina Y, Li L. (2004). BMP signaling inhibits intestinal stem cell self-renewal through suppression of Wnt-beta-catenin signaling. *Nature Genetics*, Vol.36, No.10, (October 2004), pp. 1117-1121, ISSN 1061-4036

Hill CP, Yee J, Selsted ME, Eisenberg D. (1991). Crystal structure of defensin HNP-3, an amphiphilic dimer: mechanisms of membrane permeabilization. *Science*, Vol.251, No.5000, (March 1991), pp. 1481-1485, ISSN 0036-8075

Hiratsuka T, Nakazato M, Date Y, Ashitani J, Minematsu T, Chino N, Matsukura S. (1998). Identifiation of human beta-defensin-2 in respiratory tract and plasma and its increase in bacterial pneumonia. *Biochemical Biophysical Research Communications*, Vol.249, No.3, (Auguest 1998), pp. 943-947, ISSN 0006-291X

Hornef MW, Pütsep K, Karlsson J, Refai E, Andersson M. (2004). Increased diversity of intestinal antimicrobial peptides by covalent dimer formation. *Nature Immunology*, Vol.5, No.8, (Auguest 2004), pp. 836-843, ISSN 1529-2908

Hugot JP, Chamaillard M, Zouali H, Lesage S, Cézard JP, Belaiche J, Almer S, Tysk C, O'Morain CA, Gassull M, Binder V, Finkel Y, Cortot A, Modigliani R, Laurent-Puig P, Gower-Rousseau C, Macry J, Colombel JF, Sahbatou M, Thomas G. (2001). Association of NOD2 leucine-rich repeat variants with susceptibility to Crohn's disease. *Nature*, Vol.411, No.6837, (May 2001), pp. 599-603, ISSN 0028-0836

Hugot JP. (2004). Genetic origin of IBD. *Inflammatory Bowel Diseases*, Suppl 1, (Feburary 2004), pp. S11-S15,ISSN 1078-0998

Huttner KM, Selsted ME, Ouellette AJ. (1994). Structure and diversity of themurine cryptdin gene family. *Genomics*, Vol.19, No.3, (Feburary 1994), pp. 448-453, ISSN 0888-7543

Janowitz HD, Croen EC, Sachar DB. (1998). The role of the fecal stream in Crohn's disease: an historical and analytic review. *Inflammatory Bowel Diseases*, Vol.4, No.1, (Feburary 1998), pp. 29-39, ISSN 1078-0998

Jones DE, Bevins CL. (1992). Paneth cells of the human small intestine express an antimicrobial peptide gene. *Journal of Biological Chemistry*, Vol.267, No.32, (November 1992), pp. 23216-23225, ISSN 0021-9258

Jones DE, Bevins CL. (1993). Defensin-6 mRNA in human Paneth cells: implications for antimicrobial peptides in host defense of the human bowel. *FEBS Letters*, Vol.315, No.2, (January 1993), pp. 187-192, ISSN 0014-5793

Kapel N, Benahmed N, Morali A, Svahn J, Canioni D, Goulet O, Ruemmele FM. (2009). Fecal beta-defensin-2 in children with inflammatory bowel diseases. *Journal of Pediatric Gastroenterology and Nutrition*, Vol.48, No.1, (January 2009), pp. 117-120, ISSN 0277-2116

Kelly P, Feakins R, Domizio P, Murphy J, Bevins C, Wilson J, McPhail G, Poulsom R, Dhaliwal W. (2004). Paneth cell granule depletion in the human small intestine under infective and nutritional stress. *Clinical Experimental Immunology*, Vol.135, No.2, (Feburary 2004), pp. 303-309, ISSN 0009-9104

Kobayashi KS, Chamaillard M, Ogura Y, Henegariu O, Inohara N, Nuñez G, Flavell RA. (2005). Nod2-dependent regulation of innate and adaptive immunity in the intestinal tract. *Science*, Vol.307, No.5710, (Feburary 2005), pp. 731-734, ISSN 0036-8075

Lala S, Ogura Y, Osborne C, Hor SY, Bromfield A, Davies S, Ogunbiyi O, Nuñez G, Keshav S. (2003). Crohn's disease and the NOD2 gene: a role for paneth cells. *Gastroenterology*, Vol.125, No.1, (July 2003), pp. 47-57, ISSN 0016-5085

Lehrer RI, Ferrari LG, Patterson-Delafield J, Sorrell T. (1980). Fungicidal activity of rabbit alveolar and peritoneal macrophages against Candida albicans. *Infection and Immunity*, Vol.28, No.3, (June 1980), pp. 1001-1008, ISSN 0019-9567

Lehrer RI. (2004). Primate defensins. *Nature Reviews Microbiology*, Vol.2, No.9, (Semptember 2004), pp. 727-738, ISSN 1740-1526

Leonova L, Kokryakov VN, Aleshina G, Hong T, Nguyen T, Zhao C, Waring AJ, Lehrer RI. (2001). Circular minidefensins and posttranslational generation of molecular diversity. *Journal of Leukocyte Biology*, Vol.70, No.3, (September 2001), pp. 461-464, ISSN 0741-5400

Lillard JW Jr, Boyaka PN, Chertov O, Oppenheim JJ, McGhee JR. (1999). Mechanisms for induction of acquired host immunity by neutrophil peptide defensins. *Proceedings of the National Academy of Sciences USA*, Vol.96, No.2, (January 1999), pp. 651-656, ISSN 1091-6490

Liu L, Ganz T. (1995). The pro region of human neutrophil defensin contains a motif that is essential for normal subcellular sorting. *Blood*, Vol.85, No.4, (Feburary 1995), pp. 1095-1103, ISSN 0006-4971

MacLeod RJ, Hamilton JR, Bateman A, Belcourt D, Hu J, Bennett HP, Solomon S. (1991). Corticostatic peptides cause nifedipine-sensitive volume reduction in jejunal villus enterocytes. *Proceedings of the National Academy of Sciences USA*, Vol.88, No.2, (January 1991), pp. 552-556, ISSN 1091-6490

Maisetta G, Batoni G, Esin S, Raco G, Bottai D, Favilli F, Florio W, Campa M. (2005). Susceptibility of Streptococcus mutans and Actinobacillus actinomycetemcomitans to bactericidal activity of human beta-defensin3 in biological fluids. *Antimicrobial Agents Chemotherapy*, Vol.49, No.3, (March 2005), pp. 1245-1248, ISSN 0066-4804

Mallow EB, Harris A, Salzman N, Russell JP, DeBerardinis RJ, Ruchelli E, Bevins CL. (1996). Human enteric defensins: gene structure and developmental expression. *Journal of Biological Chemistry*, Vol.271, No.8, (Feburary 1996), pp. 4038-4045, ISSN 0021-9258

Marteau P, Lepage P, Mangin I, Suau A, Doré J, Pochart P, Seksik P. (2004). Review article: gut flora and inflammatory bowel disease. *Alimentary Pharmacology Therapeutics*, Suppl 4, (October 2004), pp. 18-23, ISSN 0269-2813

Means TK, Golenbock DT, Fenton MJ. (2000). The biology of Toll-like receptors. *Cytokine Growth Factor Review*, Vol.11, No.3, (September 2000), pp. 219-232, ISSN 1359-6101

Merlin D, Yue G, Lencer WI, Selsted ME, Madara JL. (2001). Cryptdin-3 induces novel apical conductance(s) in Cl- secretory, including cystic fibrosis, epithelia. *American Journal of Physiology-Cell Physiology*, Vol.280, No.2, (Feburary 2001), pp. C296-302, ISSN 0363-6143

Nguyen TX, Cole AM, Lehrer RI. (2003). Evolution of primate theta-defensins: a serpentine path to a sweet tooth. *Peptides*, Vol.24, No.11, (November 2003), pp. 1647-1654, ISSN 0196-9781

Ogura Y, Bonen DK, Inohara N, Nicolae DL, Chen FF, Ramos R, Britton H, Moran T, Karaliuskas R, Duerr RH, Achkar JP, Brant SR, Bayless TM, Kirschner BS, Hanauer SB, Nuñez G, Cho JH. (2001). A frameshift mutation in NOD2 associated with susceptibility to Crohn's disease. *Nature*, Vol.411, No.6837, (May 2001), pp. 603-606, ISSN 0028-0836

O'Neil DA, Porter EM, Elewaut D, Anderson GM, Eckmann L, Ganz T, Kagnoff MF. (1999). Expression and regulation of the human beta-defensins hBD-1 and hBD-2 in intestinal epithelium. *Journal of Immunology*, Vol.163, No.12, (December 1999), pp. 6718-6724, ISSN 0022-1767

Ouellette AJ, Bevins CL. (2001). Paneth cell defensins and innate immunity of the small bowel. *Inflammatory Bowel Diseases*, Vol.7, No.1, (Feburary 2001), pp. 43-50,ISSN 1078-0998

Ouellette AJ, Cordell B. (1988). Accumulation of abundant messenger ribonucleic acids during postnatal development of mouse small intestine. *Gastroenterology*, Vol.94, No.1, (January 1988), pp. 114-121, ISSN 0016-5085

Ouellette AJ, Darmoul D, Tran D, Huttner KM, Yuan J, Selsted ME. (1999). Peptide localization and gene structure of cryptdin 4, a differentially expressed mouse Paneth cell alpha-defensin. *Infection and Immunity*, Vol.67, No.12, (December 1999), pp. 6643-6651, ISSN 0019-9567

Ouellette AJ, Greco RM, James M, Frederick D, Naftilan J, Fallon JT. (1989a). Developmental regulation of cryptdin, a corticostatin/defensin precursor mRNA in mouse small intestinal crypt epithelium. *Journal of Cell Biology*, Vol.108, No.5, (May 1989), pp. 1687-1695, ISSN 0021-9525

Ouellette AJ, Lualdi JC. (1990). A novel mouse gene family coding for cationic, cysteine-rich peptides. Regulation in small intestine and cells of myeloid origin. *Journal of Biological Chemistry*, Vol.265, No.17, (June 1990), pp. 9831-9837, ISSN 0021-9258

Ouellette AJ, Pravtcheva D, Ruddle FH, James M. (1989b). Localization of the cryptdin locus on mouse chromosome 8. *Genomics*, Vol.5, No.2, (Auguest 1989), pp. 233-239, ISSN 0888-7543

Ouellette AJ, Satchell DP, Hsieh MM, Hagen SJ, Selsted ME. (2000). Characterization of luminal paneth cell alpha-defensins in mouse small intestine. Attenuated antimicrobial activities of peptides with truncated amino termini. *Journal of Biological Chemistry*, Vol.275, No.43, (October 2000), pp. 33969-33973, ISSN 0021-9258

Ouellette AJ, Selsted ME. (1996). Paneth cell defensins: endogenous peptide components of intestinal host defense. *FASEB Journal*, Vol.10, No.11, (September 1996), pp. 1280-1289, ISSN 0892-6638

Ouellette AJ. (2005). Paneth cell alpha-defensins: peptide mediators of innate immunity in the small intestine. *Springer Seminars in Immunopathology*, Vol.27, No.2, (September 2005), pp. 133-146, ISSN 1863-2300

Ouellette AJ. (2006). Paneth cell alpha-defensin synthesis and function. *Current Topics in Microbiology Immunology*, Vol.306, (no date), pp. 1-25, ISSN 0070-217X

Owen SM, Rudolph DL, Wang W, Cole AM, Waring AJ, Lal RB, Lehrer RI. (2004). RC-101, a retrocyclin-1 analogue with enhanced activity against primary HIV type 1 isolates. *AIDS Research Human Retroviruses*, Vol.20, No.11, (November 2004), pp. 1157-1165, ISSN 0889-2229

Pardi A, Zhang XL, Selsted ME, Skalicky JJ, Yip PF. (1992). NMR studies of defensin antimicrobial peptides. 2. Three-dimensional structures of rabbit NP-2 and human HNP-1. *Biochemistry*, Vol.31, No.46, (November 1992), pp. 11357-11364, ISSN 0006-2960

Patil A, Hughes AL, Zhang G. (2004). Rapid evolution and diversification of mammalian alpha-defensins as revealed by comparative analysis of rodent and primate genes. *Physiology Genomics*, Vol.20, No.1, (December 2004), pp. 1-11, ISSN 1094-8341

Pinto D, Clevers H. (2005). Wnt control of stem cells and differentiation in the intestinal epithelium. *Experimental Cell Research*, Vol.306, No.2, (June 2005), pp. 357-363, ISSN 0014-4827

Porter EM, Liu L, Oren A, Anton PA, Ganz T. (1997b). Localization of human intestinal defensin 5 in Paneth cell granules. *Infection and Immunity*, Vol.65, No.6, (June 1997), pp. 2389-2395, ISSN 0019-9567

Porter EM, van Dam E, Valore EV, Ganz T. (1997a). Broad-spectrum antimicrobial activity of human intestinal defensin 5. *Infection and Immunity*, Vol.65, No.6, (June 1997), pp. 2396-2401, ISSN 0019-9567

Putsep K, Axelsson LG, Boman A, Midtvedt T, Normark S, Boman HG, Andersson M. (2000). Germ-free and colonized mice generate the same products from enteric prodefensins. *Journal of Biological Chemistry*, Vol.275, No.51, (December 2000), pp. 40478-40482, ISSN 0021-9258

Qu XD, Lloyd KC, Walsh JH, Lehrer RI. (1996). Secretion of type II phospholipase A2 and cryptdin by rat small intestinal Paneth cells. *Infection and Immunity*, Vol.64, No.12, (December 1996), pp. 5161-5165, ISSN 0019-9567

Rahman A, Fahlgren A, Sitohy B, Baranov V, Zirakzadeh A, Hammarström S, Danielsson A, Hammarström ML. (2007). Beta-defensin production by human colonic plasma cells: a new look at plasma cells in ulcerative colitis. *Inflammatory Bowel Diseases*, Vol.13, No.7, (July 2007), pp. 847-855,ISSN 1078-0998

Ramasundara M, Leach ST, Lemberg DA, Day AS. (2009). Defensins and inflammation: the role of defensins in inflammatory bowel disease. *Journal of Gastroenterology and Hepatology*, Vol.24, No. 2, (Feburary 2009), pp. 202-208, ISSN 0815-9319

Rumio C, Besusso D, Palazzo M, Selleri S, Sfondrini L, Dubini F, Ménard S, Balsari A. (2004). Degranulation of Paneth cells via toll-like receptor 9. *American Journal of Pathology*, Vol.165, No.2, (Auguest 2004), pp. 373-381, ISSN 0002-9440

Salzman NH, Chou MM, de Jong H, Liu L, Porter EM, Paterson Y. (2003). Enteric Salmonella infection inhibits Paneth cell antimicrobial peptide expression. *Infection and Immunity*, Vol.71, No.3, (March 2003), pp. 1109-1115, ISSN 0019-9567

Salzman NH, Underwood MA, Bevins CL. (2007). Paneth Cells, Defensins, and the commensal microbiota: A hypothesis on intimate interplay at the intestinal mucosa. *Seminars in Immunology*, Vol.19, No.2, (April 2007), pp. 19: 70-83, ISSN 1044-5323

Sartor RB. (2001). Intestinal microflora in human and experimental inflammatory bowel disease. *Current Opinion in Gastroenterology*, Vol.17, No.4, (July 2001), pp. 324-330, ISSN 0267-1379

Satoh Y, Habara Y, Ono K, Kanno T. (1995). Carbamylcholine- and catecholamine-induced intracellular calcium dynamics of epithelial cells in mouse ileal crypts. *Gastroenterology*, Vol.108, No.5, (May 1995), pp. 1345-1356, ISSN 0016-5085

Sawai MV, Jia HP, Liu L, Aseyev V, Wiencek JM, McCray PB Jr, Ganz T, Kearney WR, Tack BF. (2001). The NMR structure of human beta-defensin-2 reveals a novel alpha-helical segment. *Biochemistry*, Vol.40, No.13, (April 2001), pp. 3810-3816, ISSN 0006-2960

Selsted ME, Miller SI, Henschen AH, Ouellette AJ. (1992). Enteric defensins: antibiotic peptide components of intestine host defense. *Journal of Cell Biology*, Vol.118, No.4, (Auguest 1992), pp. 929-936, ISSN 0021-9525

Selsted ME, Ouellette AJ. (1995). Defensins in granules of phagocytic and non-phagocytic cells. *Trends in Cell Biology*, Vol.5, No.3, (March 1995), pp. 114-119, ISSN 0962-8924

Selsted ME, Ouellette AJ. (2005). Mammalian defensins in the antimicrobial immune response. *Nature Immunology*, Vol.6, No.6, (June 2005), pp. 551-557, ISSN 1529-2908

Sherman MP, Bennett SH, Hwang FF, Sherman J, Bevins CL. (2005). Paneth Cells and Antibacterial Host Defense in Neonatal Small Intestine. *Infection and Immunity*, Vol.73, No.9, (September 2005), pp. 6143-6146, ISSN 0019-9567

Shi J. (2007). Defensins and Paneth cells in inflammatory bowel disease. *Infammatory Bowel Diseases*, Vol.13, No.10, (October 2007), pp. 1284-1292, ISSN 1078-0998

Shirafuji Y, Tanabe H, Satchell DP, Henschen-Edman A, Wilson CL, Ouellette AJ. (2003). Structural determinants of procryptdin recognition and cleavage by matrix metalloproteinase-7. *Journal of Biological Chemistry*, Vol.278, No.10, (March 2003), pp. 7910-7919, ISSN 0021-9258

Skalicky JJ, Selsted ME, Pardi A. (1994). Structure and dynamics of the neutrophil defensins NP-2, NP-5, and HNP-1: NMR studies of amide hydrogen exchange kinetics. *Proteins*, Vol.20, No.1, (September 1994), pp. 52-67, ISSN 0887-3585

Solomon S, Hu J, Zhu Q, Belcourt D, Bennett HP, Bateman A, Antakly T. (1991). Corticostatic peptides. *Journal of Steroid Biochemistry and Molecular Biology*, Vol.40, No.1-3, (no date), pp. 391-398, ISSN 0960-0760

Sparkes RS, Kronenberg M, Heinzmann C, Daher KA, Klisak I, Ganz T, Mohandas T. (1989). Assignment of defensin gene(s) to human chromosome 8p23. *Genomics*, Vol.5, No.2, (Auguest 1989), pp. 240-244, ISSN 0888-7543

Strober W, Fuss I, Mannon P. (2007). The fundamental basis of inflammatory bowel disease. *Journal of Clinical Investigation*, Vol.117, No.3, (March 2007), pp. 514-521, ISSN 0021-9738

Tanabe H, Qu X, Weeks CS, Cummings JE, Kolusheva S, Walsh KB, Jelinek R, Vanderlick TK, Selsted ME, Ouellette AJ. (2004a). Structure-activity determinants in paneth cell alpha-defensins: loss-of-function in mouse cryptdin-4 by charge-reversal at arginine residue positions. *Journal of Biological Chemistry*, Vol.279, No.12, (March 2004), pp. 11976-11983, ISSN 0021-9258

Tanabe H, Yuan J, Zaragoza MM, Dandekar S, Henschen-Edman A, Selsted ME, Ouellette AJ. (2004b). Paneth cell alpha-defensins from rhesus macaque small intestine. *Infection and Immunity*, Vol.72, No.3, (March 2004), pp. 1470-1478, ISSN 0019-9567

Tang YQ, Yuan J, Osapay G, Osapay K, Tran D, Miller CJ, Ouellette AJ, Selsted ME. (1999). A cyclic antimicrobial peptide produced in primate leukocytes by the ligation of two truncated alpha-defensins. *Science*, Vol.286, No.5439, (October 1999), pp. 498-502, ISSN 0036-8075

Tani K, Murphy WJ, Chertov O, Salcedo R, Koh CY, Utsunomiya I, Funakoshi S, Asai O, Herrmann SH, Wang JM, Kwak LW, Oppenheim JJ. (2000). Defensins act as potent adjuvants that promote cellular and humoral immune responses in mice to a lymphoma idiotype and carrier antigens. *International Immunology*, Vol.12, No.5, (May 2000), pp. 691-700, ISSN 0953-8178

Territo MC, Ganz T, Selsted ME, Lehrer R. (1989). Monocyte-chemotactic activity of defensins from human neutrophils. *Journal of Clinical Investigation*, Vol.84, No.6, (December 1989), pp. 2017-2020, ISSN 0021-9738

Tominaga T, Fukata J, Naito Y, Nakai Y, Funakoshi S, Fujii N, Imura H. (1990). Effects of corticostatin-I on rat adrenal cells in vitro. *Journal of Endocrinology*, Vol.125, No.2, (May 1990), pp. 287-292, ISSN 0022-0795

Trabi M, Schirra HJ, Craik DJ. (2001). Three-dimensional structure of RTD-1, a cyclic antimicrobial defensin from Rhesus macaque leukocytes. *Biochemistry*, Vol.40, No.14, (April 2001), pp. 4211-4221, ISSN 0006-2960

Tran D, Tran P, Roberts K, Osapay G, Schaal J, Ouellette A, Selsted ME. (2008). Microbicidal properties and cytocidal selectivity of rhesus macaque theta defensins. *Antimicrobial Agents Chemotherapy*, Vol.52, No.3, (March 2008), pp. 944-953, ISSN 0066-4804

Tran D, Tran PA, Tang YQ, Yuan J, Cole T, Selsted ME. (2002). Homodimeric theta-defensins from rhesus macaque leukocytes: isolation, synthesis, antimicrobial activities, and bacterial binding properties of the cyclic peptides. *Journal of Biological Chemistry*, Vol.277, No.5, (Feburary 2002), pp. 3079-3084, ISSN 0021-9258

Valore EV, Ganz T. (1992). Posttranslational processing of defensins in immature human myeloid cells. *Blood*, Vol.79, No.6, (March 1992), pp. 1538-1544, ISSN 0006-4971

Valore EV, Martin E, Harwig SS, Ganz T. (1996). Intramolecular inhibition of human defensin HNP-1 by its propiece. *Journal of Clinical Investigation*, Vol.97, No.7, (April 1996), pp. 1624-1629, ISSN 0021-9738

Valore EV, Park CH, Quayle AJ, Wiles KR, McCray PB Jr, Ganz T. (1998). Human beta-defensin-1: An antimicrobial peptide of urogenital tissues. *Journal of Clinical Investigation*, Vol.101, No.8, (April 1998), pp. 1633-1642, ISSN 0021-9738

Van Es JH, Jay P, Gregorieff A, van Gijn ME, Jonkheer S, Hatzis P, Thiele A, van den Born M, Begthel H, Brabletz T, Taketo MM, Clevers H. (2005). Wnt signaling induces maturation of Paneth cells in intestinal crypts. *Nature Cell Biology*, Vol.7, No.4, (April 2005), pp. 381-386, ISSN 1476-4679

Voss E, Wehkamp J, Wehkamp K, Stange EF, Schröder JM, Harder J. (2006). NOD2/CARD15 mediates induction of the antimicrobial peptide human beta-defensin-2. *Journal of Biological Chemistry*, Vol.281, No.4, (January 2006), pp. 2005-2011, ISSN 0021-9258

Wang, W., S. M. Owen, D. L. Rudolph, A. M. Cole, T. Hong, A. J. Waring, R. B. Lal, and R. I. Lehrer. (2004). Activity of alpha- and theta-defensins against primary isolates of HIV-1. *Journal of Immunology*, Vol.173, No.1, (July 2004), pp. 515-520, ISSN 0022-1767

Wehkamp J, Chu H, Shen B, Feathers RW, Kays RJ, Lee SK, Bevins CL. (2006). Paneth cell antimicrobial peptides: Topographical distribution and quantification in human gastrointestinal tissues. *FEBS Letters*, Vol.580, No.22, (October 2006), pp. 5344-5350, ISSN 0014-5793

Wehkamp J, Fellermann K, Herrlinger KR, Baxmann S, Schmidt K, Schwind B, Duchrow M, Wohlschläger C, Feller AC, Stange EF. (2002). Human beta-defensin 2 but not beta-defensin 1 is expressed preferentially in colonic mucosa of inflammatory bowel disease. *European Journal of Gastroenterology & Hepatology*, Vol.14, No.7, (July 2002), pp. 745-752, ISSN 0954-691X

Wehkamp J, Harder J, Weichenthal M, Mueller O, Herrlinger KR, Fellermann K, Schroeder JM, Stange EF. (2003). Inducible and constitutive beta-defensins are differentially expressed in Crohn's disease and ulcerative colitis. *Inflammatory Bowel Diseases*, Vol.9, No.4, (July 2003), pp. 215-223, ISSN 1078-0998

Wehkamp J, Harder J, Weichenthal M, Schwab M, Schäffeler E, Schlee M, Herrlinger KR, Stallmach A, Noack F, Fritz P, Schröder JM, Bevins CL, Fellermann K, Stange EF. (2004). NOD2 (CARD15) mutations in Crohn's disease are associated with diminished mucosal alpha-defensin expression. *Gut,* Vol.53, No.11, (November 2004), pp. 1658-1664, ISSN 00017-5749

Wehkamp J, Salzman NH, Porter E, Nuding S, Weichenthal M, Petras RE, Shen B, Schaeffeler E, Schwab M, Linzmeier R, Feathers RW, Chu H, Lima H Jr, Fellermann K, Ganz T, Stange EF, Bevins CL. (2005). Reduced Paneth cell alpha-defensins in ileal Crohn's disease. *Proceedings of the National Academy of Sciences USA,* Vol.102, No.50, (December 2005), pp. 18129-18134, ISSN 1091-6490

Wilson CL, Ouellette AJ, Satchell DP, Ayabe T, López-Boado YS, Stratman JL, Hultgren SJ, Matrisian LM, Parks WC. (1999). Regulation of intestinal alpha-defensin activation by the metalloproteinase matrilysin in innate host defense. *Science,* Vol.286, No.5437, (October 1999), pp. 113-117, ISSN 0036-8075

Yamaguchi N, Isomoto H, Mukae H, Ishimoto H, Ohnita K, Shikuwa S, Mizuta Y, Nakazato M, Kohno S. (2009). Concentrations of alpha- and beta-defensins in plasma of patients with infammatory bowel disease. *Infammation Research,* Vol.58, No.4, (April 2009), pp. 192-197, ISSN 1023-3830

Yang D, Chen Q, Chertov O, Oppenheim JJ. (2000). Human neutrophil defensins selectively chemoattract naive T and immature dendritic cells. *Journal of Leukocyte Biology,* Vol.68, No.1, (July 2000), pp. 9-14, ISSN 0741-5400

Yang D, Chertov O, Bykovskaia SN, Chen Q, Buffo MJ, Shogan J, Anderson M, Schröder JM, Wang JM, Howard OM, Oppenheim JJ. (1999). Beta-defensins: linking innate and adaptive immunity through dendritic and T cell CCR6. *Science,* Vol.286, No.5439, (October 1999), pp. 525-528, ISSN 0036-8075

Yount NY, Wang MS, Yuan J, Banaiee N, Ouellette AJ, Selsted ME. (1995). Rat neutrophil defensins. Precursor structures and expression during neutrophilic myelopoiesis. *Journal of Immunology,* Vol.155, No.9, (November 1995), pp. 4476-4484, ISSN 0022-1767

Zasloff M. (2002). Antimicrobial peptides of multicellular organisms. (2002). *Nature,* Vol.415, No.6870, (January 2002), pp. 389-395, ISSN 0028-0836

Zhang XL, Selsted ME, Pardi A. (1992). NMR studies of defensin antimicrobial peptides. 1. Resonance assignment and secondary structure determination of rabbit NP-2 and human HNP-1. *Biochemistry,* Vol.31, No.46, (November 1992), pp. 11348-11356, ISSN 0006-2960

Zhu Q, Bateman A, Singh A, Solomon S. (1989). Isolation and biological activity of corticostatic peptides (anti-ACTH). *Endocrinology Research,* Vol.15, No.1-2, (no date), pp. 129-149, ISSN 0743-5800

Zhu Q, Singh A, Bateman A, Esch F, Solomon S. (1987). The corticostatic (anti-ACTH) and cytotoxic activity of peptides isolated from fetal, adult and tumor-bearing lung. *Journal of Steroid Biochemistry,* Vol.27, No.4-6, (no date), pp. 1017-1022, ISSN 0960-0760

Zimmermann GR, Legault P, Selsted ME, Pardi A. (1995). Solution structure of bovine neutrophil beta-defensin-12: the peptide fold of the beta-defensins is identical to that of the classical defensins. *Biochemistry,* Vol.34, No.41, (October 1995), pp. 13663-13671, ISSN 0006-2960

5

CXCL12-CXCR4 Axis in Ulcerative Colitis

Hiroshi Nakase, Minoru Matsuura,
Sakae Mikami and Tsutomu Chiba
Department of Gastroenterology and Hepatology,
Graduate School of Medicine,
Kyoto University
Japan

1. Introduction

Regulated immune responses are essential to maintain intestinal homeostasis and require direct or indirect communication among cells. Communication that occurs among cells in the absence of direct contact is often through the use of cytokines and chemokines. Ulcerative colitis (UC) and Crohn's disease (CD) are chronic intestinal inflammatory bowel diseases (IBD). IBD is characterized by increased influx of immune cells to the mucosa of genetically susceptible hosts. The characteristic increase of inflammatory infiltrate is mainly of T cells recruited to the lamina propria (LP) by a multistep process that involves the integrated interactions and effects of adhesion molecules and chemokines (1). Numerous studies in IBD patients and in animal models of colitis have demonstrated that both inflammatory chemokines and their receptors are up-regulated in settings of active inflammation (2). More importantly, blockade or absence of various chemokine receptors attenuates disease in murine models of IBD. Thus, identifying chemokines and their receptors that are involved in intestinal inflammation provide promising targets for new drug development in the treatment of IBD.

2. What is Chemokines?-Role in the pathogenesis of IBD-

Chemokines have been implicated in many fundamental immune processes, including lymphoid organogenesis, immune cell differentiation, development and positioning (3) Chemokines are small 8-12kDa cytokines that can direct the recruitment and migration of circulating leukocytes and play a critical role in the differentiation of secondary lymphoid organs. There are approximately 50 known chemokines and 20 known receptors. Chemokines are classified in 4 separate families based on the pattern of their cysteine residues(C, CC, CXC and CX3C). The CC family of chemokines contains two adjacent cysteine residues. The CXC family has two cysteine residues separated by a non-cystein amino acid, whereas the CX3C family has two cysteine residues separated by three non-cysteine amino acids. The C family has only one cysteine residue. Several reports on the relationship between IBD and chemokine have been reported. Here we will review several chemokines that have been investigated in the context of IBD and finally described CXCL12-CXCR4 axis including our data.

3. CC family of chemokines

3.1 CCL2 (MCP-1) and CCR2

CCR2 and its ligands MCP-1,-2,-3 and -4 are involved in the recruitment of monocytes, dendritic cells, and memory T cells. In the intestine, MCP-1 is produced by intestinal epithelial cells. Mice deficient in MCP-1 are protected from hapten-induced colitis, as demonstrated by reduced hitological scores of colitis and lower IL-1β, IL-12p40, and IFN-γ (4). Furthermore, CCR2-deficient mice with dextran sulfate sodium (DSS)-induced colitis had lower histological scores than wild type mice (5). The chemokine receptor antagonist TAK-779, which blocks CCR2, CCR5, and CXCR3 could reduce colonic inflammation of DSS-induced colitis (6). These data suggested that CCR2 and its ligands seemed to play a crucial role in intestinal inflammation.

3.2 CCL3 (MIP-1α), CCL4 (MIP-1β), CCL5 (RANTES) and CCR5

Expression of CCL3 is up-regulated in the colon of rats exposed to TNBS and Administration of neutralizing antibodites to CCL3 blocked massive neutrophil influx (7). Expression of RANTES is induced by TNF-α and IFN-γ and, together with its receptors CCR1 and CCR5, is up-regulated in the chronic phase of TNBS-induced colitis in rats (8).

Interestingly, RANTES was specifically expressed in non-caseating granulomas of CD patients by in situ hybridization with surrounding CD4+ T cells expressing the CCR5 ad CXCR3 receptors. CCR5 and its ligands are involved in the migration of T cells and monocytes (9). CCL5-deficient mice are less susceptible to DSS-induced colitis and the inflammation that appears in CCR5-deficient mice is characterized by increased CD4+T cell and NK1.1+ cell influx together with an up-regulation of the Th2 cytokines IL-4, IL-5 and IL-10 (4).

3.3 CCL20 and CCR6

CCL20 mediates chemotaxis of T cells, B cells and DCs (3). In the intestine, CCL20 is produced from IECs. In human IBD, CCL20 protien and RNA expression was increased in intestinal tissues of patients with CD but not those with UC. CCR6 deficient mice leads to decreased susceptibility to DSS (10) and intravital microscopic analyses showed that CCR6 blockade on T and B cells reduced their adherence to mucosal and submucosal microvessels in the course of DSS colitis. Recently, CCR6 has been identified as a key modulator of Th17 cell recruitment to the intestine (11). Taken together, these data may suggest that CCL20 and CCR6 have a chemotactic effect on T and B cells under inflammatory conditions in the colon.

3.4 CCL25 (thymus-expressed chemokine, TECK) and CCR9

CCL25 is constitutively expressed by thymic epithelial cells and IECs in the small intestine but not in the colon (12). CCL25 binds to the CCR9 expressed on T cells and IgA+ plasma cells. In the intestine, CCR9 is expressed by both αβ and γδ CD8αα+

intraepithelial lymphocytes (IELs) and these cells migrate towards CCL25. CCR9-deficient mice have a remarkable reduction of γδ IELs and administration of neutralizing antibody against CCL25 to young mice leads to decreased αβ and γδ CD8αα+ IELs, suggesting that CCL25-CCR9 pathway might be involved in the early stages of intestinal inflammation.

4. CX3CL1 (fractalkine) and CX3CR1

CX3CL1/fractalkine is a member of the CX3C chemokine family, which is expressed by epithelial cells and IECs (13). CX3CL1 can be up-regulated by TNF-α, IL-1β, LPS and IFN-γ. CX3CL1 can function as an endothelial adhesive determinant to recruit a sub-population of dendritic cells and macrophages that have high CX3CR1 expression. The association between CX3CL1 and pathogenesis of IBD remains controversial. However, Sans, et al. reported that circulating T cells and lamina propria T cells from active CD patients contained a higher proportion of CX3CR1+ cells than CD patients with inactive disease or healthy subjects (14).

5. The CXC family of Chemokines

5.1 CXCL5 (ENA-78) and CXCR2
Epithelial cell-derived neutrophil-activating peptide(ENA)-78 is a potent neutrophil chemoattractant, which is produced from IECs and LPS, TNF-α and IL-1β stimulate its production. ENA-78 shares sequence homology with CXCL-8 (IL-8). Expression of ENA-78 is induced in the colonic tissues of both patients with UC and CD (15, 16).

5.2 CXCL8 (IL-8)
IL-8 is also a neutrophil chemoattractant that is produced by macrophages, fibroblasts, epithelial cells, hepatocytes and endothelial cells (17). Up-regulation of IL-8 in the gut of both UC and CD was observed and IL-8 production appears to correlate with histological severity of disease (18). As well as ENA-78, IL-8 can bind CXCR2, although its affinity for the receptor is lower.

6. CXCL12 (SDF-1) and CXCR4

Among chemokines, CXC chemokine ligand (CXCL)12 (stromal cell-derived factor (SDF)-1/pre-B-cell-growth-stimulating factor (PBSF)) is particularly intriguing because it has been shown definitively to be involved in various developmental processes including hematopoiesis (19,20). CXCL12 was first characterized as a pre-B-cell growth-stimulating factor and and the primary physiologic receptor for CXCL12 is CXCR4, which also functions as an entry receptor for strains of HIV-1(21), The studies using mutant mice with targeted gene disruption have revealed that CXCL12 and CXCR4 are essential for B cell development and colonization of bone marrow by hematopoietic stem cells (HSCs) and myeloid lineage cells during ontogeny as well as blood vessel formation in gastrointestinal tract, cardiac ventricular septum formation, and cerebellar development (22, 23,24). Recently, it was reported that CXCL12-CXCR4 chemokine signaling is essential for the development of plasmacytoid dendritic cells (pDC), which could rapidly produces a huge amount of type I IFN (α, β) following microbial stimulation (25), This axis also play a crucial role in the development of natural killer (NK) cells, which are generated from hematopoietic stem cells and play vital roles in the innate immune response against viral infection (26). Thus, CXCL12-CXCR4 axis is widely involved in the development of immune cell. The concept of CXCL12 as being solely a constitutive chemokine was recently challenged by data from other groups that investigated immune-mediated inflammatory disorders and demonstrated its role in joint, lung, and liver inflammation (27, 28).

Nanki et al. showed that CXCL12 is highly expressed in the synovium of RA patients in contrast to patients with OA, and that anti-CD40 stimulation enhanced CXCL12 production by cultured synoviocytes from RA patients (29). Those authors hypothesized that the CD40 ligand (CD154) expressed on activated memory T cells may stimulate the production of CXCL12 by synoviocytes and increase the migration of T cells.

Thus, CXCR4/SDF-1α and its ligand CXCL12 is an important chemokine/receptor pair in various diseases, but have received very little attention in IBD.

7. How is CXCL12/CXCR4 axis involved in the pathophysiology of IBD?

Mikami, et al. investigated the role of CXCL12/CXCR4 axis in patents with IBD by analysis of CXCR4 expression on peripheral T cells (30). They demonstrated that CXCR4 expression on peripheral T cells in patients with active UC was significantly higher than that in inactive UC and controls. Moreover, a significant correlation between CXCR4 expressions and disease activity in patients with UC was observed. Hosomi, et al focused on the role of immature plasma cells in the pathophysiology of IBD (31). They demonstrated that the proportion of immature plasma cells was correlated positively with clinical activities of UC and CD and expression of CXCR3 and CXCR4 of immature plasma cells in UC patients was significantly higher than in controls. In addition, Dotan, et al. reported that CXCR4 was expressed by intestinal epithelial cells (IECs) and lamima propria cells and CXCR4 positive cells are significantly increased in lamina propria of IBD (32). Moreover, recent report indicated that evaluation of CXCR4 expression on CD4 T cells by FACS analysis could be a biomarker of Leukocytapheresis with a leukocyte removal filter (Cellsoba; Asahi Medical, Tokyo, Japan) (33). These data strongly suggested that CXCR4 positive cells could be involved in the pathophysiology of IBD.

As for expression of CXCL12 expressing cells in patients with IBD, Dotan et al. reported as follows: CXCL12 expression of normal intestinal mucosa was more limited to the surface epithelium, while the expression was enhanced and more diffuse in IBD mucosa (32). This up-regulation was specific to IBD mucosa, and did not occur in non-IBD inflammatory conditions. Moreover, in IBD, CXCL12 was significantly up-regulated in the inflamed compared to the non-inflamed epithelium and stronger expression of CXCL12 in intestinal tissues was observed in patients with UC than in those with CD. Thus, this expression was likely to be more specific in active UC patients than in CD patients,

However, using CXCL12/GFP knock-in approach, Mikami, et al. revealed that CXCL12-expressing cells were mainly observed in the perivascular sites of the normal colonic mucosa, suggesting that the CXCL12-expressing cells were morphologically considered to be pericytes (adjacent to the endothelial cell) but not epithelial cells (30). After DSS administration, gene expression of CXCL12 was strongly induced in mice with DSS-colitis, which was compatible to human IBD data reported by Dotan. In this regard, more investigation should be required to identify CXCL12 expressing cells in normal and pathogenic conditions of intestinal mucosa. However, the exact reason why CXCL12-CXCR4 signaling was specifically involved in the pathophysiology of UC remains unclear.

8. Blockade of CXCL12-CXCR4 signaling as therapeutic target of IBD

As mentioned above, this axis can be strongly involved in the pathophysiology of IBD, particularly, UC. Next question is whether or not blocking of CXCL12-CXCR4 axis can be a new therapy for IBD. Mikami, et al showed that the effect of CXCR4 antagonist (TF14016) on colitis in dextran sodium sulfate (DSS) and interleukin (IL)-10 knockout (KO) models (30).

Firstly, they examined CXCR4 expression on peripheral blood cells and CXCL12 expression of colonic tissue in mice with DSS-induced colitis. As expected, CXCR4 expression of CD4 positive cells was significantly increased after the start of DSS administration, compared with normal mice and gene expression of CXCL12 was also significantly higher in the colonic tissue of mice with DSS-induced colitis than that of normal mice. Next, they evaluated the effect of CXCR4 antagonist (TF14016) on DSS-induced colitis. TF14016 clinically and histologically attenuated intestinal inflammation of DSS-induced colitis. Interestingly, immunohistochemical analysis revealed not only the improvement of colonic inflammation but also reduction of lymphoid aggregations. They also investigated the effect of TF 14016 on cytokine production from mesenteric lymph node cells. Surprisingly, TF 14016 treatment reduced pro-inflammatory cytokine production such as TNF-α and IFN-γ but did not alter IL-10 production.

Why did not TF 14016 treatment affect IL-10 production? It should be noted that TF 14016 administration did not alter the percentage of FOXP3+CD25+T cell. This data suggested that ameliorating action of TF 14016 on DSS-induced colitis is mainly due to its inhibitory effect of CD4+CD25- T cells with increased CXCR4 expression. TF 14016 treatment also ameliorated colonic inflammation of IL-10 KO mice.

9. Conclusion

CXCL12 and CXCR4 have a constitutive and inflammatory role in the intestinal mucosa. Several human and mouse data strongly suggested that CXCL12-CXCR4 axis play a crucial role in the pathophysiology of IBD, especially UC. Therefore, we hope that therapeutic manipulation of this signaling is considered in IBD therapy.

10. References

[1] Fiocchi C. (1998) Inflammatory bowel disease: etiology and pathogenesis. Gastroenterology 115:182-205.

[2] Blumberg RS, Saubermann LJ, and Strober W. (1999) Animal models of mucosal inflammation and their relation to human inflammatory bowel disease. Curr Opin Immunol. 11:648-656.

[3] Charo IF, Ransohoff RM. (2006) The many roles of chemokines and chemokine receptors in inflammation. N Engl J Med 354:610-21.

[4] Warhurst AC, Hopkins SJ, Warhurst G. (1998) Interferon gamma induces differential upregulation of alpha and beta chemokine secretion in colonic epithelial cell lines. Gut 42:208-13.

[5] Andres PG, Beck PL, Mizoguchi E, et al. (2000) Mice with a selective deletion of the CC chemokine receptors 5 or 2 are protected from dextran sodium sulfate-mediated colitis: lack of CC chemokine receptor 5 expression results in a NK1.1+ lymphocyte-associated Th2-type immune response in the intestine. J Immunol 164:6303-6312.

[6] Tokuyama H, Ueha S, Kurachi M,.et al (2005) The simultaneous blockade of chemokine receptors CCR2, CCR5 and CXCR3 by a non-peptide chemokine receptor antagonist protects mice from dextran sodium sulfate-mediated colitis. Int Immunol 17:1023-1034.

[7] Ajuebor MN, Hogaboam CM, Le T, et al. (2004) The role of CCL3/macrophage inflammatory protein-1alpha in experimental colitis. Eur J Pharmacol 497:343-349.

[8] Ajuebor MN, Hogaboam CM, Kunkel SL, et al.,(2001) The Chemokine RANTES is a crucial mediator of the progression from acute to chronic colitis in the rat. J Immunol 166 552-558.

[9] Oki M, Ohtani H, Kinouchi Y, et al. (2005) Accumulation of CCR5+ T cells around RANTES+ granulomas in Crohn's disease: a pivotal site of Th1-shifted immune response? Lab Invest 85:137-45.

[10] Varona R, Cadenas V, Flores J, et al, (2003) CCR6 has a non-redundant role in the development of inflammatory bowel disease. Eur J Immunol 33:2937-46.

[11] Wang C, Kang SC, Lee J, et al. (2009) The Role of CCR6 in migration of Th17 cells and regulation of effector T-cell balance in the gut. Mucosal Immunol 2:173-83.

[12] Wurbel MA, Phillippe JM, Nguyen C, et al, (2000) The chemokine TECK is expressed by thymic and intestinal epithelial cells and attracts double- and single-positive thymocytes expressing the TECK receptor CCR9. Eur J Immunol 30: 262-71.

[13] Muehlhoefer A, Saubermann LJ, GU X et al. (2000) Fractalkine is an epithelial and endothelial cell-derived chemoattractant for intraepithelial lymphocytes in the small intestinal mucosa. J Immunol 164: 3368-76.

[14] Sans M, Danes S, de la Motte C, et al (2007) Enhanced recruitment of CX3CR1+ T cells by mucosal endothelial cell-derived fractalkine in inflammatory bowel disease. Gastroenterology;132:139-53.

[15] Keats S, Keats AC, Mizoguchi E, et al. (1997) Enterocytes are the primary source of the chemokine ENA-78 in normal colon and ulcerative colitis. Am J Physiol 273: G75-82.

[16] Z'Graggen K, Walz A, Mazzucchelli L. et al. (1997) The C-X-C chemokine ENA-78 i preferentially expressed in intestinal epithelium in inflammatory bowel disease. Gastroenterology 113: 808-816.

[17] Baggiolini M, Walz A, Kunkel SL. (1989) Neutrophil-activating peptide-1/interleukin 8, a novel cytokine that activates neutrophils. J Clin Invest 84:1045-1049.

[18] Daig R, Andus T, Aschenbrenner E, et al. (1996) Increased interleukin-8 expression in the colon mucosa of patients with inflammatory bowel disease. Gut 38: 216-222.

[19] Nagasawa T, Hirota S, Tachibana K et al. (1996) Defects of B-cell lymphopoiesis and bone-marrow myelopoiesis in mice lacking the CXC chemokine PBSF/SDF-1. Nature 382 (6592): 635-8.

[20] Nagasawa T. (2000) A chemokine, SDF-1/PBSF, and its receptor, CXC chemokine receptor 4, as mediators of hematopoiesis. Int J Hematol. 72:408-11.

[21] Bleul CC, Farzan M, Choe H, (1996) The lymphocyte chemoattractant SDF-1 is a ligand for LESTR/fusin and blocks HIV-1 entry. Nature.; 382(6594):829-33.

[22] Tachibana K, Hirota S, Iizasa H, et al (1998) The chemokine recepotor CXCR4 is essential for vascularization of the gastrointestinal tract Nature 393(6685) 591-594.23 23 Zou YR, Kottmann AH, Kuroda M, Taniuchi I, Littman DR.

[23] Zou YR, Kottman AH, Kuroda M, et al. (1998) Function fo the chemokine receptor CXCR4 in haematopoiesis ans in cerebellar development. Nature 393 (6685):595-9.

[24] Egawa T, Kawabata K, Kawamoto H, et al. (2001) The earliest stages of B cell development require a chemokine stromal cell-derived factor/pre-B cell growth-stimulating factor. Immunity. 15:323-34.

[25] Kohara H, Omatsu Y, Sugiyama T, et al. (2007) Development of plasmacytoid dendritic cells in bone marrow stromal cell niches requires CXCL12-CXCR4 chemokine signaling Blood. 110:4153-60.

[26] Noda M, Omatsu Y, Sugiyama T, et al. (2011) CXCL12-CXCR4 chemokine signaling is essential for NK-cell development in adult mice. Blood. 117:451-8.

[27] Phillips RJ, Burdick MD, (2004) Circulating fibrocytes traffic to the lungs in J Clin Invest 114:438-446:

[28] Wald O, Pappo O, Safdi R, et al. (2004) Involvement of the CXCL12/CXCR4 pathway in the advanced liver disease that is associated with hepatitis C virus or hepatitis B virus. Eur J Immuno 34:1164-1174.).

[29] Nanki T, Hayashida K, El-Gabalawy HS, et al.(2000) Stromal cell-derived factor-1 CXC chemokine receptor 4 interactions play a central role in CD4+T cell accumulation in rheumatoid arthritis synovium J Immunol 165:6590-6598.

[30] Mikami S, Nakase H, Yamamoto S, et al. (2008) Blockade of CXCL12/CXCR4 axis ameliorates murine experimental colitis J Pharmacol Exp Ther 327 383-392

[31] Hosomi S, Oshitani N, Kamata N,. et al. (2011) Increased numbers of immature plasma cells in peripheral blood specifically overexpress chemokine receptor CXCR3 and CXCR4 in patients with ulcerative colitis. Clin Exp Immunol. 163:215-24.

[32] Dotan I, Werner L, Vigodman S, et al. (2010) CXCL12 is a constitutive and inflammatory chemokine in the intestinal immune system. Inflamm Bowel Dis. 16:583-92.

[33] Nakase H, Mikami S, Chiba T. (2009) Alteration of CXCR4 expression and Th1/Th2 balance of peripheral CD4-positive T cells can be a biomarker for leukocytapheresis therapy for patients with refractory ulcerative colitis. Inflamm Bowel Dis 15:963-4

6

Enteric Nervous System Abnormalities in Ulcerative Colitis

Carla Cirillo, Giovanni Sarnelli and Rosario Cuomo
University of Naples "Federico II"
Italy

1. Introduction

Ulcerative colitis (UC) is a chronic non-specific inflammatory disease affecting the mucosa and the submucosa of the colon, and is characterized by alterations of gut functions which influence the clinical symptoms (Fiocchi, 1998; Reddy et al., 1991; Spriggs et al., 1951). Although reports showed morpho-functional abnormalities of the enteric nervous system in UC patients, the available literature is still heterogeneous and confusing.

UC-related intestinal inflammation causes structural and functional changes to the enteric nervous system and its cellular components (neurons and glial cells), which could be directly related to the development of the disease and its associated symptoms (Geboes & Collins, 1998; Lakhan & Kirchgessner, 2010; Lomax et al., 2005; Villanacci et al., 2008).

UC-related alteration in the enteric nervous system can be categorised into two groups: a) the alterations that occur in the structural morphology of the system, and b) those that occur in the level of enteric transmitters released by neurons and glial cells (Lakhan & Kirchgessner, 2010). Routine pathology of UC reports describe: 1) hypertrophy, hyperplasia and axonal damage of nerve fibres (Cook & Dixon, 1973; Geboes, 1993); 2) a normal aspect, hypertrophy, hyperplasia or damage of neuronal cell bodies (Belai et al., 1997; Siemers & Dobbins, 1974; Strobach et al., 1990); 3) glial cells hyperplasia (Antonius et al., 1960); 4) a variable increase of glial cells number (Geboes et al., 1992; Koretz et al., 1987); and 5) ganglioneuritis (Ohlsson et al., 2007).

Besides structural changes, disruption in the function of neurons and glial cells is reported in patients with UC: defective neuronal control of epithelial secretion, increased excitability of enteric neurons, alteration in synaptic transmission, and variablility in the expression of neuronal and glial-derived factors (vasoactive intestinal peptide, inducible nitric oxide synthase and other mediators in neuronal cell bodies; S100B protein, glial fibrillary acidic protein and other factors in glial cells) (Lomax et al., 2005).

The aim of this chapter is to illustrate the new insights into the pathophysiology of UC, providing an exhaustive overview of the current knowledge of the role of the enteric nervous system during gut inflammation.

Initially, we describe the morphology and the basic physiological functions of the enteric nervous system and its cellular components, neurons and glial cells, respectively. Then, a more extensive part is dedicated to the modifications of the enteric nervous system in UC. Besides the well documented role of enteric neurons, attention is also focused on the involvement of glial network in the complex scenario of intestinal inflammation, on which there is accumulating evidence in recent years. Finally, the implication of the enteric nervous system in the control of the gut immune system during inflammation is described in the last part of the chapter, as recently hypothesized.

2. The Enteric Nervous System: Morphological and functional features

The Enteric nervous System (ENS) is a collection of neurons in the gastrointestinal (GI) tract, and constitutes the "brain in the gut", since it has the unique ability to control several GI functions, such as exocrine and endocrine secretions, motility, blood flow and immune/inflammatory processes, independent of the central nervous system (Goyal & Hirano, 1996). In the ENS, the nerve-cell bodies are grouped into small ganglia that are connected by nerve bundles forming two major layers embedded in the gut wall, the myenteric plexus (or Auerbach's plexus) and the submucosal plexus (or Meissner's plexus) (Goyal & Hirano, 1996). The myenteric plexus lies between the longitudinal and circular muscle and extends the entire length of the gut. This layer primarily provides motor innervations to the two muscle layers, and secretomotor innervations to the mucosa. The submucosal plexus, located between the mucosa and circular muscle (Furness & Costa 1980; Grundy et al., 2006), is best developed in the small intestine, where it plays an important role in the control of secretion. Both these components contain functionally different neurons (about 100 millions) and four to ten times more glial cells, together organized in ganglia (Goyal & Hirano, 1996; Hoff et al., 2008). Neurons and glial cells of the ENS are derived from stem cells in the neuronal crest, a transient structure present during embryonic development (Dupin et al., 2006).

2.1 Enteric neurons
Although up to eight morphologic forms of neurons have been identified in the ENS, there are two main types: type I neurons, that have many club-shaped processes and a single long process, and type II neurons, that are multipolar and have many long, smooth processes (Furness & Costa, 1980). Functionally, enteric neurons can be classified into primary afferent neurons, interneurons and motor neurons, synaptically linked to each other in microcircuits (Furness & Costa, 1980). Moreover, there is a general classification between neurons of the submucosal plexus and neurons of the myenteric plexus: while the first ones predominantly innervate the mucosa and regulate secretion, absorption and blood flow, the second ones are primarily involved in the control of intestinal motility (Brookes, 2001). Enteric neurons are also known to control mucosal development and function as well as some aspects of the local immune system within the gut. This fine regulation of several and different functions is possible because enteric neurons are in close proximity to other cells present in the gut wall (mucosal immune cells and epithelial cells) and also secrete a wide range of neurotransmitters.

The chemical neuro-mediators of the ENS were initially thought to be limited to neurotransmitters such as acetylcholine and serotonin, but, subsequently, purines, such as ATP, amino acids, such as γ-aminobutyric acid, and peptides, such as vasoactive intestinal polypeptide (VIP) and neuropeptide Y (NPY), were identified (Gershon et al., 1994). More recently, nitric oxide (NO) has emerged as an important neurotransmitter in the ENS (Bogers et al., 1994). Overall, more than 20 candidate neurotransmitters have now been identified in enteric neurons, and most neurons contain several of them (Gershon et al., 1994). Distinctive patterns of co-localization of mediators appear to identify sets of neurons that perform distinct functions (Costa & Brookes, 1994; Gershon et al., 1994). Although neurotransmitter functions have been clearly defined for only a few of these mediators such acetylcholine, substance P (SP), VIP, NPY and NO, it is well known that a wide variety of neurons that perform different functions may use the same neurotransmitter.

2.2 Enteric Glial Cells (EGC)

Morphologically, EGC are small cells with a 'star-like' appearance (Hoff et al., 2008) containing intracellular arrays of 10 nm filaments made up of glial fibrillary acidic protein (GFAP) (Bjorklund et al., 1984; Endo & Kobayashi, 1987; Hoff et al., 2008; Mestres et al., 1992). These cells envelop enteric neuronal cell bodies and axon bundles (Gershon & Rothman, 1991), as well as intestinal blood vessels (Bjorklund et al., 1984; Geboes et al., 1992), and extend their processes into the intestinal mucosa (Bush et al., 1998; Jessen & Mirsky, 1980). Though, phenotypically comparable to the astrocytes in the central nervous system, EGC account for other similiar functions, such as the regulation of gut homeostasis, as well as inflammatory responses (Broussard et al., 1993; Gershon & Rothman, 1991). Since their first description by Dogiel in 1899, EGC have been assumed to be the most abundant cell type in the ENS (Gabella, 1981). At present, the S100B protein and GFAP, together with more recently identified markers such as Sox 10, are commonly used to identify EGC in the human gut (Bjorklund et al., 1984; Cirillo et al., 2009a; Esposito et al., 2007; Ferri et al., 1982; Hoff et al., 2008). Functionally, EGC have been traditionally considered as a mechanical support for enteric neurons since they release a wide range of factors responsible for the development, survival and differentiation of peripheral neurons (Laranjeira & Pachnis, 2009). Like their counterpart in the brain, EGC, in physiological conditions, constitutively express major histocompatibility complex (MHC) class I molecules, whereas MHC class II expression is sparsely detectable (Geboes et al., 1992; Koretz et al., 1987). In recent years, this restrictive view has been changed to one of a more articulate and complex nature, since EGC are involved in the maintenance of intestinal homeostasis (Bassotti et al., 2007; Van Landeghem et al., 2009). Indeed, these cells control intestinal epithelial barrier functions, such as permeability, via the release of GSNO (S-nitrosoglutathione) as well as the regulation of expression of zonulin-1 and occludin (Neunlist et al., 2008; Savidge et al., 2007a).

Besides the well documented 'protective role', EGC are also activated by means of inflammatory insults and they directly contribute to an inflammatory condition by antigen presentation and by promoting the release of pro-inflammatory cytokines in the gut milieu, thus making them the initiators of immune responses (Cabarrocas, 2003; Cirillo et al., 2009a; Esposito et al., 2007; Neunlist et al., 2008; Savidge et al., 2007b). This ability of EGC to be atigen presenting cell is due to the expression of MHC class II molecule, in the presence of pro-inflammatory stimuli, as recently demonstrated (Cirillo et al., 2009a). Therefore, EGC act as 'receptors' for cytokines and may themselves produce cytokines, such as interleukin-6 and interleukin-1-beta (Murakami et al., 2009; Ruhl et al., 2001). In addition, EGC express the inducible form of nitric oxide synthase (iNOS) and L-arginine, the machinery required for the time-delayed and micromolar release of nitric oxide (NO), one of the most important pro-inflammatory mediators within the gut (Aoki et al., 1991; Cirillo et al., 2009b; Nagahama et al., 2001).

2.2.1 EGC markers: GFAP and S100B protein

Mature EGC are rich in the intermediate filament protein GFAP (Eng et al., 2000; Jessen & Mirsky, 1980). In animals, two classes of EGC can be distinguished, namely the GFAP positive and GFAP negative groups and this ratio is under control of pro-inflammatory cytokines (von Boyen et al., 2004). GFAP expression is modulated by cell differentiation, inflammation and injury (Eng et al., 2000), indicating that the level of this filament matches with the functional state of EGC. Increased GFAP expression has been observed in inflammation or inflammatory diseases of the gut, such as UC (Bradley et al., 1997; Cornet et al., 2001).

S100B is an easily diffusible protein that is a homodimer of β subunit (Baudier et al., 1986). It belongs to the S100 protein family that includes more than 20 EF-hand Ca^{2+}/Zn^{2+}-binding proteins (Haimoto et al., 1987; Sugimura et al., 1989; Zimmer & Van Eldik, 1987). In the human gut, among S100 proteins, only the S100B protein is specifically and physiologically expressed by EGC (Cirillo et al., 2009a; Cirillo et al., 2009b; Esposito et al., 2007), while other members, such as S100A8, S100A9 and S100A12 are found in phagocytes and in intestinal epithelial cells in patients affected by inflammatory bowel disease (Leach et al., 2007; Pietzsch & Hoppmann, 2009). Recent findings have demonstrated that aberrant expression of S100B correlates with the degree of the gut inflammation (Cirillo et al., 2009b; Esposito et al., 2007). The search for a specific S100B signalling receptor has demonstrated that, in micromolar concentrations, this protein may accumulate at the RAGE (receptor for advanced glycation endproducts) site on target cells, such as immune cells (Adami et al., 2004; Hofmann et al., 1999; Schmidt et al., 2001). Such interaction leads to the activation of a signalling cascade resulting in the transcription of different pro-inflammatory cytokines and iNOS protein. S100B can, thus, be considered as a diffusible pro-inflammatory cytokine which gains access to the extracellular space especially at immune-inflammatory reaction sites in the gut (Adami et al., 2001; Cirillo et al., 2009a; Cirillo et al., 2009b; Esposito et al., 2007; Petrova et al., 2000).

3. Role of enteric neurons in UC

Inflammation is well known to affect gut functions, since it leads to persistent changes in enteric nerves thus resulting in dismotility, hypersensitivity and dysfunction. Data obtained from intestinal biopsies from UC patients, or on animal models of UC, have consistently suggested a role of neuro-inflammation in the generation of symptoms associated with the disease (Beyak & Vanner, 2005; Geboes & Collins, 1998). Neuronal abnormalities strongly illustrate the impact of inflammatory signals generated within the gut mucosa on the ENS. In this context, the neuronal regeneration represents a challenging concept and studies aiming to the identification of progenitor-like cells in the ENS are crucial (Kruger et al., 2002).

3.1 Structural changes

To understand the relationship between the intestinal inflammation that characterizes UC and structural abnormalities to the enteric neurons, animal models of colitis are routinely used. This enables us to elucidate the mechanisms underlying gut dysfuctions, which would be rather difficult to observe in humans. The most commonly used models to induce colitis are characterized by intracolonic administration of 1) trinitrobenzene sulfonic acid (TNBS) or 2) 2,4-dinitrobenzene-sulfonic acid (DNBS) or 3) *Trichinella spiralis* (T. Spiralis) infection in the animal.

In guinea pigs, it has been described that the number of myenteric neurons per ganglion is significantly decreased in TNBS-induced colitis (Linden et al., 2005). In this experimental model, the observed decrease in myenteric neurons was not associated with a decrease in any particular subpopulation of neurons, suggesting a severe loss of neurons that occur during the onset of colitis. In addition, the neurotoxic insult is followed by a rapid regeneration of the axons from the surviving neurons. These data are confirmed in a rat model of TNBS-induced colitis, in which there is a significant loss of myenteric neurons as a result of an increased rate of apoptosis (Sarnelli et al., 2009). Similar changes are reported in another model of chemically-induced colitis in rats, with DNBS administration, which is characterized by a significant decrease of neuronal cells in the myenteric plexus of the ENS (Sanovic et al., 1999; Hawkins et al., 1997). As confirmed by histopathological assessment, in this model, compared to the TNBS-induced model, the neuronal damages are more similar to those observed in UC patients. Significant neuronal death is also observed in T. spiralis induced colitis in mice and rats (Auli et al., 2008). Intracolonic administration of T. spiralis larvae in rats causes colitis with features similar to UC, notably with inflammation predominantly limited to the colonic mucosa (Auli et al., 2008). Interestingly, in this animal model of colitis, the authors also provide information about the subpopulation of neurons affected by inflammation, describing that there is a significant decrease especially in the number of nitric oxide synthase (NOS)-immunoreactive neurons in the myenteric plexus of infected rats, with consequent changes in intestinal motility.

In humans, abnormalities of the neuronal components of the ENS reported in UC patients include hyperplasia or increased number of neuronal cell bodies, mainly in the ganglia of the submucosal plexus, neuronal cell damage, and neuronal hypertrophy. In addition, hypertrophy of the neuronal cell bodies in the submucosal plexus seems to be common in UC patients (Mottet, 1971; Van Patter et al., 1954). Neuronal hyperplasia of the myenteric plexus is also reported for UC but the data available in the literature is rare and may have been complicated by difficulties in the differential diagnosis between granulomatous colitis and genuine UC (Okamoto, 1964; Storsteen et al., 1953). Neuronal cell hyperplasia is certainly more frequently reported for Crohn's disease and seems more common with a significant, statistical difference when compared with UC. In addition to hypertrophy and hyperplasia of neuronal cell bodies, signs of degeneration have been described occasionally in areas of the inflamed gut in UC patients (Oehmichen & Reiffersscheid, 1977; Rienmann & Schmidt, 1982).

Also neuronal synapses appear to be altered in patients with UC. This is because of an increased synaptophysin (a synaptic vesicle protein involved in synapse formation but without a well defined functional role) immunoreactivity, compared to samples from normal mucosa and from cases with non-specific colitis, in which mucosal fibres are rare and usually small (Strobach et al., 1990). Submucosal and myenteric nerve fibre hypertrophy is uncommon in UC patients. Ultra-structural studies of UC and control samples have shown that, in both submucosal and myenteric layers, the nerve fibres or axons appear as swollen, empty, lucent structures, with large membrane-bound vacuoles, swollen mitochondria and concentrated neurofibrils (Dvorak et al., 1980). These changes can be focal or diffuse and can affect all axons in one nerve bundle or just few of them. This data supports the hypothesis of a correlation between the neural hyperplasia and the inflammatory reaction in UC patients. It appears, thus, that UC is characterized by two types of structural neuronal abnormalities: damage and hyperplasia of neurons in all parts of the ENS, related to inflammation.

Changes in the chemical coding of myenteric neurons are described in UC patients (Neunlist et al., 2003). Immunohistochemical characterization of neurons in the myenteric plexus revealed that alterations occur in the proportion of choline acetyltransferase (ChAT)/negative (-ve), ChAT/SP-ve, and SP-ve populations in UC patients compared to the intestinal tissues from control subjects. These changes have similar features in inflamed and non-inflamed areas of the gut in UC patients. The use of a combination of antibodies against ChAT, VIP and SP enabled the identification of transmitter co-localisation in colonic myenteric neurons, showing five distinct subpopulations (ChAT-ve, ChAT/SP-ve, ChAT/VIP-ve, VIP-ve, and SP-ve). The largest neuronal population identified in the myenteric plexus of UC patients is ChAT immunoreactive and hence of cholinergic nature. VIP formed 9% of the total neuronal population. Most of the SP+ve neurons co-localize with ChAT. In UC patients, there is a threefold increase in the proportion of myenteric neurons immunoreactive for SP, compared to control subjects, whereas the proportion of ChAT+ve and VIP+ve neurons was not affected. The increase in SP observed in the inflamed gut of UC patients is a hallmark of the disease pathology. Moreover, an increase in the density of SP immunoreactive fibres and SP content in UC patients, especially in the lamina propria has been reported (Goldin et al., 1989; Keranen et al., 1995; Vento et al., 2001). At present, no data are available to address the questions of whether the changes in SP observed in myenteric neurons of UC patients are the result of transductional, post-transductional, or even alterations in peptide transport. In this context, changes in mRNA levels for SP receptors are observed in UC patients (Goede et al., 2000) but it is not known whether SP mRNA is increased in myenteric neurons or whether degradation of SP is altered in this inflammatory disease. The increase in SP+ve neurons observed in UC patients occurs primarily in the population of ChAT-ve neurons detected in control subjects. In fact, the total proportion of ChAT+ve neurons is not modified in UC patients compared with control subjects, and the increase in the proportion of ChAT/SP-ve neurons is equivalent to the decrease in the proportion of the ChAT-ve population observed in UC patients. What might be the clinical relevance of the SP increase in UC? Firstly, SP may play an important role in the pathophysiology of UC (Holzer, 1998). In fact, there is increased expression of SP binding sites in UC as well as an increase in neurokinin 1 (NK-1) receptor mRNA (Goede et al., 2000; Mantyh et al., 1995). Confirming the involvement of NK-1 in the modulation of gut inflammation, in an animal model of colitis, the administration of NK-1 antagonist reduced colonic inflammation (Stucchi et al., 2000). In the same animal model, inflammation induced an increase in SP synthesis in myenteric neurons. Moreover, a decrease in neutral endopeptidase activity (the enzyme which degrades SP) was observed in T. spiralis-infected intestine in conjunction with increased SP levels (Hwang et al., 1993). These combined effects result in an increased SP levels and down-regulation of endopeptidase activity, which could significantly increase SP that might contribute to uncontrolled intestinal inflammation in UC. A surprising finding is that alterations in the neurochemical code of myenteric neurons occur in similar proportions in inflamed and non-inflamed areas of UC patients, as mentioned above. SP induction during UC in non-inflamed and inflamed areas could be due to an increase in inflammatory cytokines such as interleukin-1beta, which have been observed during UC in the intestine (Fiocchi, 1998). In fact, interleukin-1beta induces increased SP expression in rat myenteric fibres (Hurst et al., 1993). In summary, marked changes in the neurochemical coding of myenteric neurons characterize UC. ChAT-ve neurons can be considered as the putative neuronal population exhibiting neural plasticity by expressing different levels of SP. Therefore, this remodelling in UC occurs as a shift from mainly cholinergic to more peptidergic innervation. Similar changes in neurochemical coding were also observed in the least affected sites of inflammation. This effect may constitute part of the neuronal basis for the altered motility observed during UC.

Another important neuropeptide, calcitonin gene-related peptide (CGRP), is involved in inflammatory processes and is regulated by nerve growth factor (NGF) (Linsday & Harmar, 1989). In inflammatory bowel disease, NGF and its high affinity receptor (trkA) are highly over-expressed in the inflamed tissues (Di Mola et al., 2000). Studies have shown that neuropeptides, like CGRP (Reinshagen et al., 1998), are protective in acute (Reinshagen et al., 1994) and chronic (Reinshagen et al., 1996) models of experimental colitis. As a result, the protective effect of neurotrophic factors can partly be explained by a specific modulation of neuropeptide expression during inflammation. Therefore, in an experimental model of inflammation of the rat gut, NGF and neurotrophin-3 seem to have a protective effect. When these neurotrophic factors are experimentally and selectively blocked during colitis, this leads to a significant increase in inflammation (Reinshagen et al., 2000).

3.2 Functional changes

Abnormalities of the enteric neurons during the course of inflammation leads to altered intestinal functions. Three major groups of functional neuronal changes are observed in UC patients: 1) defects in the neuronal control of epithelial secretion, 2) increased excitability of enteric neurons and 3) alteration in synaptic transmission (Lomax et al., 2005). Due to their localization within the intestine, changes in enteric neurons reflect in the alterations of a broad range of functions that are orchestrated by the other cell types (epithelial, immune, endocrine cells) residing the gut wall. Specifically, the five primary targets of the enteric neurons are 1) smooth muscle cells responsible for motility; 2) mucosal secretory cells; 3) endocrine cells; 4) the microvasculature that maintains mucosal blood flow during intestinal secretion and 5) the immunomodulatory and inflammatory cells that are involved in mucosal immunologic, allergic and inflammatory responses (Goyal & Hirano, 1996).

A number of electrophysiological studies have been performed in animal models of colitis in order to elucidate the mechanisms underlying inflammation-induced changes in enteric neuronal functions in UC patients (Lakhan & Kirchgessner, 2010). Independent of the method used to induce colitis, the type of enteric neurons most dramatically affected by inflammation is the after-hyperpolarizing (AH) neurons. The AH neurons physiologically work as intrinsic primary afferent neurons in the myenteric plexus and control intestinal peristalsis, mucosal secretion and vasodilatation. While in normal conditions these neurons very rarely receive fast synaptic inputs, in course of inflammation more AH neurons receive fast synaptic inputs, exhibit increased excitability, depolarized membrane potential, reduced AH potential amplitude and duration along with increased input resistance (Lennon et al., 1991; Yoshida et al., 1988). AH neurons characteristically receive slow excitatory postsynaptic potentials in the normal non inflamed intestine, but increased excitation (long-term hyperexcitability) occurs in AH neurons during the course of inflammation (Qualman et al., 1984). This pathological phenomenon indicates that a brief synaptic activation can trigger a long period of hyperexcitability in AH neurons after they have been exposed to an inflamed environment, thus suggesting that perturbation of the sensory component of intrinsic motor reflexes may occur during inflammation and that increased neuronal excitation may contribute to the altered motility, pain and discomfort associated with intestinal inflammation in UC patients. The mechanisms responsible for the changes in excitability are not yet understood, but it is postulated that they involve a persistent alteration in channel expression and/or a continuous release of inflammatory mediators in the intestinal milieu.

Together with neuronal hyperexcitability, alterations in sympathetic neural activity, with consequent impact on the functions of the ENS, are reported in UC patients (May & Goyal, 1994). In animal models of colitis, the decrease in the release of noradrenaline from sympathetic varicosities due to inhibition of N-type voltage-gated Ca^{2+} current in postganglionic sympathetic neurons, has been reported in both inflamed and un-inflamed regions of the gut (Ikeda et al., 1982). However, at present, how an alteration of sympathetic function contributes to the pathogenesis of UC has not yet been fully understood.

As described above, UC is also characterized by nerve fibre hypertrophy and hyperplasia, but it is not clear whether these alterations have functional consequences or which functional changes they might induce in the inflamed gut of UC patients. Some of the fibres with a prominent appearance on routinely stained slides may indeed not be functional. The swollen aspect of the axons observed with ultra structural studies might correspond with the thickened appearance of the fibres reported in some immunohistochemical studies while in fact these fibres are damaged and hence not functional.

4. Role of Enteric Glial Cells in UC

It is widely known that EGC display many morphological and functional similarities with astrocytes in the brain, which are essential to maintain homeostasis in the central nervous system. Emerging reports indicate a regulatory role of EGC in the gut (Bassotti et al., 2007; Neunlist et al., 2008; Van Landeghem et al., 2009). From *in vivo* studies, we now know that the selective ablation of the glial network, carried out by using chemical methods, leading to intestinal inflammation that is associated with the alteration of mucosal barrier integrity (Bush et al., 1998; Savidge et al., 2007). Moreover, animal models in which the ablation of EGCs was auto-immune mediated, demonstrated that these cells are also capable of immune functions *in vivo* (Cornet et al., 2001). Additional studies have demonstrated that EGC directly affect intestinal epithelial barrier integrity via the release of factors such as transforming growth factor-beta, S-nitrosogluthatione and glial-derived neurotrophic factor (GDNF) (Neunlist et al., 2007; Savidge et al., 2007; von Boyen et al., 2011), thus confirming the crucial role played by EGC in the regulation of gut homeostasis. Given the ability of EGC to modulate the intestinal barrier functions and to mediate immune responses *in vivo*, it has also been claimed that these cells are involved in inflammatory bowel disease (Cirillo et al., 2009b; Cornet et al., 2001; Neunlist et al., 2007; Neunlist et al., 2008). Several studies have underlined the involvement of EGC in intestinal inflammation during which both mucosal and motor functions are altered (Cirillo et al., 2009b; Cornet et al., 2001; Sethi & Sarna, 1991). Indeed, changes in EGC architecture, together with impaired expression of EGC-derived factors, are reported in UC patients. Among the glial-derived mediators, GFAP, S100B protein and GDNF are up-regulated in UC patients (Cirillo et al., 2009; Cornet et al., 2001; Steinkamp et al., 2003; von Boyen et al., 2011).

Confirming the involvement of EGC in the intestinal inflammatory scenario, immunohistochemical studies also revealed an increase in MHC class II membranous expression on EGC and glial sheaths of nerve fibres in the mucosa and submucosa of UC patients. This increased and aberrant expression is present in both macroscopically involved and uninvolved areas, in the colon and ileum, and correlates with the increased MHC class II expression on epithelial cells. The enhanced MHC class II expression on the EGC is positively correlated with the local intensity of the cellular inflammatory infiltrate, especially with the increased infiltration of T lymphocytes.

4.1 Neuro-glial crosstalk in UC

Morpho-functional changes in EGC observed in UC patients could also be a major link between the alterations in neuronal functions described above. Indeed, EGC have been shown to control neuronal functions which alter the course of gut inflammation.

Various observations indicate that EGC may promote neuronal survival by directly regulating substrate supply (Cabarrocas et al., 2003; Nagahama et al., 2001). They also appear to regulate perineuronal homeostasis (Cabarrocas et al., 2004). For example, EGC are the only cell type in the ENS that express glutamine synthetase, which might be involved in the detoxification of glutamate and γ-aminobutyric acid. Selective ablation of cycling EGC is also associated with a moderate degeneration of myenteric neurons but not in neuronal content of SP. Changes in enteric neuron phenotype and intestinal functions are described in a transgenic mouse model of EGC disruption. In this experimental model, in which immune alteration of EGC was induced in adult animals, EGC abnormalities induce changes in both the neurochemical coding of enteric neurons and in intestinal motor and mucosal functions. In this adoptive transfer model, however no overt clinical signs were observed. This minor disruption of EGC is characterized by a decrease in GFAP expression both at the protein and mRNA level. Alteration of GFAP expression is not associated with intestinal inflammation, as detected by histological assessment. While it has been reported that acute intestinal inflammation is usually associated with an increase in GFAP expression, as well as proliferation of EGC (Bradley et al., 1997, von Boyen et al., 2004), the absence of intestinal inflammation reported in the mentioned study could be due to the fact that EGC disruption was not profound enough to cause severe inflammation as the number of GFAP structures was not affected. In addition, in this mouse model of EGC disruption, the number of enteric neurons per ganglion from the submucosal and myenteric layers is not modified compared to the control animals, suggesting that neuronal cell loss did not occur at this stage. In contrast, the neurochemical coding in both enteric layers is altered and these changes in the phenotype affect different cell populations of the ENS. The mechanism responsible for these modifications however remains to be explored. Similar to the central nervous system, astrocytes are well known synthesizers of various neurotrophic factors (NT-3, GDNF, NGF) that are involved in the regulation of enteric neuromediator expression (De Giorgio et al., 2000; Saffrey et al., 2000). In the same way, enteric neurons have also been shown to express neurotrophin receptors (De Giorgio et al., 2000). Therefore, alterations in EGC could result from altered neurotrophic factor synthesis.

Apart from the involvement of other neurotrophic factors, alterations in EGC induce motor changes both *in vivo* and *in vitro*, with a corresponding decrease in intestinal motility. These changes in motility could be correlated with the decrease in NOS immunoreactivity in myenteric neurons, which are notoriously recognized to be inhibitory motor neurons

(Kunze & Furness, 1999). Together with changes in NO expression, the delayed transit observed in transgenic mice may be the result of the alterations in neurotrophic factors, such as neurotrophins or from modifications in EGC of the spinal cord as extrinsic neuronal pathways can modulate GI functions (Cabarrocas et al., 2003; Coulie et al., 2000; Parkman et al., 2003). As mentioned above, EGC are also involved in the regulation of intestinal paracellular permeability. It is conceivable that the decrease in VIPergic submucosal neurons observed when EGC are ablated could be partly responsible for the increased permeability, since the activation of VIPergic neurons decreases paracellular permeability (Neunlist et al., 2003). In summary, EGC are involved in the regulation of GI functions, such as intestinal motility and permeability, and participate in the control of the neurochemical phenotype of enteric neurons.

4.2 S100B expression in UC

It is clear that EGC directly participate in the chronic mucosal inflammation in UC. EGC perform this role via the release of several mediators. Among these, S100B protein plays a crucial role in UC (Cirillo et al., 2009b). More specifically, a study performed in both UC patients and control subjects demonstrates that in the rectal mucosa of UC patients there is an increased S100B immunoreactivity, together with a significant increase in S100B mRNA, protein expression and secretion. This up-regulation is associated with enhanced NO production through the specific induction of iNOS protein. This correlation is very interesting, since a growing body of evidence indicates that UC is characterized by abnormal mucosal NO production in response to iNOS induction by pro-inflammatory cytokines (Linehan et al., 2005; Menchen et al., 2004). Within the human gut, the ability of EGC to specifically modulate NO production through S100B protein seems to play a pivotal role. In fact, it is described that the application of exogenous S100B, in micromolar concentrations, induces a significant and concentration-dependent increase in NO production, through the induction of iNOS expression, in the human non-inflamed rectal mucosa of control subjects. It's interesting that micromolar concentrations of S100B mediate a significant NO increase in UC patients, as well as in the rectal mucosa of control subjects. This finding suggests that EGC are able to mediate mucosal NO-dependent inflammatory responses by increasing S100B protein level within the intestinal milieu. Once released, S100B acts as extracellular ligand for cell surface receptor RAGE (receptor for advanced glycation endproducts) on targeted cells, by triggering pro-inflammatory signals that lead to NO production. It has been previously demonstrated that other members of S100 proteins family (i.e. S100A12) play a role during intestinal inflammation via RAGE interaction (Foell et al., 2003). More specifically, the S100A12/RAGE-mediated pathway affect immune cell-derived NO production. The specificity of EGC activation induced by inflammation is confirmed by the fact that, in an *in vitro* model of gut inflammation, S100B mRNA, protein expression and release are significantly increased, simultaneously with an enhanced NO production. These findings indicate that EGC are able to recognize inflammatory stimuli and that, once activated, they produce and release S100B contributing to the induction of iNOS. In addition, EGC activation observed in the inflamed gut mucosa of UC patients is not reduced by the administration of cortisone suggesting that this phenomenon occurs via a steroid-insensitive mechanism and that it is not secondary to immune system activation. These findings, together with the recent demonstration that EGC express MHC class II molecule when stimulated (Cirillo et al., 2009) pave the way to look at this cell population as primary effectors and not as secondary targets during inflammatory responses within the gut.

5. ENS-immune system cross-talk in UC

The gut is also home to the largest component of the immune system. The interaction between ENS and immune system remains an important topic and considerable progress has been achieved to shed some light on the neuro-immune axis in the human gut. Although the immunomodulatory role of the ENS remains to be clarified, it is conceivable that chronic gut inflammation is characterized by altered ENS-immune system cross-talk. It has been known for some time that the ENS and mucosal immune systems have the ability to regulate one another's functions. For example, in experimental animal models of colitis it has been reported that the vagal anti-inflammatory pathway plays a crucial role in the control of gut inflammation and that the ENS is probably involved in this phenomenon as a player in the 'final step' (Ghia et al., 2006; Tracey, 2007).

Neurons in the ENS are found in close proximity to immune cells in the mucosa. The two systems even share several chemical mediators, such as SP. Neuronal activation can lead to degranulation of mast cells and influx of neutrophils, thereby recruiting elements of innate immunity to the area. Lymphocytes express receptors for neuropeptides released by enteric nerves, and stimulation of these cells with SP or VIP can induce their differentiation and alter their production of immunoglobulins. SP receptor antagonists therefore reduce inflammation and gut infiltration with neutrophils. As enteric neurons are closely co-localized to macrophages, as well as B- and T-lymphocytes in the gut wall, these neurons seem to exacerbate inflammation by stimulating the release of cytokines in the latter directly by releasing VIP (Goyal & Hirano, 1996) from their terminals. Similarly, VIP secretion of neurons can influence IgA synthesis, by stimulating B-lymphocytes, and increase secretion in enterocytes directly by releasing VIP from varicosities close to epithelial crypt cells (Pascual et al., 1994). After stimulation, primary afferent neurons, originating from the dorsal root ganglia, cause submucosal vasodilatation by releasing CGRP (Holzer et al., 1995). The vasodilatation enhances the recruitment of neutrophils from blood into the gut tissue. Additionally, the ENS modulates vasodilatation indirectly by degranulation of mast cells, whose mediators contribute to vasodilatation. As several non-neuronal cells, including epithelial and immune cells, express neurotrophin high and low affinity receptors (Levi Montalcini et al., 1996), there must be additional pathways for neurotrophic factors to modulate gut inflammation.

Signalling between immune cells and enteric neurons can also evoke alterations in gut functions. Linden et al. indicated that the hyperexcitability of intrinsic primary afferent neurons of inflamed guinea pig colon may be secondary to the activation of cyclooxygenase-2 and also for the production of prostaglandins (Linden et al., 2004). This increase in prostaglandins may be underlying factor responsible for some of the changes in neuronal properties observed at sites of gut inflammation. These changes can occur in non-involved regions during episodes of intestinal inflammation. Several studies indicate that the loss of neurons is associated with the appearance of eosinophilic and neutrophilic infiltrates into myenteric ganglia, suggesting that it might be mediated by interactions with the mucosal immune system (Sanovic et al., 199). Myenteric ganglionitis, associated with infiltrates of lymphocytes, such as plasma cells and mast cells, is frequently observed in UC patients and in experimental models of colitis (De Giorgio & Camilleri 2004; Tornblom et al., 2002).

Following TNBS colitis, eosinophils and T cells are commonly found adjacent to myenteric ganglia. This indicates a specific targeting of enteric ganglia by immune components (Pontell et al., 2009). Eosinophils are first observed adjacent to myenteric ganglia at six hours, and T cells are observed at twenty-four hours. Interestingly, no eosinophils and T lymphocytes are associated with myenteric ganglia in normal intestine. Thus, their presence in elevated numbers is an indication of ganglionitis and suggestive of neuropathology.

Recently, it has been demonstrated that NPY, which is produced by enteric neurons, plays an important role in initiating and modulating gut inflammation and in regulating immune system functions (Chandrasekharan et al., 2008; Hassani et al., 2005; Wheway et al., 2007). NPY has been shown to have the capacity to activate macrophages, stimulate the production of various cytokines such as tumor necrosis factor-α, and affect T-helper1 function (Chandrasekharan et al., 2008; Dimitrijevic et al., 2005; Sung et al., 1991; Wheway et al., 2007). Confirming the role played by NPY, a marked increase in both the mucosal NPY expression in experimental colitis and plasma levels of NPY in UC patients has been observed (Chandrasekharan et al., 2008). These results indicate that NPY can promote inflammation and is related to the pathogenesis of UC. Therefore, it has been postulated that, targeting or blocking NPY may be beneficial for the treatment of UC. In this context, recently, it has been demonstrated that the administration of NPY antisense oligodeoxynucleotides ameliorates the significantly established experimental colitis, suggesting that antisense oligodeoxynucleotides may be a useful therapeutic approach for the treatment of UC.

6. Conclusion

In the recent years, there is increasing evidence highlighting the crucial role played by ENS in intestinal inflammation, as demonstrated by the growing numbers of studies looking at both morphological and functional alterations in the ENS and its cellular elements, neurons and glial cells. These observations are the results of investigations carried out in both experimental animal models and in intestinal tissues of patients with inflammatory bowel disease. Although morpho-functional abnormalities of the ENS of UC patients have been consistently reported, additional studies are necessary to better understand the changes in the enteric cells, including neurons (of both submucosal and myenteric layers) and glial cells, which control gut functions, such as colonic motility and secretion, in the inflamed gut. This approach will help to prevent enteric neuropathies associated with inflammation and pave the way to future therapeutic options. Targeting neuronal and/or glial alterations during the course of inflammation may represent a novel approach to diminish the entity of tissue damage as well as the lack of long-term effectiveness of classical immunosuppressant agents used in the treatment of UC. Moreover, additional studies investigating the relationship between ENS and immune cells are warranted in order to carry out an in-depth assessment of the role of neurons, glial cells and their derived factors in the modulation of immune/inflammatory responses in the human gut, in light of establishment of new therapeutic approaches towards the treatment of gut inflammatory diseases.

One of the main questions that still need to be addressed to is whether the alterations of the ENS precede or are secondary to the inflammatory process within the gut. This will hopefully help to predict the disease outcome in UC, that until now remains a challenge, and for better understanding of the pathogenesis of this disease.

In conclusion, the complex interactions of the ENS and the other systems during gut inflammation require a broad perspective from neurophysiology, biochemistry and immunology to completely understand the regulation of inflammatory processes involved in UC. Therefore, important progress in this field can only be achieved by interdisciplinary approaches. Further research in this direction needs to be done for the discovery of long-lasting, effective treatment for inflammatory diseases of the gut.

7. References

Adami, C., Bianchi, R., Pula, G. & Donato, R. S100B-stimulated NO production by BV-2 microglia is independent of RAGE transducing activity but dependent on RAGE extracellular domain. *Biochimica et Biophysica Acta*, Vol. 1742, No. 1-3, (December 2004), pp. 169-177, ISSN 0006-3002

Adami, C., Sorci, G., Blasi, E., Agneletti, A.L., Bistoni, F. & Donato, R. S100B expression in and effects on microglia. *Glia*, Vol. 33, No. 2, (February 2001), pp. 131-142, ISSN 1098-1136

Antonius, J.I., Gump, F.E., Lattes, R. & Lepore, M. A study of certain microscopic features in regional enteritis, and their possible prognostic significance. *Gastroenterology*, Vol. 38, (June 1960), pp. 889–905, ISSN 0016-5085

Aoki, E., Semba, R. & Kashiwamata, S. Evidence for the presence of L-arginine in the glial components of the peripheral nervous system. *Brain Research*, Vol. 559, No. 1, (September 1991), pp. 159-162, ISSN 0006-8993

Auli, M., Nasser, Y., Ho, W., Burgueno, J.F., Keenan, C.M., Romero, C., Sharkey, K.A. & Fernandez, E. Neuromuscolar changes in a rat model of colitis. *Autonomic Neuroscience*, Vol. 141, No. 1-2, (August 2008), pp. 10-21, ISSN 1566-0702

Bassotti, G., Villanacci, V., Antonelli, E., Morelli, A. & Salerni, B. Enteric glial cells: new players in gastrointestinal motility? *Laboratory Investigation*, Vol. 87, No. 7, (July 2007), pp. 628-632, ISSN 0023-6837

Baudier, J., Glasser, N. & Gerard, D. Ions binding to S100 proteins. I. Calcium- and zinc-binding properties of bovine brain S100 alpha alpha, S100a (alpha beta), and S100b (beta beta) protein: Zn2+ regulates Ca2+ binding on S100b protein. *The Journal of Biological Chemistry*, Vol. 261, No. 18, (June 1986), pp. 8192-8203, ISSN 0021-9258

Belai, A., Boulos, P.B., Robson, T. & Burnstock, G. Neurochemical coding in the small intestine of patients with Crohn's disease. *Gut*, Vol. 40, No. 6, (June 1997), pp. 767–674, ISSN 0017-5749

Beyak, M.J. & Vanner, S. Inflammation-induced hyperexcitability of nociceptive gastrointestinal DRG neurones: the role of voltage-gated ion channels. *Neurogastroenterology and Motility*, Vol. 17, No. 2, (April 2005), pp. 175-186, ISSN 1365-2982

Bjorklund, H., Dahl, D. & Seiger, A. Neurofilament and glial fibrillary acid protein-related immunoreactivity in rodent enteric nervous system. *Neuroscience*, Vol. 12, No. 1, (May 1984), pp. 277-287, ISSN 0306-4522

Bogers, J.J., Timmermans, J.P., Scheuermann, D.W., Pelckmans, P.A., Mayer, B. & van Marck, E.A. Localization of nitric oxide synthase in enteric neurons of the porcine and human ileocaecal junction. *Annals of Anatomy*, Vol. 176, No. 2, (April 1994), pp. 131-135, ISSN 0940-9602

Bradley, J.S. Jr, Parr, E.J. & Sharkey, K.A. Effects of inflammation on cell proliferation in the myenteric plexus of the guinea-pig ileum. *Cell and Tissue Research*, Vol. 289, No. 3, (September 1997), pp. 455–461, ISSN 0302-766X

Brookes, S.J. Classes of enteric nerve cells in the guinea-pig small intestine. *The Anatomical Record*, Vol. 262, No. 1, (January 2001), pp. 58-70, ISSN 1097-0185

Broussard, D.L., Bannerman, P.G.C., Tang, C.M., Hardy, M. & Pleasure, D. Electrophysiologic and molecular properties of cultured enteric glia. *Journal of Neuroscience Research*, Vol. 34, No. 1, (January 1993), pp. 24–31, ISSN 1097-4547

Bush, T.G., Savidge, T.C., Freeman, T.C., Cox, H.J., Campbell, E.A., Mucke, L., Johnson, M.H. & Sofroniew, M. Fulminant jejuno-ileitis following ablation of enteric glia in adult transgenic mice. *Cell*, Vol. 93, No. 2, (April 1998), pp. 189-201, ISSN 0092-8674

Cabarrocas, J., Bauer, J., Piaggio, E., Liblau, R. & Lassmann, H. Effective and selective immune surveillance of the brain by MHC class I-restricted cytotoxic T lymphocytes. *European Journal of Immunology*, Vol. 33, No. 5, (May 2003), pp. 1174–1192, ISSN 1521-4141

Cabarrocas, J., Savidge, T.C. & Liblau, R.S. Role of enteric glial cells in inflammatory bowel disease. *Glia*, Vol. 41, No. 1, (January 2003), pp. 81–93, ISSN 1098-1136

Chandrasekharan, B., Bala, V., Kolachal,a V.L., Vijay-Kumar, M., Jones, D., Gewirtz, A.T., Sitaraman, S.V. & Srinivasan, S. Targeted deletion of neuropeptide Y (NPY) modulates experimental colitis. *PLoS ONE*, Vol. 3, No. 10, (October 2008), p. e3304, ISSN 1932-6203

Cirillo, C., Sarnelli, G., Mango, A., Esposito, I. & Cuomo, R. (2009). Effect of pro-inflammatory stimuli on cellular activation and nitric oxide production in primary cultures of human enteric glia. *Proceedings of Digestive Disease Week 2009*, p. A4, Chicago, Illinois, USA, May 30-June 4, 2009

Cirillo, C., Sarnelli, G., Esposito, G., Grosso, M., Petruzzelli, R., Izzo, P., Calì, G., D'Armiento, F.P., Rocco, A., Nardone, G., Iuvone, T., Steardo, L. & Cuomo, R. Increased mucosal nitric oxide production in ulcerative colitis is mediated in part by the enteroglial-derived S100B protein. *Neurogastroenterology and Motility*, Vol. 21, No. 11, (November 2009), pp. 1209–e112, ISSN 1365-2982

Cook, M.G. & Dixon, M.F. An analysis of the reliability of detection and diagnostic value of various pathological features in Crohns's disease and ulcerative colitis. *Gut*, Vol. 14, No. 4, (April 1973), pp. 255–262, ISSN 0017-5749

Cornet, A., Savidge, T.C., Cabarrocas, J., Deng, W.L., Colombel, J.F., Lassmann, H., Desreumaux, P. & Liblau, R.S. Enterocolitis induced by autoimmune targeting of enteric glial cells: a possible mechanism in Crohn's disease? *Proceedings of the National Academy of Sciences of U S A*, Vol. 98, No. 23, (November 2001), pp. 13306-13311, ISSN 1091-6490

Costa, M. & Brookes, S.J. (1995). The enteric nervous system and its extrinsic connections. In: *Textbook of gastroenterology* 3rd ed., Yamada, T., Alpers, D.H., Laine, L., Owyang, C., Powell, D.W, pp. 11–35, Lippincott-Williams and Wilkins, ISBN 9780781728614, Philadelphia, USA

Coulie, B., Szarka, L.A., Camilleri, M., Burton, D.D., McKinzie, S., Stambler, N. & Cedarbaum, J.M. Recombinant human neurotrophic factors accelerate colonic transit and relieve constipation in humans. *Gastroenterology*, Vol. 119, No. 1, (July 2000), pp. 41-50, ISSN 0016-5085

De Giorgio, R., Arakawa, J., Wetmore, C.J. & Sternini, C. Neurotrophin-3 and neurotrophin receptor immunoreactivity in peptidergic enteric neurones. *Peptides*, Vol. 21, No. 9, (September 2000), pp. 1421–1426, ISSN 0196-9781

De Giorgio, R. & Camilleri, M. Human enteric neuropathies: morphology and molecular pathology. *Neurogastroenterology and Motility*, Vol. 16, No. 5, (October 2004), pp. 515-531, ISSN 1365-2982

Dimitrijevic, M., Stanojevic, S., Vujic, V., Beck-Sickinger, A. & von Horsten, S. Neuropeptide Y and its receptor subtypes specifically modulate rat peritoneal macrophage function in vitro: counter regulation through Y1 and Y2/5 receptors. *Regulatory Peptides* Vol. 124, No. 1-3, (January 2005), pp. 163–172, 0167-0115

Di Mola, F.F., Friess, H., Zhu, Z.W., Koliopanos, A., Bley, T., Di Sebastiano, P., Innocenti, P., Zimmermann, A. & Büchler, M.W. Nerve growth factor and Trk high af nity receptor (TrkA) gene expression in inflammatory bowel disease. *Gut*, Vol. 46, No. 5, (May 2000), pp. 670–678, ISSN 0017-5749

Dogiel, A.S. Uber den Bau der Ganglien in den Geflechten des Darmes und der Gallenblase des Menschen und der Saugethiere. *Zeitschrift für Naturforschung B*, Vol. 5, (1899), pp. 130-158, ISSN 0932-0776

Dupin, E., Creuzet, S. & Le Douarin, N.M. The contribution of the neural crest to the vertebrate body. *Advances in Experimental Medicine and Biology*, Vol. 589, (2006), pp. 96-119, ISSN 0065-2598

Dvorak, A.M., Osage, J.E., Monahan, R.A. & Dickersin, G.R. Crohn's disease: transmission electron microscopic studies. III. Target tissues proliferation of and injury to smooth muscle and the autonomic nervous system. *Human Pathology*, Vol. 11, No. 6, (November 1980), pp. 620-634, ISSN 0046-8177

Endo, Y. & Kobayashi, S. A scanning electron microscope study on the autonomic ground plexus in the lamina propria mucosae of the guinea-pig small intestine. *Archivum histologicum Japonicum*, Vol. 50, No. 3, (July 1987), pp. 243-250, ISSN 0004-0681

Eng, L.F., Ghirnikar, R.S. &, Lee, Y.L. Glial fibrillary acidic protein: GFAP-thirty-one years [1969-2000]. *Neurochemical Research*, Vol. 25, No. 9-10, (October 2000); pp. 1439-1451, ISSN 0364-3190

Esposito, G., Cirillo, C., Sarnelli, G., De Filippis, D., D'Armiento, F.P., Rocco, A., Nardone, G., Petruzzelli, R., Grosso, M., Izzo, P., Iuvone, T. & Cuomo, R. Enteric Glial-Derived S100B Protein Stimulates Nitric Oxide Production in Celiac Disease. *Gastroenterology*, Vol. 133, No. 3, (September 2007), pp. 918-925, ISSN 0016-5085

Ferri, G.L., Probert, L., Cocchia, D., Michetti, F., Marangos, P.J. & Polak, J.M. Evidence for the presence of S-100 protein in the glial component of the human enteric nervous system. *Nature*, Vol. 297, No. 5865, (June 1982), pp. 409-410, ISSN 0028-0836

Fiocchi, C. Inflammatory bowel disease: etiology and pathogenesis. *Gastroenterology*, Vol. 115, No. 1, (July 1998), pp. 182-205, ISNN 0016-5085

Foell, D., Kucharzik, T., Kraft, M., Vogl, T., Sorg, C., Domschke, W. & Roth, J. Neutrophil derived human S100A12 (EN-RAGE) is strongly expressed during chronic active inflammatory bowel disease. *Gut*, Vol. 52, No. 6, (June 2003), pp. 847–853, ISSN 0017-5749

Furness, J.B. & Costa, M. Types of nerves in the enteric nervous system. *Neuroscience*, Vol. 5, No. 1, (1980), pp. 1-20, ISSN 0306-4522

Gabella, G. Ultrastructure of the nerve plexuses of the mammalian intestine: the enteric glial cells. *Neuroscience*, Vol. 6, No. 3, (1981), pp. 425-436, ISSN 0306-4522

Geboes, K. & Collins, S. Structural abnormalities of the nervous system in Crohn's disease and ulcerative colitis. *Neurogastroenterology and Motility*, Vol. 10, No. 3, (June 1998), pp. 189-202, ISSN 1365-2982

Geboes, K., Rutgeerts, P., Ectors, N., Mebis, J., Penninckx, F., Vantrappen, G. & Desmet, V.J. Major histocompatibility class II expression on the small intestinal nervous system in Crohn's disease. *Gastroenterology*, Vol. 103, No. 2, (August 1992), pp. 439–447, ISNN 0016-5085

Geboes, K. Immunopathological studies on the small intestinal intramural nervous system and of intramural vessels in Crohn's disease. *Verhandelingen - Koninklijke Academie voor Geneeskunde van België*, Vol. 55, No. 4, (1993), pp. 267–303, ISSN 0300-9017

Gershon, M.D., Kirchgessner, A.L. & Wade, P.R. (1994). Functional anatomy of the enteric nervous system, In: *Physiology of the gastrointestinal tract* 3rd ed., Johnson, L.R., ISBN 978-0-12-088394-3, pp. 381-422, Raven press, New York, USA

Gershon, M.D. & Rothman, T.P. Enteric glia. *Glia*, Vol. 4, No. 2, (1991), pp. 195–204, ISSN 1098-1136

Ghia, J.E., Blennerhassett, P., Kumar-Ondiveeran, H., Verdu, E.F. & Collins, S.M. The vagus nerve: a tonic inhibitory influence associated with inflammatory bowel disease in a murine model. *Gastroenterology*, Vol. 131, No. 4, (October 2006), pp. 1122-1130, ISSN 0016-5085

Goldin, E., Karmeli, F., Selinger, Z. & Rachmilewitz, D. Colonic substance P levels are increased in ulcerative colitis and decreased in chronic severe constipation. *Digestive Diseases and Sciences*, Vol. 34, No. 5, (May 1989), pp. 754–757, ISSN 0163-2116

Goode, T., O'Connell, J., Anton, P., Wong, H., Reeve, J., O'Sullivan, G.C., Collins, J.K. & Shanahan, F. Neurokinin-1 receptor expression in inflammatory bowel disease: molecular quantitation and localisation. *Gut*, Vol. 47, No. 3, (September 2000), pp. 387–396, ISSN 0017-5749

Goyal, R.K. & Hirano, I. The enteric nervous system. *The New England Journal of Medicine*, Vol. 334, No. 17, (April 1996), pp. 1106-1115, ISSN 0028-4793

Grundy, D., Al-Chaer, E.D., Aziz, Q., Collins, S.M., Ke, M., Taché, Y. & Wood, J.D. Fundamentals of neurogastroenterology: basic science. *Gastroenterology*, Vol. 130, No. 5, (April 2006), pp 1391-1411, ISSN 0016-5085

Haimoto, H., Hosoda, S. & Kato, K. Differential distribution of immuno-reactive S100α and S100β proteins in normal non-nervous human tissue. *Laboratory Investigation*, Vol. 57, No. 5, (November 1987), pp. 489-498, ISSN 0023-6837

Hassani, H., Lucas, G., Rozell, B. & Ernfors, P. Attenuation of acute experimental colitis by preventing NPY Y1 receptor signaling. *American Journal of Physiology. Gastrointestinal and Liver Physiology*, Vol. 288: No. 3, (March 2005), pp. G550–G556, ISSN 0193-1857

Hawkins, J.V., Emmel, E.L., Feuer, J.J., Nedelman, M.A., Harvey, C.J., Klein, H.J., Rozmiarek, H., Kennedy, A.R., Lichtenstein, G.R. & Billings, P.C. Protease activity in a hapten-induced model of ulcerative colitis in rats. *Digestive Disease Science*, Vol. 42, No. 9, (September 1997), pp. 1969-1980, ISSN 0163-2116

Hoff, S., Zeller, F., von Weyhern, C.W., Wegner, M., Schemann, M., Michel, K. &, Rühl, A. Quantitative assessment of glial cells in the human and guinea pig enteric nervous system with an anti-Sox8/9/10 antibody. *The Journal of Comparative Neurology*, Vol. 509, No. 4, (August 2008), pp. 356-371, ISSN 0021-9967

Hofmann, M.A., Drury, S., Fu, C., Qu, W., Taguchi, A., Lu, Y., Avila, C., Kambham, N., Bierhaus, A., Nawroth, P., Neurath, M.F., Slattery, T., Beach, D., McClary, J., Nagashima, M., Morser, J., Stern, D. & Schmidt, A.M. RAGE mediates a novel pro-inflammatory axis: A central cell surface receptor for S100/calgranulin polypeptides. *Cell*, Vol. 97, No. 7, (June 1999), pp. 889-901, ISSN 0092-8674

Holzer, P., Wachter, C., Heinemann, A., Jocic, M., Lippe, I.T. & Herbert, M.K. Sensory nerves, nitric oxide and NANC vasodilatation. *Archives Internationales de Pharmacodynamie et de Therapie*, Vol. 329, No. 1, (January-February 1995), pp. 67–79, ISSN 0003-9780

Holzer, P. Implications of tachykinins and calcitonin gene-related peptide in inflammatory bowel disease. *Digestion*, Vol. 59, No. 4, (July-August1998), pp. 269–283, ISSN 0012-2823

Hurst, S.M., Stanisz, A.M., Sharkey, K.A. & Collins, S.M. Interleukin 1 beta-induced increase in substance P in rat myenteric plexus. *Gastroenterology*, Vol. 105, No. 6, (December 1993), pp. 1754–1760, ISSN 0016-5085

Hwang, L., Leichter, R., Okamoto, A., Payan, D., Collins, S.M, & Bunnett, N.W. Downregulation of neutral endopeptidase (EC 3.4.24.11) in the inflamed rat intestine. *American Journal of Physiology*, Vol. 264, No. 4, (April 1993), pp. G735–743, ISSN 0193-1857

Ikeda, S.I., Makishita, H., Oguchi, K., Yanagisawa, N. & Nagata, T. Gastrointestinal amyloid deposition in familial amyloid polyneuropathy. *Neurology*, Vol. 32, No. 12, (December 1982), pp. 1364-1368, ISSN 0028-3878

Jessen, K.R. & Mirsky, R. Glial cells in the enteric nervous system contain glial fibrillary acidic protein. *Nature*, Vol. 286, No. 5774, (August 1980), pp. 736–737, ISSN 0028-0836

Keranen, U., Kiviluoto, T., Jarvinen, H., Bäck, N., Kivilaakso, E. & Soinila, S. Changes in substance P-immunoreactive innervation of human colon associated with ulcerative colitis. *Digestive Diseases and Sciences*, Vol. 40, No. 10, (October 1995), pp. 2250–2258, ISSN 0163-2116

Koretz, K., Momburg, F., Otto, H.F. & Moller, P. Sequential induction of MHC antigens on autochthonous cells of ileum affected by Crohn's disease. *The American Journal of Pathology*, Vol. 129, No. 3, (December 1987), pp. 493–502, ISSN 0002-9440

Kruger, G.M., Mosher, J.T., Bixby, S., Joseph, N., Iwashita, T. & Morrison, S.J. Neural crest stem cells persist in the adult gut but undergo changes in self-renewal, neuronal subtype potential, and factor responsiveness. *Neuron*, Vol. 35, No. 4, (August 2002), pp. 657-669, ISSN 0896-6273

Kunze, W.A. & Furness, J.B. The enteric nervous system and regulation of intestinal motility. *Annual Review of Physiology*, Vol. 61, (1999), pp. 117–42, ISSN 0066-4278

Lakhan, S.E., & Kirchgessner, A. Neuroinflammation in inflammatory bowel disease. *Journal of Neuroinflammation*, Vol. 7, No. 37, (July 2010), ISSN 1742-2094

Laranjeira, C. & Pachnis, V. Enteric nervous system development: Recent progress and future challenges. *Autonomic Neuroscience*, Vol. 151, No. 1, (November 2009), pp. 61-69, ISSN 1566-0702

Leach, S.T., Yang, Z., Messina, I., Song, C., Geczy, C.L., Cunningham, A.M. & Day, A.S. Serum and mucosal S100 proteins, calprotectin (S100A8/S100A9) and S100A12, are elevated at diagnosis in children with inflammatory bowel disease. *Scandinavian Journal of Gastroenterology*, Vol. 42, No. 11, (November 2007), pp. 1321-1331, ISSN 0036-5521

Lennon, V.A., Sas, D.F., Busk, M.F., Scheithauer, B,, Malagelada, J.R., Camilleri, M., Miller, L.J. Enteric neuronal autoantibodies in pseudoobstruction with small-cell lung carcinoma. *Gastroenterology*, Vol. 100, No.1, (January 1991), pp. 137-142, ISSN 0016-5085

Levi Montalcini, R., Skaper, S.D., Dal Toso, R., Petrelli, L. & Leon, A. Nerve growth factor: from neurotrophi n to neurokine. *Trends in Neurosciences*, Vol. 19, No. 11, (November 1996), pp. 514–520, ISSN 0166-2236

Linden, D.R., Couvrette, J.M., Ciolino, A., McQuoid, C., Blaszyk, H., Sharkey, K.A. & Mawe, G.M. Indiscriminate loss of myenteric neurones in the TNBS-inflamed guinea-pig distal colon. *Neurogastroenterology and Motility*, Vol. 17, No. 5, (October 2005), pp. 751-760, ISSN 1365-2982

Linden, D.R., Sharkey, K.A., Ho, W. & Mawe, G.M. Cyclooxygenase-2 contributes to dysmotility and enhanced excitability of myenteric AH neurones in the inflamed guinea pig distal colon. *The Journal of Physiology*, Vol. 15, No. 557, (May 2004), pp. 191-205, ISSN 0022-3751

Linehan, J.D., Kolios, G., Valatas, V., Robertson, D.A. & Westwick, J. Effect of corticosteroids on nitric oxide production in inflammatory bowel disease: are leukocytes the site of action? *American Journal of Physiology. Gastrointestinal and Liver Physiology*, Vol. 288, No. 2, (Febrauary 2005), pp. G261–267, ISSN 0193-1857

Lindsay, R.M. & Harmar, A.J. Nerve growth factor regulates expression of neuropeptide genes in adult sensory neurons. *Nature*, Vol. 337, No. 6205, (January 1989), pp. 362–364, ISSN 0028-0836

Lomax, A.E., Fernández, E. & Sharkey, K.A. Plasticity of the enteric nervous system during intestinal inflammation. *Neurogastroenterology and Motility*, Vol. 17, No. 1, (February 2005), pp. 4-15, ISSN 1365-2982

Mantyh, C.R., Vigna, S.R., Bollinger, R.R., Mantyh, P.W., Maggio, J.E. & Pappas, T.N. Differential expression of substance P receptors in patients with Crohn's disease and ulcerative colitis. *Gastroenterology*, Vol. 109, No. 3, (September 1995), pp. 850–860, ISSN 0016-5085

May, R.J. & Goyal, R.K. (1994). Effects of diabetes mellitus on the digestive system. In: *Joslin's diabetes mellitus* 13th ed., Kahn, C.R. & Weir, G.C., pp. 921-954, Lea & Febiger, ISBN 0812117530, Philadelphia, USA

Menchen, L., Colon, A.L., Madrigal, J.L., Beltrán, L., Botella, S., Lizasoain, I., Leza, J.C., Moro, M.A., Menchén, P., Cos, E. & Lorenzo, P. Activity of inducible and neuronal nitric oxide synthases in colonic mucosa predicts progression of ulcerative colitis. *American Journal of Gastroenterology*, Vol. 99, No. 7, (September 2004), pp. 1756–1764, ISSN 0002-9270

Mestres, P., Diener, M. & Rummel, W. Electron microscopy of the mucosal plexus of the rat colon. *Acta Anatomica* [Basel], Vol. 143, No. 4, (1992), pp. 275-282, ISSN 0365-0332

Mottet, N.K. Histopathologic spectrum of regional enteritis and ulcerative colitis. *Major Problems in Pathology*, Vol. 2, (February 1971), pp. 1-249, ISSN 0076-2881

Murakami, M., Ohta, T. & Ito, S. Lipopolysaccharides enhance the action of bradykinin in enteric neurons via secretion of interleukin-1beta from enteric glial cells. *Journal of Neuroscience Research*, Vol. 87, No. 9, (July 2009), pp. 2095-2104, ISSN 1097-4547

Nagahama, M., Semba, R., Tsuzuki, M. & Aoki, E. L-arginine immunoreactive enteric glial cells in the enteric nervous system of rat ileum. *Biological Signals and Receptors*, Vol. 10, No. 5, (September-October 2001), pp. 336–340, ISSN 1422-4933

Neunlist, M., Aubert, P., Toquet, C., Oreshkova, T., Barouk, J., Lehur, P.A., Schemann, M. & Galmiche, J.P. Changes in chemical coding of myenteric neurones in ulcerative colitis. *Gut*, Vol. 52, No. 1, (January 2003), pp. 84-90, ISSN 0017-5749

Neunlist, M., Toumi, F. Oreschkova, T., Denis, M., Leborgne, J., Laboisse, C.L., Galmiche, J.P. & Jarry, A. Human ENS regulates the intestinal epithelial barrier permeability and a tight junction-associated protein ZO-1 via VIPergic pathways. *American Journal of Physiology*, Vol. 285, No. 5, (November 2003), pp. G1028–1036, ISSN 0193-1857

Neunlist, M., Van Landeghem, L., Bourreille, A. & Savidge, T. Neuro-glial crosstalk in inflammatory bowel disease. *Journal of Internal Medicine*, Vol. 263, No. 6, (June 2008), pp. 577-583, ISSN 1365-2796

Oehmichen, M. & Reiffersscheid, P. Intramural ganglion cell degeneration in inflammatory bowel disease. *Digestion*, Vol. 15, No. 6, (1977), pp. 482-496, ISSN 0012-2823

Ohlsson, B., Veress, B., Lindgren, S. & Sundkvist, G. Enteric ganglioneuritis and abnormal interstitial cells of Cajal: features of inflammatory bowel disease. *Inflammatory Bowel Disease*, Vol. 13, No. 6, (June 2007), pp. 721–726, ISSN 1078-0998

Okamoto, E. Morphological studies on the myenteric plexus of the colon in chronic ulcerative colitis: a preliminary report. *Medical journal of Osaka University*, Vol. 15, (June 1964), pp. 85-106, ISSN 0030-6169

Parkman, H.P., Rao, S.S., Reynolds, J.C., Schiller, L.R., Wald, A., Miner, P.B., Lembo, A.J., Gordon, J.M., Drossman, D.A., Waltzman, L., Stambler, N. & Cedarbaum, J.M., Functional Constipation Study Investigators. Neurotrophin-3 improves functional constipation. *American Journal of Gastroenterology*, Vol. 98, No. 6, (June 2003), pp. 1338–1347, ISSN 0002-9270

Pascual, D.W., Kiyono, H. & McGhee, J.R. The enteric nervous and immune systems: interactions for mucosal immunity and inflammation. *Immunomethods*, Vol. 5, No. 1, (August 1994), pp. 56–72, ISSN 1058-6687

Petrova, T.V., Hu, J. & Van Eldik L.J. Modulation of glial activation by astrocyte-derived protein S100B: differential responses of astrocyte and microglial cultures. *Brain Research*, Vol. 853, No. 1, (January 2000), pp. 74-80, ISSN 0006-8993

Pietzsch, J. & Hoppmann, S. Human S100A12: a novel key player in inflammation? *Amino Acids*, Vol. 36, No. 3, (March 2009), pp. 381-389, ISSN 1438-2199

Pontell, L., Castelucci, P., Bagyánszki, M., Jovic, T., Thacker, M., Nurgali, K., Bron, R. & Furness, J.B. Structural changes in the epithelium of the small intestine and immune cell infiltration of enteric ganglia following acute mucosal damage and local inflammation. *Virchows Archive*, Vol. 455, No. 1, (July 2009), pp. 55-65, ISSN 0945-6317

Qualman, S.J., Haupt, H.M., Yang, P. & Hamilton, S.R. Esophageal Lewy bodies associated with ganglion cell loss in achalasia: similarity to Parkinson's disease. *Gastroenterology*, Vol. 87, No. 4, (October 1984), pp. 848-856, ISSN 0016-5085

Reddy, S.N., Bazzochi, G., Chan, S., Akashi, K., Villanueva-Meyer, J., Yanni, G., Mena, I. & Snape, W.J. Colonic motility and transit in health and ulcerative colitis. *Gastroenterology*, Vol. 101, No. 5, (November 1991), pp. 1289–1297, ISSN 0016-5085

Rienmann, J.F. & Schmidt, H. Ultrastructural changes in the gut autonomic nervous system following laxative abuse and in other conditions. *Scandinavian Journal of Gastroenterology*, Vol. 71, (1982), pp. 111-124, ISSN 0036-5521

Reinshagen, M., Patel, A., Sottili, M., Nast, C., Davis, W., Mueller, K. & Eysselein, V. Protective function of extrinsic sensory neurons in acute rabbit experimental colitis. *Gastroenterology*, Vol. 106, No. 5, (May 1994), pp. 1208-1214, ISSN 0016-5085

Reinshagen, M., Patel, A., Sottili, M., French, S., Sternini, C. & Eysselein, V.E. Action of sensory neurons in an experimental rat colitis model of injury and repair. *American Journal of Physiology*, Vol. 270, No. 1, (January 1996), pp. G79 –86, ISSN 0193-1857

Reinshagen, M., Flamig, G., Ernst, S., Geerling, I., Wong, H., Walsh, J.H., Eysselein, V.E. & Adler, G. Calcitonin gene-relate d peptide mediates the protective effect of sensory nerves in a model of colonic injury. *The Journal of Pharmacology and Experimental Therapeutics*, Vol. 286, No. 2, (August 1998), pp. 657–661, ISSN 0022-3565

Reinshagen, M., Rohm, H., Steinkamp, M., Lieb, K., Geerling, I., Von Herbay, A., Flämig, G., Eysselein, V.E. & Adler, G. Protective role of neurotrophins in experimental inflammation of the rat gut. *Gastroenterology*, Vol. 119, No. 2, (August 2000), pp. 368–376, ISSN 0016-5085

Ruhl, A., Franzke, S., Collins, S.M. & Stremmel, W. Interleukin-6 expression and regulation in rat enteric glial cells. *American Journal of Physioliogy. Gastrointestinal and Liver Physiology*, Vol. 280, No. 6, (June 2001), pp. G1163-1171, ISSN 0193-1857

Saffrey, M.J., Wardhaugh, T., Walker, T., Daisley, J. & Silva, A.T. Trophic actions of neurotrophin-3 on postnatal rat myenteric neurones in vitro. *Neuroscience Letters*, Vol. 278, No. 3, (January 2000), pp. 133–136, ISSN 0304-3940

Sanovic, S., Lamb, D.P. & Blennerhassett, M.G. Damage to the enteric nervous system in experimental colitis. *American Journal of Pathology*, Vol. 155, No. 4, (October 1999), pp. 1051-1057, ISSN 0002-9440

Sarnelli, G., De Giorgio, R., Gentile, F., Calì, G., Grandone, I., Rocco, A., Cosenza, V., Cuomo, R. & D'Argenio, G. Myenteric neuronal loss in rats with experimental colitis: role of tissue transglutaminase-induced apoptosis. *Digestive and Liver Diseases*, Vol. 41, No. 3, (March 2009), pp. 185-193, ISSN 1590-8658

Savidge, T.C., Newman, P., Pothoulakis, C., Ruhl, A., Neunlist, M., Bourreille, A., Hurst, R. & Sofroniew, M.V. Enteric glia regulate intestinal barrier function and inflammation via release of S-nitrosoglutathione. *Gastroenterology*, Vol. 132, No. 4, (April 2007), pp. 1344-1358, ISSN 0016-5085

Savidge, T.C., Sofroniew, M.V. & Neunlist, M. Starring roles for astroglia in barrier pathologies of gut and brain. *Laboratory Investigation*, Vol. 87, No. 8, (August 2007), pp. 731-736, ISSN 0023-6837

Schmidt, A.M., Yan, S.D., Yan, S.F. & Stern, D.M. The multiligand receptor RAGE as a progression factor amplifying immune and inflammatory responses. *Journal of Clinical Investigation*, Vol. 108, No. 7 (October 2001), pp. 949-955, ISSN 00219738

Sethi, A.K. & Sarna, S.K. Colonic motor activity in acute colitis in conscious dogs. *Gastroenterology*, Vol. 100, No. 4, (April 1991), pp. 954–963, ISSN 0016-5085

Siemers, P.T. & Dobbins, W. The Meissner plexus in Crohn's disease of the colon. *Surgery, gynecology & obstetrics*, Vol. 138, No. 1, (January 1974), pp. 39–42, ISSN 0039-6087

Spriggs, E.A., Code, C.F., Bargen, J.A., Curtiss, R.K. & Hightower, N.C. Motility of the pelvic colon and rectum of normal persons and patients with ulcerative colitis. *Gastroenterology*, Vol. 19, No. 3, (November 1951), pp. 480–491, ISSN 0016-5085

Steinkamp, M., Geerling, I., Seufferlein, T., von Boyen, G., Egger, B., Grossmann, J., Ludwig, L., Adler, G. & Reinshagen, M. Glial-derived neurotrophic factor regulates apoptosis in colonic epithelial cells. *Gastroenterology*, Vol. 124, No. 7, (June 2003), pp. 1748-1757, ISSN 0016-5085

Storsteen, K.A., Kernohan, J.W.& Bargen, J.A. The myenteric plexus in chronic ulcerative colitis. *Surgery, gynecology & obstetrics*, Vol. 97, No. 3, (September 1953), pp. 335-343, ISSN 0039-6087

Strobach, R.S., Ross, A., Markin, R.S., Zetterman, R.K. & Linder, J. Neural patterns in inflammatory bowel disease: an immunohistochemical survey. *Modern Pathology*, Vol. 3, No. 4, (July 1990), pp. 488–493, ISSN 0893-3952

Stucchi, A.F., Shofe, S., Leeman, S., Materne, O., Beer, E., McClung, J., Shebani, K., Moore, F., O'Brien, M. & Becker, J.M. NK-1 antagonist reduces colonic inflammation and oxidative stress in dextran sulfate-induced colitis in rats. *American Journal of Physioliogy*, Vol. 279, No. 6, (December 2000), pp. G1298–1306, ISSN 0193-1857

Sugimura, K., Haimoto, H., Nagura, H., Kato, K. & Takahashi, A. Immunohistochemical differential distribution of S-100 alpha and S-100 beta in the peripheral nervous system of the rat. *Muscle & Nerve*, Vol. 12, No. 11, (November 1989), pp. 929-935, ISSN 1097-4598

Sung, C.P., Arleth, A.J. & Feuerstein, G.Z. Neuropeptide Y upregulates the adhesiveness of human endothelial cells for leukocytes. *Circulation Research*, Vol. 68, No. 1, (January 1991), pp. 314–318, ISSN 0009-7300

Törnblom, H., Lindberg, G., Nyberg, B. & Veress, B. Full-thickness biopsy of the jejunum reveals inflammation and enteric neuropathy in irritable bowel syndrome. *Gastroenterology*, Vol. 123, No. 6, (December 2002), pp. 1972-1979, ISSN 0016-5085

Tracey, K.J. Physiology and immunology of the cholinergic antiinflammatory pathway. *Journal of Clinical Investigation*, Vol. 117, No 2, (February 2007), pp. 289-296, ISSN 00219738

Van Landeghem, L., Mahé, M.M., Teusan, R., Léger, J., Guisle, I., Houlgatte, R. & Neunlist, M. Regulation of intestinal epithelial cells transcriptome by enteric glial cells: impact on intestinal epithelial barrier functions. *BMC Genomics*, Vol. 10, (November 2009), p. 507, ISSN 1471-2164

Van Patter, W.N., Bargen, J.A,, Dockerty, M.C., Feldmann, W.H., Mayo, C.W. & Waugh, J.M. Regional enteritis. *Gastroenterology*, Vol. 26, No. 3, (March 1954), pp. 347-351, ISSN 0016-5085

Vento, P., Kiviluoto, T., Keranen, U., Järvinen, H.J., Kivilaakso, E. & Soinila, S. Quantitative comparison of growth-associated protein-43 and substance P in ulcerative colitis.

Journal of Histochemistry and Cytochemistry, Vol. 49, No. 6, (June 2001), pp. 749–758, ISSN 1121-760X

Villanacci, V., Bassotti, G., Nascimbeni, R., Antonelli, E., Cadei, M., Fisogni, S., Salerni, B. &, Geboes, K. Enteric nervous system abnormalities in inflammatory bowel diseases. *Neurogastroenterology and Motility*, Vol. 20, No. 9, (September 2008), pp. 1009-1016, ISSN 1350-1925

von Boyen, G.B., Schulte, N., Pflüger, C., Spaniol, U., Hartmann, C. & Steinkamp, M. Distribution of enteric glia and GDNF during gut inflammation. BMC *Gastroenterology*, Vol. 11, (January 2011), p. 3.

von Boyen, G.B., Steinkamp, M., Reinshagen, M., Schäfer, K.H., Adler, G. & Kirsch, J. Proinflammatory cytokines increase glial fibrillary acidic protein expression in enteric glia. *Gut*, Vol. 53, No. 4, (February 2004), pp. 222-228, ISSN 0017-5749

Wheway, J., Herzog, H. & Mackay, F. NPY and receptors in immune and inflammatory disease. *Current Topics in Medicinal Chemistry*, Vol. 7, No. 17, (2007), pp. 1743–1752, ISSN 1568-0266

Yoshida, M.M., Krishnamurthy, S., Wattchow, D.A., Furness, J.B. & Schuffler, M.D. Megacolon in myotonic dystrophy caused by a degenerative neuropathy of the myenteric plexus. *Gastroenterology*, Vol. 95, No. 3, (September 1988), pp. 820-827, ISSN 0016-5085

Zimmer, D.B. & Van Eldik, L.J. Tissue distribution of rat S100α and S100 β and S100 binding proteins. *American Journal of Physiology*, Vol. 252, No. 3, (March 1987), pp. 285-289, ISSN 0193-1857

7

Molecular Determinants in Ulcerative Colitis – Epigenetics and Telomere Dysfunction

Ramesh P. Arasaradnam[1,2] and Chuka U. Nwokolo[1]
[1]Department of Gastroenterology, University Hospital Coventry & Warwickshire,
Coventry
[2]Clinical Sciences Research Institute, University of Warwick, Coventry
United Kingdom

1. Introduction

Ulcerative colitis (UC) is a chronic relapsing disease which runs a rather unpredictable clinical course. It usually starts in the 2nd or 3rd decade of life and is associated with an increased risk of bowel cancer. Unlike Crohn's disease, there is a relative paucity of basic science research as to the molecular determinants that govern mucosal inflammation and subsequent risk of developing colon cancer. Genetic linkage studies in inflammatory bowel disease (IBD) traditionally have focussed on candidate genes and haplotypes in at risk individuals but emerging evidence would also suggest the importance of epigenetics. Epigenetics is the heritable alteration in gene expression but without alteration in DNA sequence. Consequently the human epigenomic project has now been established. In this chapter we will discuss emerging epigenetic changes in UC and also newer molecular targets that have come to the fore such as telomere dysfunction which, may be used as putative biomarkers.

One of the more common epigenetic alterations includes DNA methylation of the gene promoter. Much work has focussed on colon cancer but our group and others have identified gene promoter DNA hypermethylation in individuals with UC. Critically these epigenetic markings affect key tumour suppressor genes which, are then silenced as a result of hypermethylation. This therefore may be a potential pathway by which those with UC develop colon cancer and will be explored in further detail in this chapter.

Similarly telomere dysfunction has been well studied in colon cancer and the ageing population but lacking in those with UC. Telomeres are the end of chromosomes and are long at birth but get shorter with age. At a critical length the telomere signals the end of a cell's life (apoptosis) but some cells can escape death and instead become neoplastic. There is reduction in telomerase enzyme (key regulator in telomere length) in UC as well as alteration in key telomere binding proteins (TBP). One such protein is TRF2 which is a protein that helps protect telomeres from degrading with age and inflammation thus delaying the inevitable changes described earlier. Patients with ulcerative colitis appear to have a shortage of this protein and the longer the duration of the disease the less the protein. There is also a suggestion that it may also be altered with therapy (immune-modulating) drugs used to treat UC. TRF2 may yet provide a candidate protein for a biomarker which we will discuss together with the role of other TBPs and its relationship with UC disease activity.

This chapter will cover in detail a literature review and summary of current and developing work in our lab and others using the headings outlined below:

2. Epigenetics

Epigenetic alterations are heritable alterations in gene expression not mediated by alteration in DNA sequence i.e. the message is altered but not the gene itself [Jaenisch et al 2003]. Such changes include DNA methylation and are among the most common molecular alterations in human cancers including colorectal cancer. Other epigenetic changes include histone acytelation and protein ubiquitination. For the purpose of this chapter we will concentrate on DNA methylation as it is the most common epigenetic marking and has demonstrable changes in UC.

DNA methylation involves the addition of a methyl group to the carbon-5 position of cytosine residues and is the only common covalent modification of human DNA. It occurs almost exclusively at cytosines that are followed immediately by guanine (CpG dinucleotides). The majority of the genome displays a depletion of CpG dinucleotides and those that are present are nearly always methylated. Conversely, small stretches of DNA known as *CpG islands* (usually located within the promoter regions of human genes), whilst rich in CpG dinucleotides, are nearly always **free** of methylation. Methylation of CpGs within these *islands* are associated with transcriptional inactivation of the corresponding gene, which, appears to be tissue specific. In colon cancer (CRC) for example, aberrant methylation resulting in gene silencing can occur in important tumour suppressor genes such as $p16^{INK4a}$ [Merlo et al 1995]. Both genomic DNA hypomethylation as well as gene specific (promoter) hypermethylation have been observed in CRC. DNA methylation is vital in controlling gene transcription through histone modification. Such conformational changes can induce either activation through acetylation for example or repression due to methylation of a histone residue – Figure 1.

Although the methylation profile within the human genome is as yet undetermined, it is estimated that 70% of CpG dinucleotides are methylated in mammals. Hypermethylation in gene promoter regions are associated with transcriptional silencing which is at least as common as inactivation of tumour suppressor genes through DNA mutations [Jones et al 2002]. Aberrant hypermethylation is thought to be an early event in CRC as it is detectable in early precursor lesions e.g. Aberrant Crypt Foci (ACF). Such aberrant changes can occur in chronically inflamed tissue which, if involves key tumour suppressor genes may have deleterious effects.

2.1 Age related DNA methylation

Genomic loss of methylation has been known to occur with ageing. This phenomenon has yet to be shown in the *normal* ageing colon until recently [Arasaradnam 2007]. Most of the attention surrounding DNA methylation has been centred on gene specific methylation. In the colon, age related methylation accounts for 70% of aberrant gene specific methylation events. This process is thought to be a non-stochastic i.e. predictable event and is tissue specific. For example, methylation of the *ESR1* (tumour suppressor gene) promoter has been shown to increase with age in normal human colon and is present also in adenomas thus supporting the idea that epigenetic gene silencing is an early event [Issa et al 1994]. Thus it is apparent that methylation homeostasis is perturbed with ageing but it is not known if ageing is accelerated as a result of if there are consequential effects on other factors such as telomere attrition for example (discussed later).

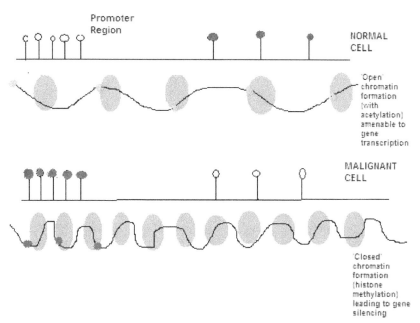

Fig. 1. A stretch of genomic DNA in normal and malignant cell. The white pins denote unmethylated CpG sites within the promoter region of normal cells which become methylated (red pins) during malignant transformation. Conversely, globally the remaining CpG dinucleotides are methylated in the normal cell (red pins) and unmethylated in malignancy (white pin). The nucleosome (DNA and histones) shown as grey ovals depicts the open and closed formation which affects gene transcription either through acetylation (green dots) which results in activation or repression due to methylation of certain histone residues (pink dots)

In the aged, as with chronic inflammation (e.g. ulcerative colitis), a critical threshold of random accumulation of somatic mutations is thought to be reached leading to the development of cancer. However it is more likely due to a combination of effects such as cumulative mutational load, epigenetic gene silencing, telomere dysfunction and even altered stromal environment [dePinho, 2000]. The perceived key genes regulating this process have been studied but with inconsistent results.

2.2 Influence of dietary factors on DNA methylation
Epigenetic changes such as DNA methylation are potentially reversible and gene expression can be re-established. The active ingredient in Green Tea (EGCG) provides a good example of reversal of aberrant methylation with a dietary food component reaffirming the role of diet in cancer prevention. The concept of dietary intervention gained further momentum following evidence in animal models and epidemiological studies in humans showing that folate status can modulate risk of development of colorectal adenoma and cancer. The role of folate in UC is discussed further in section 2.3.1. For detailed review on mechanisms of diet influencing epigenetics specifically colorectal carcinogenesis please see reference [Arasaradnam et al 2008].

2.3 DNA methylation in UC

Altered DNA methyl transferase (DNMT) activity, histone modification and exogenous insults such as diet have been postulated to result in genomic DNA methylation but their relative importance in human colonic disease is not well understood (Wilson et al. 2007). Apart from folate, little is known if environmental factors or lifestyle factors for example smoking patterns, alcohol consumption and diet could influence genomic DNA methylation. Furthermore, it would also be important to determine genomic DNA methylation in other colonic disease groups – chronic mucosal inflammation, including those which predispose to increased risk of CRC e.g. ulcerative colitis.

2.3.1 DNA global methylation

UC is a chronic inflammatory condition with an increased risk of developing CRC (Crohn, Ginzburg et al. 1984; Ransohoff 1988) especially in those diagnosed at a younger age and with greater extent of disease (Ekbom et al. 1990). Genomic instability has been proposed as a likely explanation for the observed UC associated CRC risk. Examples of molecular determinants used to assess risk in UC include cellular proliferation, genomic DNA methylation (Gloria et al. 1996, Arasaradnam et al 2010) and microsatellite instability (Tahara, Inoue et al. 2005) amongst others.

We have shown that using tritium labelled experiments, 3[H] dCTP incorporation into DNA was lower in UC patients compared to age and sex matched controls (Arasaradnam et al 2010). In other words, there was relative genomic hypermethylation in UC subjects compared with healthy controls. This finding is in contrast with the only other report a decade ago of genomic hypomethylation in UC patients (Gloria et al. 1996). Here the authors report genomic hypomethylation in 26 patients with UC compared to 11 controls using the methyl acceptance assay. This assay has several limitations (indirect, semi-quantitative and prone to false positives due to damaged DNA templates) (Pufulete et al. 2005). They also speculate that low levels of S-Adenosyl Methionine (SAM); universal methyl donor in active UC coupled by increased cell proliferation may impair DNA methylation status. Conversely we have shown that although folate status was lower in UC subjects, it was still within the normal reference range. Apart from the different methods employed to quantify genomic DNA methylation, the other significant difference was in the proportion of UC patients with active disease. The SCAI is a validated scoring system used to identify patients that have relapsed after being in remission (Walmsley et al. 1998) . Of note in our study, 5 patients (20%) had active disease as opposed to 12 (50%) in the study by Gloria et al - this is likely to be an important contributory factor especially as rectal mucosal cells have been shown to undergo increased cellular proliferation (Gloria et al. 1996) when disease is active and hence incur greater DNA damage. Interestingly, no association was seen with age at diagnosis, duration of disease and number of flares with genomic DNA methylation.

Although red cell folate levels of UC patients in our study were lower than controls, it was within normal limits. Previous work (Spiers A et al unpublished) has shown good correlation between red cell folate status and mucosal folate levels. Lower levels of folate have been attributed to variation in dietary intake, interaction with certain medications (sulphapyridines) and increased cell proliferation (Biasco 2005). The normal folate level and relative hypermethylation profile in UC patients (mainly quiescent/ mild disease and with significantly lower total leucocyte count than controls) may be a consequence of lower rectal cell proliferation and increased cell renewal hence altering the genomic DNA methylation profile favourably. A further novel finding is that almost 16% of variability in genomic DNA methylation between UC subjects and controls could be explained by BMI alone (Arasaradnam 2007). Thus lower BMI is associated with genomic hypermethylation which provides support for existing evidence of increasing body fatness being associated with increased colon cancer risk (Friedenreich et al. 2006).

The lower folate status and relative genomic hypermethylation observed in UC subjects corroborate a recent report showing a protective effect of low folate status on risk of CRC (Van Guelpen et al. 2006). The biological role of folate and DNA methylation in UC is not as clear as initially thought and the question of its protective role against CRC, if any, remains unclear (Arasaradnam 2010).

2.3.2 Gene specific methylation in UC

Epigenetic studies especially in colon carcinogenesis have focussed mainly on gene specific methylation. This is not remarkable as gene specific hypermethylation can result in reduced gene expression/ silencing with consequent detriment to the colonocyte, particularly, if key genes such as tumour suppressor genes (*APC*, *p53*, *p16^{INK4a}*, *p14^{ARF}* and *ESR-1*) are involved (Issa et al. 1994; Merlo et al. 1995; Esteller 2002). Indeed, most genes hypermethylated in tumours originate from the gastrointestinal tract – oesophagus, stomach and colon with significantly less reported in other tumour types e.g. ovarian (Esteller et al. 2001). CpG island methylation affects several genes including tumour suppressor genes (*p16^{INK4a}*, *p14^{ARF}*, *APC*, *p53*), silencing of DNA mismatch repair genes (*hMLH1*, *O^6-MGMT*), possible loss of function of apoptosis genes (*DAPK*, *APAF-1*) and altered carcinogen metabolism (*GSTP1*) (Esteller 2002).

Most studies in UC have considered DNA hypermethylation of two genes – Oestrogen receptor gene (*ESR-1*) and Tumour suppressor gene candidate 3 (*N-33*) – both putative tumour suppressor genes. *ESR-1* which is located on chromosome 6 has been shown to be hypermethylated in the colonic mucosa of those with CRC and to a lesser extent in normal individuals (Ahuja et al. 1998). In cell culture, de-methylation of *ESR-1* has been shown to suppress growth and hence has been proposed to be putative tumour suppressor gene (Issa et al. 1994). *N-33*, also a putative tumour suppressor gene is located on chromosome 8 and has been shown in vitro to result in growth suppression of cancer cells. One small study has shown hypermethylation of *N-33* in both tumour tissue as well as in the normal colon (Ahuja et al. 1998). Moreover promoter hypermethylation of both these genes have been shown to be age related.

Little is known about the mucosal inflammatory effect of UC on gene specific methylation. Using the COBRA assay, Issa and colleagues found higher methylation of *ESR-1* in 12 UC subjects with high grade dysplasia or cancer compared with 6 UC patients without dysplasia. In that study, methylation levels were comparable for UC patients without dysplasia and healthy controls (n = 5). A later study by Tominaga et al (2005), also using the COBRA method, reported higher levels of *ESR-1* methylation in the neoplastic epithelium of UC patients compared with non-neoplastic tissue (25% vs 4% respectively). There were also higher levels of methylation in the distal colon compared with the proximal colon but only in UC patients with neoplasia. No healthy controls were used. Table 1 summarises the studies on gene specific methylation in UC.

Specifically promoter gene methylation for both *ESR-1* and *N-33* were significantly higher in the macroscopically normal epithelium of UC subjects compared with age and sex matched controls (Arasaradnam et al 2010). There was no evidence of dysplasia (confirmed histologically) and importantly on subsequent follow up at three years, no cancers were identified. A smaller study by Issa et al. showed no difference in *ESR-1* methylation between controls (n = 5) and UC subjects without dysplasia (n = 6). This lack of a difference may be explained by the relatively small sample size (only 6 UC patients without dysplasia and 5 controls) compared with the study by Arasaradnam et al. which recruited 68 patients (24 UC subjects and 44 age and sex matched controls). Furthermore, the clinical characteristics of the UC subjects in the study by Issa et al. were not described in detail. For example, it is not known whether the UC subjects without dysplasia had less active, less extensive disease and shorter duration of disease compared with those with dysplasia. Importantly no relationship between age at diagnosis, disease duration, number of flare-ups, SCCAI score or disease extent with promoter methylation of *ESR-1* or *N-33* was identified (Arasaradnam et al 2010).

Study Characteristics	(Issa, Ahuja et al. 2001)	(Fujii, Tominaga et al. 2005)	(Tominaga, Fujii et al. 2005)	(Arasaradnam et al. 2010)
Gene	*ESR-1*, p16, hMLH, CSPG2	*ESR-1*	*ESR-1*	*ESR-1, MYOD-1, N-33*
Sample size	21	30	18	68
Patient Characteristics	12-HGD/cancer 6– No Dysplasia 5 - controls	13 with cancer 17 without cancer	8 with cancer 10 without cancer	24 UC 44 age & sex matched controls
Assay Method	COBRA	MSP	COBRA	COBRA
Findings	Higher methylation of *ESR-1*, P16 & CSPG2 in UC with HGD/cancer. Controls had similar levels to UC with dysplasia	Higher *ESR-1* methylation in UC with cancer compared to without.	Higher *ESR-1* methylation in UC with cancer compared to without. Methylation gradient in colon only for those with cancer	Higher *ESR-1*, N33 methylation compared to controls. Lower methylation for *MYOD-1*. Less smokers among UC
Relationship to UC disease characteristics	-	No relationship between *ESR-1* and inflammatory activity	No relationship between *ESR-1* and inflammatory activity	No relationship btw *ESR-1, MYOD-1, N-33* and disease activity, duration, SCAI score, no. of flares or site.

HGD = High Grade Dysplasia; MSP = Methylation Sensitive PCR (MSP is a sensitive method to detect methylation but is not quantitative)

Table 1. Summary of studies on gene specific methylation in UC.

The findings of CpG hypermethylation of the putative tumour suppressor genes *N-33* and *ESR-1* in normal tissue suggests that inactivation through methylation of these specific putative tumour suppressor genes may not be associated with development of CRC in UC patients. The functional role of *N-33* in UC remains unknown as yet.

2.3.3 DNA methylation in UC and colon cancer
The central pathway (normal epithelium→adenoma→carcinoma) are a result of linear accumulation of genetic mutations and/or chromosomal instability in the wnt signalling pathway. Mutation of the *APC* gene and resultant truncated APC products are unable to bind to β-catenin resulting in Wnt signalling dysfunction – the latter involved in progression

of most sporadic and certain hereditary CRC. It should be noted however that APC inactivation is not always the first genetic event and that *k-Ras* mutations which have been observed in normal colonic mucosa as well as in aberrant crypt foci may precede this (Jan Willem 2000). CpG methylation is thought to be an early event and may even initiate tumourogenesis since it is detected in precursor lesions such as Aberrant Crypt Foci (ACF) and adenomatous polyps (Goelz et al. 1985). Consequently Esteller et al (2000) has proposed the role of tumour suppressor gene silencing through hypermethylation early in the pathway.

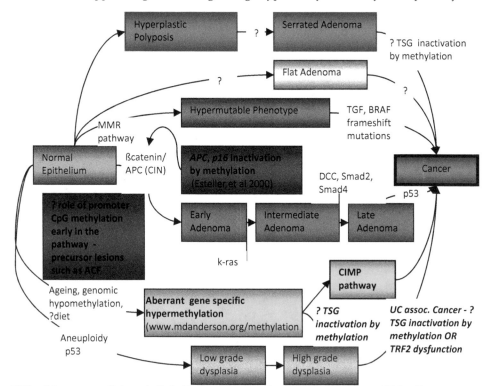

APC = Adenomatous Polyposis Coli; CIMP = CpG island methylator phenotype; CIN = Chromosomal Instability; DCC = Deleted in Colon cancer; Smad = mothers against decapentaplegic homolog 2,4; MMR = Mismatch Repair; TGF = Tumour Growth Factor; BRAF = (v-raf) oncogene homolog B1; TSG = Tumour Suppressor Gene; UC = Ulcerative colitis; TRF2 = Telomere Repeat Binding Factor

Fig. 2. Schematic model for genetic alterations in the development of CRC – modified from Fearnhead et al 2001. Incorporates updates of the model to demonstrate possible roles for methylation/ telomere dysfunction in the UC - CRC pathway

Although not well understood, certain genes appear susceptible to silencing through hypermethylation. A subset of genes which have particularly high methylation levels have been identified in sporadic colon cancers and hence the term CpG island methylator phenotype (CIMP) has been coined. Certain subsets of hyperplastic polyps (although the precise genetic alterations are unknown) appear to have potential for malignant transformation through the hyperplastic polyp→serrated adenoma→adenocarcinoma sequence. This has been coined the 'methylator pathway' (Jass 2004). Similarly, the genetic alterations in the progression of flat adenomas (Paris type 0/11 clinical classification) to cancer remain elusive. In ulcerative colitis associated cancers unlike sporadic cancers, p53 mutations appear to be an early event. It is not clear what triggers the progression from high grade dysplasia to cancer but it is possible that aberrant methylation of tumour suppressor genes or telomere dysfunction could initiate this – see proposed pathway in Figure 2.

3. Telomere and telomere binding proteins

Chromosome instability in colon epithelial cells and peripheral blood lymphocytes (PBLs) has been described in ulcerative colitis (Loeb et al 1999). Telomeres are specialized structures that cap and protect chromosome ends. They are made up of a specific sequence of DNA repeats and form a T-loop structure which is stabilized by telomere associated proteins. Disruption of the T-loop structure causes the telomere to be recognised as a DNA double strand break, activates the DNA repair mechanism leading to telomere fusions and chromosome instability usually followed by apoptosis or senescence (Karlseder 2003). Telomere shortening occurs with each cell division and as a result of cellular stress. This causes depletion of telomeric repeats and telomere binding proteins threatening the stability of the T-loop structure. Telomere dysfunction also follows decreased expression of the telomere proteins which bind double stranded DNA. This causes disruption of the T-loop structure without significant telomere shortening and is known as telomere uncapping (Ben-Porath et al 2004). Dysfunction can also occur with loss of the 3' overhang, a single stranded stretch of DNA at the very end of the telomere protected by proteins known as telomere binding proteins such as TRF1, TRF2, TPP1, TIN2, RAP1 like POT-1 (15)(4,16). These proteins have been described to influence telomere maintenance (de Lange 2005) – Figure 3.

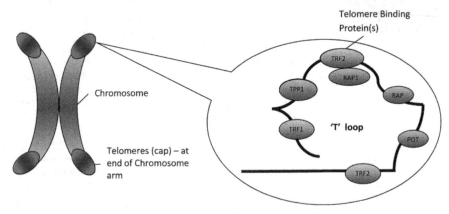

Fig. 3. Telomere caps at the end of chromosomes. Magnified view showing 'T' loop structure of 'Shelterin complex comprising the Telomere binding proteins

3.1 Telomere dysfunction in UC

The two main forms of inflammatory bowel disease (IBD), ulcerative colitis (UC) and Crohn's disease (CD), are characterised by chronic intestinal inflammation and risk of progression to colon cancer (Ransohoff 1988). One proposed cause of the latter characteristic is chromosome instability, since the rearrangement of genetic material can lead to activation of oncogenes, loss of tumour suppressor genes and other changes that lead to uncontrolled cell growth.

Since genomic instability in peripheral blood mononuclear cells (PBMCs) has been used as a biomarker for global cancer risk in a number of diseases (Cottliar et al 2000), the latter observation suggests the possibility of a chromosome instability syndrome in UC that could affect all tissues. One possible cause of chromosome instability aside from genomic DNA methylation is telomere dysfunction. In eukaryotic cells, telomeres are maintained by telomerase and the sub complex of telomere binding proteins. The chromosome instability observed in UC PBMC includes telomere fusions, suggesting the involvement of these structures in its generation. Other observations linking telomeres and UC include decreased telomerase in the colitic colonic mucosa (Ussleman et al 2001), colitis-like ulcerations of the bowel in the telomerase knockout mouse (Lee et al 1998) and shortened telomeres in UC patients showing evidence of dysplasia (Arasaradnam et al 2009). Furthermore telomere shortening is not accelerated in peripheral blood mononuclear cells of UC patients compared with controls and therefore cannot be the mechanism by which chromosome instability arises in these cells (Getliffe et al 2005). Of particular note is the observation in rectal fibroblasts of UC patients showing slower telomere shortening particularly in those with late onset UC. This suggests those who develop UC later in life perhaps have more efficient anti-oxidant systems that protect against telomere damage. (Getliffe et al 2006)

3.2 Role of telomere binding proteins (TBPs) in UC

The telosome/shelterin complex consists of important regulatory telomere binding proteins to include TPP1 (tripeptidyl peptidase1 - formerly PTOP/PIP1/TINT1), POT1 (protection of telomere 1), TIN2 (TRF1 interacting nuclear factor 2), RAP1 (repressor activator protein), TRF1 (telomere repeat binding factor 1) and TRF2 (de Lange 2005).Telomere repeat binding factor 2 (TRF2) is a double stranded DNA binding protein which stabilizes the telomere T-loop. Cells lacking functional TRF2 have an extremely striking chromosome instability phenotype including frequent telomere fusions and erosion of the 3' overhang, but no significant telomere shortening (de Lange 2002). Therefore decreased expression of TRF2 in UC peripheral mononuclear cells, might explain the chromosome instability observed in these cells. More recent data also suggests that aside from maintaining telomeres, TRF2 may also be involved in the repair of DNA damage, including that which occurs at dysfunctional telomeres (Bradshaw et al 2005).

3.2.1 Telomere Repeat Binding Factor 2 (TRF2)

TRF2 mRNA expression is significantly decreased in activated T lymphocytes in both UC and CD, suggesting possible telomeric deficiency of this protein which could lead to destabilisation of the T-loop structure in these cells (da Silva et al 2010). This telomere dysfunction could then cause activation of DNA damage response to repair what is perceived as a double strand break resulting in the telomere fusions previously observed in UC PBMCs. Thus decreased TRF2 mRNA levels in circulating T lymphocytes in IBD could be a putative bio-marker for potential active or refractory disease. It is uncertain if similar changes are present in the cells of the colonic mucosa in IBD where chromosomal abnormalities are thought to precede dysplasia and malignant change.

The finding of low levels of TRF2 in IBD T lymphocytes makes it unlikely that this protein has a significant role in DNA repair mechanisms in this disease. An alternative explanation is that the cells have entered a phase of early senescence hence there is down regulation of telomere binding proteins (Risqué et al 2011). Telomere attrition has been demonstrated in colonic epithelium of patients with ulcerative colitis which, could potentially initiate senescence (Risque et al 2008).

Senescence is thought to act as a tumour suppressor forcing cells to undergo apoptosis rather than uncontrolled cellular proliferation which leads to cancer. mRNA expression levels of RAP1 for example is lower in activated T lymphocytes in UC (da silva et al 2010). RAP1 is closely regulated by TRF2 which in turn is stabilised by TIN2 to form a bridge across telomeric DNA. The reduced RAP1 expression in activated T lymphocytes hints at premature cellular senescence in circulating activated lymphocytes. It is yet unknown if these findings are replicated at mucosal level. Of interest is the observation of a positive association between RAP1 gene expression with 5 – aminosalicylate therapy (da silva et al 2010). It is possible that 5 - aminosalicylate therapy may help stabilise the RAP1/ TRF2/ TIN2 sub complex by increasing its expression thus providing better telomere dynamics in UC. This in turn may explain the clinical observation of the protective effect of 5 - aminosalicylate therapy in UC associated cancer providing further support for its chemo-prophylactic use (Rubin et al 2006). It is evident that the telomeric milieu at the chromosome end zone is intricately balanced with telomerase and telomere binding factors being the key players. The precise role and function of individual telomere binding proteins are largely unknown but it is clear that its coordinated interaction with telomere DNA is vital to maintaining telomere stability. Perturbance, as a result of local (mucosal) inflammation within this delicate sub complex of telomere proteins will, not surprisingly cause telomere dysfunction.

4. Conclusion

Further evaluation to measure *N-33* expression (at mRNA and protein level) as well as to evaluate further epigenetic marking of tumour suppressor genes in larger UC cohorts including those with dysplasia and UC associated cancer are required. This will help elucidate further the role of DNA methylation in particular within the UC-CRC pathway. Additionally, studies to determine associations with habitual dietary intake are required – the latter being an important variable given the modifiable effect of diet on DNA methylation. Finally the role of TBPs in particular mucosal TRF2 in UC patients in the clinical setting of progressive dysplasia and colon cancer will be vital to elucidate its role as a putative biomarker of cancer risk.

5. References

Ahuja, N., Q. Li, et al. (1998). Aging and DNA methylation in colorectal mucosa and cancer. *Cancer Res* 58(23): 5489-94.

Arasaradnam RP (2007). Dietary factors and mucosal biomarkers of colon cancer risk. British Library, London (PhD thesis)

Arasaradnam RP, Commane D, Bradburn D, Mathers JC (2008). A Review of dietary factors and its influence on DNA methylation in colorectla carcinogenesis. *Epigenetics* Jul-Aug;3(4):193-8.

Arasaradnam RP, Khoo KTJ, Bardburn M et al.(2009) Telomere attrition in colorectal mucosa of patients with Ulcerative Colitis (abs). *Gut* ;A100:257

Arasaradnam RP (2010). The conundrum of folate and colorectal cancer (CRC) risk. *Eur J Clin Nutr*. Dec; 64(12):1501

Arasaradnam RP, Khoo KTJ, Bradburn M, Mathers JC, Kelly S (2010). DNA methylation of ESR-1 and N-33 in colorectal mucosa of patients with Ulcerative colitis (UC). *Epigenetics* Jul;5(5):422-6

Ben-Porath I, Weinberg RA (2004). When cells get stressed: an integrative view of cellular senescence. *J Clin Invest* ;113:8-13.

Biasco, G. and M. C. Di Marco (2005). Folate and prevention of colorectal cancer in ulcerative colitis. *Eur J Cancer Prev* 14(4): 395-8.

Bradshaw PS, Stavropoulos DJ, Meyn MS (2005). Human telomeric protein TRF2 associates with genomic double-strand breaks as an early response to DNA damage. *Nat Genet*; 37:193-7.

Crohn, B. B., L. Ginzburg, et al. (1984). Landmark article Oct 15, 1932. Regional ileitis. A pathological and clinical entity. By Burril B. Crohn, Leon Ginzburg, and Gordon D. Oppenheimer. *JAMA* 251(1): 73-9.

Cottliar A, Fundia A, Boerr L, et al (2000). High frequencies of telomeric associations, chromosome aberrations, and sister chromatid exchanges in ulcerative colitis. *Am J Gastroenterol* ;95:2301-7.

da Silva N, Arasaradnam R, Getliffe K et al (2010). Altered mRNA expression of telomere binding proteins (TPP1, POT1, RAP1, TRF1, TRF2) in Ulcerative colitis and Crohn's disease. *Dig Liver Dis* 42(8):544-8

de Lange T (2005). Shelterin: the protein complex that shapes and safeguards human telomeres. *Genes Dev* 15;19(18):2100-10

de Lange T(2002). Protection of mammalian telomeres. *Oncogene* ;21:532-40.

DePinho, R. A. (2000). The age of cancer. *Nature* 408(6809): 248-254.

Ekbom, A., C. Helmick, et al. (1990). Ulcerative colitis and colorectal cancer. A population-based study. *N Engl J Med* 323(18): 1228-33.

Esteller, M., A. Sparks, et al. (2000). Analysis of Adenomatous Polyposis Coli Promoter Hypermethylation in Human Cancer. *Cancer Res* 60(16): 4366-4371.

Esteller, M., P. G. Corn, et al. (2001). A Gene Hypermethylation Profile of Human Cancer. *Cancer Res* 61(8): 3225-3229.

Esteller, M. (2002). CpG island hypermethylation and tumor suppressor genes: a booming present, a brighter future. *Oncogene* 21(35): 5427-40.

Fearnhead, N. S., M. P. Britton, et al. (2001). The ABC of APC 10.1093/hmg/10.7.721. *Hum. Mol. Genet.* 10(7): 721-733.

Friedenreich, C., T. Norat, et al. (2006). Physical Activity and Risk of Colon and Rectal Cancers: The European Prospective Investigation into Cancer and Nutrition. *Cancer Epidemiol Biomarkers Prev* 15(12): 2398-2407.

Fujii, S., K. Tominaga, et al. (2005). Methylation of the oestrogen receptor gene in non-neoplastic epithelium as a marker of colorectal neoplasia risk in longstanding and extensive ulcerative colitis. *Gut* 54(9): 1287-1292.

Getliffe KM, Al Dulaimi D, Martin-Ruiz C, et al (2005). Mononuclear telomere dynamics and telomerase activity in inflammatory bowel disease: effect of drugs and smoking. *Aliment Pharmacol Ther*; 21:121-31.

Getliffe KM, Martin-Ruiz C, Passos JF, von-Zglinicki, Nwokolo C (2006). Extended lifespan and long telomeres in rectal fibroblasts from late-onset ulcerative colitis patients. *Eur J Gastroenterol Hepatol* 18(2):133-41

Gloria, L., M. Cravo, et al. (1996). DNA hypomethylation and proliferative activity are increased in the rectal mucosa of patients with long-standing ulcerative colitis. *Cancer* 78(11): 2300-6.

Goelz, S. E., B. Vogelstein, et al. (1985). Hypomethylation of DNA from benign and malignant human colon neoplasms. *Science* 228(4696): 187-90.

Issa, J. P., Y. L. Ottaviano, et al. (1994). Methylation of the oestrogen receptor CpG island links ageing and neoplasia in human colon. *Nat Genet* 7(4): 536-40.

Issa, J.-P. J., N. Ahuja, et al. (2001). Accelerated Age-related CpG Island Methylation in Ulcerative Colitis. *Cancer Res* 61(9): 3573-3577.

Jaenisch, R. and A. Bird (2003) Epigenetic regulation of gene expression: how the genome integrates intrinsic and environmental signals. *Nat Genet*. 2003;245-254

Jan Willem, A. (2000). Molecular interactions in the Vogelstein model of colorectal carcinoma. *The Journal of Pathology* 190(4): 412-416.

Jass, J. R. (2004). Hyperplastic polyps and colorectal cancer: is there a link? *Clin Gastroenterol Hepatol* 2(1): 1-8.

Jones, P. A. and S. B. Baylin (2002). The Fundamental Role of Epigenetic events in Cancer. *Nature Reviews Genetics* 3(6): 415-428.

Karlseder J (2003). Telomere repeat binding factors: keeping the ends in check. *Cancer Lett*; 194:189-97

Lee HW, Blasco MA, Gottlieb GJ, et al (1998). Essential role of mouse telomerase in highly proliferative organs. *Nature*; 392:569-74.

Loeb KR, Loeb LA (1999). Genetic instability and the mutator phenotype. Studies in ulcerative colitis. *Am J Pathol* ; 154:1621-6.

Merlo, A., J. G. Herman, et al. (1995). 5' CpG island methylation is associated with transcriptional silencing of the tumour suppressor p16/CDKN2/MTS1 in human cancers. *Nat Med* 1(7): 686-92.

Pufulete, M., R. Al-Ghnaniem, et al. (2005). Effect of folic acid supplementation on genomic DNA methylation in patients with colorectal adenoma. *Gut* 54(5): 648-653.

Ransohoff, D. F. (1988). Colon cancer in ulcerative colitis. *Gastroenterology* 94(4): 1089-91.

Risques RA, Lai LA, Brentall TA et al (2008). Ulcerative Colitis is a disease of accelerated colon ageing: evidence of from telomere attrition and DNA damage. *Gastroenterology*; 135:410-8

Risques RA, Lai LA, Himmetolgu C et al (2011). Ulcerative colitis associated colorectal cancer arises in a field of short telomeres, senescence and inflammation. *Cancer Res*. 2011 Mar 1;71(5):1669-79.

Rubin DT, LoSavio A, Yadron N et al (2006). Aminosalicylate therapy in the prevention of dysplasia and colorectal cancer in ulcerative colitis. *Clin Gastroenterol Hepatol*; 4(11):1346-50

Tahara, T., N. Inoue, et al. (2005). Clinical significance of microsatellite instability in the inflamed mucosa for the prediction of colonic neoplasms in patients with ulcerative colitis. *Journal of Gastroenterology and Hepatology* 20(5): 710-715.

Tominaga, K., S. Fujii, et al. (2005). Prediction of Colorectal Neoplasia by Quantitative Methylation Analysis of Estrogen Receptor Gene in Nonneoplastic Epithelium from Patients with Ulcerative Colitis. *Clin Cancer Res* 11(24): 8880-8885.

Usselmann B, Newbold M, Morris AG, et al (2001). Deficiency of colonic telomerase in ulcerative colitis. *Am J Gastroenterol*; 96:1106-12.

Van Guelpen, B., J. Hultdin, et al. (2006). Low folate levels may protect against colorectal cancer. *Gut* 55(10): 1461-1466.

Walmsley, R. S., R. C. S. Ayres, et al. (1998). A simple clinical colitis activity index. *Gut* 43(1): 29-32.

Wilson, A. S., B. E. Power, et al. (2007). DNA hypomethylation and human diseases. *Biochimica et Biophysica Acta (BBA) - Reviews on Cancer* 1775(1): 138-162.

8

Role of Interferon-γ-Inducible Protein (IP)-10/ (IP-10/CXCL10) in Ulcerative Colitis; A Review of the Present Status

Kenji Suzuki[1], Hiroyuki Yoneyama[2] and Hitoshi Asakura[3]
[1]*Department of Medicine III, Niigata University Medical and Dental Hospital,*
[2]*Stelic Institute of Regenerative Medicine, Stelic Institute & Co.,*
[3]*The Koukann Clinics*
Japan

1. Introduction

Ulcerative colitis (UC) is a chronic, relapsing inflammatory bowel disease (IBD) affecting the colonic mucosa; it is of unknown etiology (Baumgart & Carding, 2007). UC clinically displays bloody diarrhea, abdominal pain and weight loss, and often leads to a severe outcome since the therapeutic approaches, including corticosteroid and 5-aminosalicylic acid, are not always successful in inducing long-term remission (Baumgart & Sandborn, 2007). Although the incidence of UC varies from 1 to 15 per 100,000 population in different locations, it increases year by year. Moreover, UC generally acts upon young people, and approximately 30% of patients with UC will undergo colectomy in the course of their life-times (Stewenius et al., 1996). Thus, UC is a serious disease affecting the quality of life for a long period.

It is now considered that IBD is not a simple inflammatory disease but a rather complicated disorder of intestinal components including epithelial cells, immune cells, neural cells, and extracellular matrix. Particular types of microbes, environmental factors including sanitary conditions and food, and genetic factors are also suggested to be involved (Xavier & Podolsky, 2007; Kaser et al., 2010;Asakura & Suzuki, 2010). Global approaches are therefore needed to reveal the pathogenesis of IBD, and to develop new therapeutic approaches for IBD as well.

Chemokines have taken great attention since their discovery, because this family of chemotactic cytokines is intimately involved in the pathogenesis of many important human diseases. Developing new therapeutic approaches targeting several chemokines have been tried (Viola & Luster, 2008).

In this chapter, we will review the role of interferon-γ-inducible protein (IP)-10 (IP-10/CXCL10) in the colon of normal condition and UC, introducing our recent findings about the effect of neutralization of IP-10 on animal models of UC. We also discuss about the possibility of clinical application of antagonist therapies targeting IP-10.

2. Chemokines and chemokine receptors

Chemokines are small 8-12 kDa proteins with 20 to 70 percent homology in amino acid sequence, are relatively resistant to inactivation, and have a long half-life in vivo (Rossi &

Zlotnik, 2000). They can direct the recruitment and migration of circulating leukocytes and play a critical role in the differentiation of secondary lymphoid organs. At present approximately 50 chemokines and 20 chemokine receptors are known. The chemokine system is characterized by redundancy (Mantovani,1999). A single chemokine can interact with several different chemokine receptors and a single chemokine receptor can respond to multiple chemokines. No chemokine is uniquely active on one leukocyte population, and usually a given leukocyte population has receptors for and responds to different molecules.

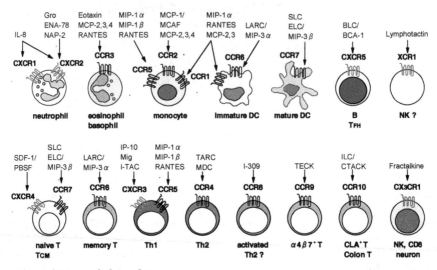

Fig. 1. Chemokines and chemokine receptors

Chemokines are classified into four families on the basis of the pattern of the first two of four cysteine residues of the ligands (Rossi & Zlotnik, 2000). The CXC family (α chemokine) has two cysteine residues separated by a non-cysteine amino acid. The CC family (β chemokine) contains two adjacent cysteine residues. The CX3C family (γ chemokine) has two cysteine residues separated by three non-cysteine amino acids, whereas the C family (δ chemokine) has only one cysteine residue.

Chemokine receptors are G-protein-coupled receptors possessing a seven transmembrane domain that upon binding to calcium influx and activation of several downstream targets including the PI3 kinase pathway (Rossi & Zlotnik, 2000). Based on the chemokine class they bind, the receptors have been named CXCR1, 2, 3, 4 and 5 (bind CXC chemokines); CCR1 through CCR10 (bind CC chemokines); XCR1 (binds the C chemokine, Lymphotactin); and CX3CR1 (binds the CX3C chemokine, fractalkine or neurotactin).

Schematically, CXC chemokines are active on polymorphonuclear neutrophis (PMNs) and T and B cells. IL-8 is a typical CXC chemokine that acts on PMNs. An essential structural element of CXC chemokine for neutrophil activation is a Glu-Leu-Arg (ELR) motif in the 5'-structure of the protein. Thus CXC chemokines are divided into two groups; ELR motif chemokine and non-ELR motif chemokine. In contrast, CC chemokines exert their action on multiple leukocyte subtypes, including monocytes, basophils, eosinophils, T cells, dendritic cells and natural killer (NK) cells, but they are generally inactive on PMNs. The representative CC chemokines, eotaxins, are active selectively on eosinophils and basophils.

Lymphotactin is a C chemokine, and fractalkine is a CX3C chemokine. They both act on T cells and NK cells, and fractalkine is also active on monocytes.

Thus chemokines facilitate leukocyte migration and positioning to sites of tissue damage as well as other process such as angiogenesis and leukocyte degradation (Mackay, 2001). Chemokines and their receptors also important in dendritic cell maturation, B and T cell development, Th1 and Th2 responses, infections, angiogenesis, wound healing and tumor growth as well as metastasis (Rossi & Zlotnik, 2000).

Chemokines can be divided into two categories: inducible inflammatory chemokines are produced by activated cells and recruit leukocytes in response to physiological stress, whereas homeostatic chemokines are constitutively produced and involved in maintaining basal leukocyte trafficking as well as the architecture of secondary lymphoid organs (Gerard & Rollins, 2001).

Recent advance of clinical and basic research have revealed that several diseases are associated with inappropriate activation of the chemokine-chemokine receptor network, and they include cardiovascular disease, allergic inflammatory disease, transplantation, neuroinflammation, cancer and HIV-associated disease (Gerard, & Rollins, 2001).

Unlike cytokines, which have pleiotropic effects, chemokines target specific leukocyte subsets and, in some settings, may only attract these cells without activating them. Antagonism of a single chemokine ligand or receptor would be expected to have a relatively circumscribed effect, thereby endowing the antagonism with a limited side effect profile (Gerard & Rollins, 2001; Viola & Luster, 2008; Nishimura et al., 2009).

Type of inflammation	Main target cells	Chemokine	Chemokine receptor
Acute inflammation	Neutrophil	CXCL1 (GROα), CXCL2 (GROβ), CXCL8 (IL-8)	CXCR2, CXCR1
	Monocyte	CCL2 (MCP-1)	CCR2
Th1–type inflammation	Monocyte	CCL2 (MCP-1), CCL4 (MIP-1β),CCL5 (RANTES), CX3CL1(Fractalkine)	CCR2, CCR5, CCR1, CCR3, CX3CR1
	Th1 cell	CXCL9 (Mig), CXCL10 (IP-10), CXCL11 (I-TAC)	CXCR3
	CD8+ T cell	CCL3 (MIP-1αS), CCL4 (MIP-1β), CXCL9 (Mig), CXCL10 (IP-10)	CCR5, CCR1, CXCR3
	B cell	CXCL13 (BCA-1)	CXCR5
Th2-type inflammation	Th2 cell	CCL17 (TARC), CCL22 (MDC), CCL1 (I-309)	CCR4, CCR8
	Eosinophil	CCL11 (Eotaxin), CCL26 (Eotaxin-3)	CCR3
	Mast cell	CCL2 (MCP-1), CCL11 (Eotaxin), CXCL10 (IP-10)	CCR2, CCR3, CXCR3
	B cell	CXCL13 (BCA-1)	CXCR5
Th17- type inflammation	Th17, DC	CCL20 (MIP-3α)	CCR6

* modified from Viola & Luster, 2008

Table 1. The type of inflammation and chemokine/chemokine receptor system

3. Interferon-γ-inducible protein (IP)-10 and its receptor CXCR3

Luster et al. initially identified human IFN-γ-inducible protein of 10 kDa (IP-10/CXCL10) as an early response gene induced by IFN-γ in U937 cells (a monocyte-like cell line) (Luster et al, 1985). IP-10 is secreted by a diverse range of tissue under proinflammatory conditions (Nevelle et al., 1997; Farber, 1997). It is a key mediator of the interferon response, preferentially attracts activated Th1 lymphocytes to sites of inflammation, and is an inhibitor of angiogenesis (Taub et al., 1993). IP-10 is constitutively expressed at low levels in thymic, splenic, and lymph node stroma. However, its expression can be highly induced in endothelial cells, keratinocytes, fibroblasts mesangial cells, astrocytes, monocytes, and neutrophils by stimulation with IFN-α, IFN-β, IFN-γ, or LPS and in T cells by antigen activation.

Dufour et al. have generated mice deficient in IP-10 by targeted gene deletion mutagenesis (Dufour et al., 2002). IP-10-/- mice showed no overt developmental or morphological abnormalities, and fertile. Immunophenotyping of leukocyte subsets were similar between wild-type and IP-10-/- mice. In contrast, immunological analysis revealed a role for IP-10 in both the generation of effector T cells and their delivery to sites of tissue inflammation.

Although described above chemokines and chemokine receptors are redundant in their action on target cells (Mantovani, 1999), IP-10 is somewhat atypical, in that it specifically activates a single receptor, CXCR3 (Loetscher et al., 1996). While CXCR3 binds two other interferon-γ-induced, angiostatic CXC chemokines: monokine induced by interferon-γ (Mig:CXCL9) and interferon-inducible T cell α chemoattractant (I-TAC; CXCL11) (Loetscher et al, 1996; Cole et al.,1998), it is becoming clear that they exhibit unique expression patterns in vivo, and several data support the concept that these three chemokines may have nonredundant function in vivo (Dufour et al., 2002; Khan et al, 2000). Crystal structures of IP-10 revealed that IP-10 's action may involve oligomerization of the protein, and that IP-10 shares the ability to bind to cell surface glycosaminoglycan (GAGs) with most, if not all, chemokines (Swaminathan et al.,2003; Luster et al., 1995). Chemokine-GAG interactions can promote chemokine oligomerization (Hoogewerf et al., 1997)), and the formation of immobilized chemokine gradients (Tanaka et al.,1993) , which are likely to be important for chemokine action.

It has been reported that the expression of IP-10 was elevated in several diseases such as UC (Uguccioni et al., 1999), hepatitis (Narumi et al, 1998), multiple slcerosis (Sorensen et al., 2002), and Sjoegren's syndrome (Ogawa et al., 2002), suggesting the involvement of IP-10 in the development of these diseases.

4. IP-10 and other chemokines in ulcerative colitis

UC is a chronic relapsing disease of unknown etiology with a prominent leukocyte infiltrate, which is confined to the mucosa and submucosa of the colon and contributes largely to the tissue damage (Baumgart & Carding, 2007; Xavier & Podolsky, 2007). The disease usually involves the rectum and extends proximally to involve all or part of the colon (Baumgart & Sandborn, 2007). Proximal spread occurs in continuity without areas of uninvolved mucosa. The affected regions exhibit a mixture of acute and chronic inflammatory aspects accompanied by massive infiltration of macrophages, neutrophils, eosinophils, T cells, and plasma cells. The neutrophils invade the epithelium, usually in the crypts, giving rise to cryptitis and, ultimately, to crypt abscess. The following two major histological findings suggest chronicity of UC (Friedman & Blumberg, 2010). The first is basal plasma cytosis; multiple basal lymphoid aggregates are observed in some patients. The second is the distorted crypt architecture of the colon; crypts may be bifid and reduced in number, often with a gap between the crypt bases and the muscularis mucosae. The immune system seems to be shifted to atypical Th2 dominance, with coexistence of Th1 response.

The recruitment and activation of leukocytes in inflamed tissues is a complex process driven by chemokines and possibly other attractants that induces cell adhesion and locomotion (Luster, 1998). Chemokines may play a central role in UC because chemokines are relatively resitant to inactivation in vivo, compared with other chemoattractants such as leukotriene B4, N-formyl-methionyl-leucyl-phenylalanin, and peptide activating factor, which have shorter half-lives (MacDermott et al., 1998). Furthermore, chemokines are produced by a wide variety of different cell types after stimulation by proinflammatory cytokines. The ability of chemokines to activate cells to produce destructive molecules also makes them excellent candidates to be involved in the perpetuation of UC (MacDermott et al., 1998).

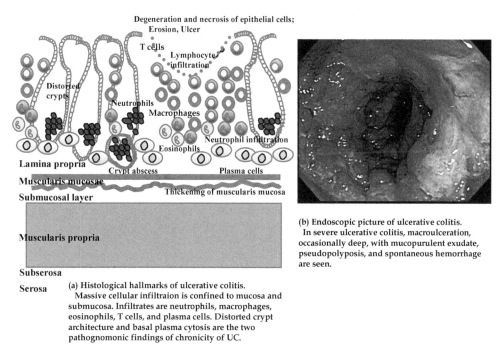

(b) Endoscopic picture of ulcerative colitis. In severe ulcerative colitis, macroulceration, occasionally deep, with mucopurulent exudate, pseudopolyposis, and spontaneous hemorrhage are seen.

(a) Histological hallmarks of ulcerative colitis. Massive cellular infiltraion is confined to mucosa and submucosa. Infiltrates are neutrophils, macrophages, eosinophils, T cells, and plasma cells. Distorted crypt architecture and basal plasma cytosis are the two pathognomonic findings of chronicity of UC.

Fig. 2. Histological features and endoscopic findings of ulcerative colitis

Studies have demonstrated that IL-8, MCP-1, and ENA-78 are highly expressed in the intestinal mucosa in areas of UC as well as Crohn disease. Neutrophils and macrophages in the inflamed intestine synthesize and secrete large amounts of chemokines in patients with UC. Increased chemokine expression has also been observed in colonic epithelial cells, endothelial cells and smooth muscle cells (MacDermott, 1999).

Several studies have reported increased expression of IP-10 in the mucosa of patients with UC and pouchitis (Uguccioni, 1999; Helwig, 2004; Autschbach, 2002; Grimm & Doe, 1996). However, there is a controversy about the source of IP-10 in the colonic mucosa; whether epithelial cells or immune cells. Generally, IP-10 is secreted by neutrophils, monocytes, fibroblasts, keratinocytes, dendritic cells, and epithelial cells. Dwinell et al. and Shibahara et al. have reported that human intestinal epithelial cell lines produce chemoattractants including IP-10 for IEL, and such chemokine production is regulated by proinflammatory cytokines such as IFN-γ (Dwinell et al., 2001, Shibahara et al., 2001). Intestinal subepithelial myofibroblasts have been also reported to produce IP-10 (Inatomi et al., 2005).

5. IP-10 in animal models of IBD

Mechanistic studies of IBD are difficult to perform in humans, hence animal models have been developed to analyse and develop new therapeutic approaches.

IL-10$^{-/-}$ mice spontaneously develop colitis at ~ 3 months of age (Kuhn et al., 1993). This murine disease is similar to that seen in human Crohn disease with small intestine and colon disease localization, chronic mucosal inflammation, alterations in mucosal architecture, bowel-wall thickening, and a chronic progressive disease course. However, this murine model differs from human Crohn disease, because colitis in IL-10$^{-/-}$ mice does not yield focal granulomatous, or transmural inflammation.

Singh et al. administered rabbit anti-IP-10 polyclonal IgG antibody to IL-10$^{-/-}$ mice by i.p. injection every 3 days at the onset of asymptomatic colitis (Singh, U.P. et al., 2003). They monitored serum amyloid A protein and IL-6 levels every other week, and determined the onset. mRNA expression analysis shows upregulated IP-10 and CXCR3 in the inflamed colon of IL-10$^{-/-}$ mouse, while IP-10 is predominantly expressed in the mesenteric lymph nodes (MLNs). Neutralization of IP-10 ameliorated the severity of colitis along with decrease of SAA and several inflammatory cytokines. In their additional report, they showed that IP-10 is largely produced by CD4$^+$ T cells in the mesenteric lymph nodes and lamina propria during colitis, and that IP-10 blockade decreased the number of CD4$^+$ CXCL10$^+$ cells in MLNs and lamina propria of IL10$^{-/-}$ mice (Singh et al., 2007). These results suggest intestinal inflammation is driven by the presence of CD4$^+$ CXCR3$^+$ T cells and cells that produce IP-10.

In confirmation, Hyun et al. have shown that anti-IP-10 antibody treatment can mitigate colitis in IL-10$^{-/-}$ mice through decreased trafficking of Th1 cells (Hyun et al, 2007) , with administration of hamster antimurine CXCL10 monoclonal antibody (1F11). They also revealed that CXCL10 blockade specifically decreased recruitment of transferred Th1 cells into MLNs and colon of IL-10$^{-/-}$ mice. These data suggest that IP-10/CXCL10 plays a dual role in colitis development by enhancing Th1 cell generation in inductive sites (MLNs) and promoting effector cell recruitment to inflamed tissue (effector sites; colon).

6. Our recent findings about IP-10

IBD consists of two major forms: UC and Crohn disease. Crohn disease is suggested to be mediated by Th1/Th17-associated cytokines such as IL-23, IL-12, IL-17, and IFN-γ that are overproduced by macrophages and Th1/Th17 cells of the intestine (Strober & Fuss, 2011). Th17 cells are important in host defense against bacterial and fungal infections, in particular at mucosal surfaces (Ouyang, W. et al., 2008). Among many IBD animal models, colitis observed in both IL-10$^{-/-}$ mice and Rag2$^{-/-}$ mice reconstituted with CD4$^+$CD45RB^{high}T cells has been characterized as a Th1/Th17-dependent disease, mimicking Crohn disease.

In contrast, Th2-cytokines have been linked to UC, and UC is regarded as an atypical Th2 disease with coexistence of Th1 type (Strober & Fuss, 2011). Okayasu et al. have reported a murine colitis model induced by administration of dextran sulphate sodium (DSS) as a model for UC (Okayasu et al., 1990). Additionally, we have esatablished a new chronic colitis using murine AIDS virus, which we termed MAIDS colitis, as a UC model (Suzuki et al.,1997).

Thus, to reveal the involvement of IP-10 in pathophysiology of UC, these two animal models; DSS colitis and MAIDS colitis, are ideal for mechanistic study using neutralizing anti-IP-10 antibody.

6.1 Blockade of IP-10 ameliorated acute colitis and enhances crypt cell survival

We have revealed that the endogenously produced chemokine IP-10 regulates crypt cell proliferation (Sasaki et al., 2002). IP-10 was constitutively expressed by basal crypts in normal mouse colon, but the expression of IP-10 as well as CXCR3 was enhanced in the proliferative zone during acute phase of the colitis after oral administration of DSS. Neutralization of IP-10 with mouse monoclonal anti-IP-10 antibody protected mice from epithelial ulceration by promoting crypt cell survival without evidence of altered immune cell infiltration. Furthermore, recombinant IP-10 administration into normal mice inhibited intestinal epithelial cell proliferation. These findings suggest that IP-10 negatively regulates crypt cell growth to maintain intestinal homeostasis in an acute DSS colitis by enhancing crypt cell survival.

Besides colonic crypt epithelial cells, IP-10 is also active on non-leukocytes/T cells such as endothelial cells and fibroblasts. Campanella et al. have recently reported that IP-10 can inhibit endothelial proliferation through a CXCR3-independent mechanism (Campanella et al., 2010). They speculate that the ability of IP-10 to inhibit endothelial cell proliferation is more associated with its binding to glycosaminoglycans than its binding to CXCR3.

We should further reveal the exact molecular mechanism how IP-10 could down regulate crypt cell proliferation.

6.2 Blockade of IP-10 ameliorated pancreatitis-like injury of mice with MAIDS

The LP-BM5 murine leukemia virus (MuLV) is a retrovirus that is known to induce profound immunodeficiency with splenomegaly and generalized lymphadenopathy in susceptible strains of mice, and occasionally brings about lymphoid malignancy (Mosier et al., 1985). Resembling the severe immunodeficiency with human acquired immunodeficiency syndrome (AIDS), the virus-infected mice have been studied as a mouse model of AIDS, termed murine AIDS (MAIDS) (Jolicoeur 1991). Based on the findings that systemic exocrinopathy resembling Sjoegren's syndrome was induced in salivary glands and lacrimal glands as well as in the pancreas, we proposed that MAIDS mice could be an animal model for Sjoegren's syndrome as well as AIDS (Suzuki et al., 1993). The pancreas-infiltrating cells comprise both Th1 and Th2 type CD4+ T cells, although with a predominance of Th2 over Th1. Thus, the pancreatic lesions of MAIDS mice have some similarities to autoimmune-related chronic pancreatitis, especially the lesions associated with Sjoegren's syndrome (Watanabe et al., 2003).

We administered anti-IP-10 monoclonal antibody to MAIDS mice, and showed that anti-IP-10 administration ameliorated the pancreatic lesions by blocking the cellular infiltration of CD4+ T cells and IFN-γ+ Mac-1+ cells into the pancreas (Kawauchi et al., 2006).

6.3 Blockade of IP-10 ameliorated MAIDS colitis

Systemic exocrinopathy resembling Sjoegren's syndrome and autoimmune pancreatitis-like pancreatic lesions were induced in mice with MAIDS, but colitis was not observed in MAIDS mice (Suzuki et al., 1993). In contrast, nude mice inoculated with lymph node cells from mice with MAIDS developed chronic inflammatory bowel disease-like colitis, which we termed MAIDS colitis (Suzuki et al., 1997). The precise mechanism of pathogenesis of the colitis remains largely unknown, however, regulatory T cells (Treg) deficiency might play a role in its development because there are some reports of colitis modulated by Treg (Izcue et al., 2006). We demonstrated that the pathological lesions of MAIDS colitis resembled ulcerative colitis and that the major populations of colon-infiltrating cells in MAIDS colitis were Mac1+ macrophages and CD4+ T cells with polarized immune responses toward Th2 (Suriki et al., 2000). Thus, MAIDS colitis could serve as an animal model for UC.

Using our MAIDS colitis, we examined the effect of IP-10 blockade (Suzuki et al., 2007). Anti-IP-10 antibody treatment reduced the number of colon infiltrating cells when compared to those mice given a control antibody. The treatment made the length of the crypt of the colon greater than control antibody. The number of Ki67+ proliferating epithelial cells was increased by the anti-IP-10 antibody treatment. Terminal deoxynucleotidyl transferase-mediated dUTP nick-end labelling (TUNEL)+ apoptotic cells were observed in the epithelial cells of the luminal tops of crypts in control MAIDS colitis, whereas TUNEL+ apoptotic epithelial cells were rarely observed with anti-IP-10 antibody treatment. In summary, blockade of IP-10 attenuated MAIDS colitis through blocking cellular trafficking and protecting intestinal epithelial cells, suggesting that IP-10 plays a key role in the development of UC as well as in chronic MAIDS colitis.

6.4 Our hypothesis of the role of IP-10 in UC, and theoretical therapeutic approach

From our research findings about blockade of IP-10 for UC animal models, we propose the hypothesis of the role of IP-10 in UC as follows (Fig. 3.).

In normal condition, naive T cells are activated by dendritic cells through IP-10 in mesenteric lymph nodes (inductive site) where they immediately express CXCR3 and differentiate into Th1 effector cells. IP-10 is constitutively expressed in normal colon, and promotes colonic recruitment of Th1 cells from blood vessels (Fig. 3a). Colonic epithelial cell regeneration and proliferation are regulated by a net balance between positive regulating factors and negative regulating factors (Podolsky, 1999). Several growth factors such as epidermal growth factor (EGF), keratinocyte growth factor (KGF), and hepatocyte growth factor (HGF) are typical positive regulating factors for intestinal epithelial proliferation and regeneration. They are secreted from both the local epithelial cells and the mesenchymal cells. In contrast, TGF-β is a typical negative regulator which inhibit proliferation of intestinal epithelial cells. Additionally, as we described above, we found that IP-10 is another negative regulator of crypt epithelial proliferation (Sasaki et al., 2002). In normal intestine, the net balance between these two factors is well balanced, and normal intestinal epithelial renewing is maintained (Fig. 3a).

In UC, IP-10 production is increased in both the mesenteric lymph nodes and the diseased colon, and more Th1 cells are differentiated and recruited into the effector site of colon (Fig. 3b). In the colon of patients with UC, IP-10, a negative regulator for epithelial proliferation, is relatively over produced against positive regulators such as HGF (Fig. 3b). We have reported previously that intrinsic HGF is over produced in the colon of mice with DSS colitis (Hanawa, et al., 2006). In UC, net balance between positive and negative regulators are shifted toward negative ones, and colonic epithelial proliferation and regeneration are inhibited (Fig. 3b).

Thus IP-10 plays two roles in the pathophysiology of UC: First, IP-10 is a chemokine which differentiates naive T cells into Th1 cells, and recruits them into the inflamed colon. Second, it is a negative regulator for intestinal epithelial proliferation and regeneration (Fig. 3b).

Therefore, theoretically, blocking IP-10 is an ideal therapeutic approach for UC as we reported using two mouse models (Sasaki et al., 2002; Suzuki et al., 2007).

We think that blockade of IP-10 promotes crypt epithelial cell proliferation and regeneration as well as inhibiting differentiation of Th1 cells and their trafficking into the diseased colon (Fig. 3c).

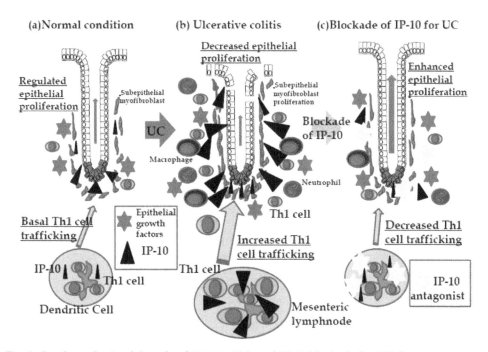

Fig. 3. Our hypothesis of the role of IP-10 in UC, and IP-10 blockade for UC therapy

CXCR3 is a receptor for IP-10, and IP-10/CXCR3 axis plays a critical role in pathophysiology in several diseases including IBD (Singh et al., 2007; Groom & Luster, 2011).

Several clinical trials using CXCR 3 antagonists are now under investigation for psoriasis, rheumatoid arthritis, and nephritis (Singh et al., 2007).

CXCR3 respond not only for IP-10, but also for Mig and I-TAC. In addition, IP-10 exerts its effects through at least two systems such as CXCR3 and CXCR3-independent mechanism (Campanella et al., 2010).

Therefore, we think that blockade of IP-10 using anti-human-IP-10 monoclonal antibody is a realistic strategy for the development of a new therapy targeting IP-10 for UC.

7. Application of antagonist therapies targeting IP-10 for UC

Chemokine and chemokine receptors are central to the inflammatory process and are attractive therapeutic targets. Several approaches are being pursued simultaneously, including antibodies to chemokines or their receptors, small molecule inhibitors of chemokine receptors modified chemokine antagonists, and inhibitors of chemokine presentation or higher-order structure (Viola & Luster, 2008). Schall and Proudfoot propose that inappropriate target selection and ineffective dosing, not the 'redundancy' of the chemokine system, are the main barriers to the use of chemokine receptor antagonists as anti-inflammatory therapies (Schall & Proudfoot, 2011).

Recently, Phase 2, multi-dose, double-blind, placebo-controlled, randomized, multicenter study of MDX-1100 (anti-CXCL10 human monoclonal antibody) has been completed for patients with moderately-to-severely active UC (ClinicalTrials.gov Web;

http://www.clinicaltrials.gov/ct2/show/NCT00656890?term=MDX-1100&rank=2).
We are looking forward to seeing all the data about this proof-of-concept study.

8. Conclusion

As shown in this review, several important clinical and experimental data suggest that IP-10 plays a critical role in the pathophysiology in UC, and it is an attractive therapeutic target. IP-10 is unique not only for its chemoattractant feature for activated Th1 cells, but also for its negative regulator activity for crypt epithelial cell cycle. Regulation of IP-10 could become a novel therapeutic approach for UC, which has both anti-inflammatory feature and facilitating ability of crypt epithelial cell regeneration.

9. Acknowledgments

The authors thank Drs. Yokoyama, J., Kawauchi, Y., Honda, J.(Niigata University Medical and Dental Hospital), Sukumaran, V., and Professor Watanabe, K. (Niigata Unviersity of Pharmacy and Applied Life Sciences) for their contribution to the research. This work was supported in part by grants-in-aid for Science Research, from the Ministry of Education, Culture, Sports, Science and Technology; the Ministry of Health Welfare and Labor of Japan; the Japan Science and Technology Agency, Japan.

10. References

Asakura., H., and Suzuki, K. (2010) Immunomodulation by foods and microbes in Crohn disease and ulcerative colitis, In: *Dietary components and immune funciton*, Watson, R.R., Zibadi, S., and Preedy, V.R., pp. 657, Humana Press, ISBN978-1-60761-060-1, New York

Autschbach, F., Giese, T., Gassler, N., Sido, B., Heuschen, G., Heuschen, U., Zuna, I., Schulz, P., Weckauf, H., Berger, I., Otto, H. F., and Meuer, S.C. (2002) Cytokine/chemokine messenger-RNA expression profiles in ulcerative colitis and Crohn's disease. Virchows Arch *441*, 500-513.

Baumgart, D.C., and Carding, S.R.(2007) Inflammatory bowel disease: cause and immunobiology. Lancet, *369*, 1627-40.

Baumgart, D., and Sandborn, W.J. (2007) Inflammatory bowel disease: clinical aspects and established and evolving therapies. Lancet *369*, 1641-57.

Campanella, G.S.V., Colvin, R.A., and Luster, A.D. (2010) CXCL10 can inhibit endothelial cell proliferation independently of CXCR3. PLoS ONE *5*, e12700.

Cole, K.E., Strick, C.A., Paradis, T.J., Ogborne, K.T., Loetscher, M., Gladue, R.P., Lin, W., Boyd, J.G., Moser, B., Wood, D.E., Sahagan, B.G., and Neote, K. (1998) Interferon-inducible T cell alpha chemoattractant (I-TAC): a novel non-ELR CXC chemokine with potent activity on activated T cells through selective high affinity binding to CXCR3. J Exp Med *187*, 2009-2021.

Dufour, J.H., Dziejman, M., Liu, M.T., Leung, J.H., Lane, T.E., Luster, A.D. (2002) IFN-g-inducible protein 10 (IP-10; CXCL 10)-deficient mice reveal a role for IP-10 in effector T cell generation and trafficking. J Immunol *168*, 3195-3204.

Dwinell, M.B., Lugering, N., Eckmann, L., and Kagnoff, M.F. (2001) Regulated production of interferon-inducible T-cell chemoattractants by human intestinal epithelial cells. Gastroenterol *120*, 49-59.

Farber, J.M. (1997) Mig and IP-10: CXC chemokines that target lymphocytes. J Leukoc Biol *61*, 246-257.

Friedman, S., and Blumberg, R.S. (2010) Inflammatory bowel disease, *In: Harrison's Gastroenterology and Hepatology*, Longo, D., and Fauci, A.S., pp. 174, McGraw Hill, ISBN978-0-07-166333-5, New York

Gerard, C., and Rollins B.J. (2001) Chemokines and disease. Nat Immunol 2, 108-115.

Grimm, M.C., and Doe, W.F. (1996) Chemokines in inflammatory bowel disease mucosa: expression of RANTES, macrophage inflammatory protein (MIP)-1a, MIP-1b, and g-interferon-inducible protein-10 by macrophages, lymphocytes, endothelial cells, and granulomas. Inflamm Bowel Dis 2, 88-96.

Groom, J.R., and Luster, A.D. (2011) CXCR3 in T cell function. Exp Cell Res *317*, 620-631.

Hanawa, T., Suzuki, K., Kawauchi, Y., Takamura, M., Yoneyama, H., Han, G.D., Kawachi, H., Shimizu, F., Asakura, H., Miyazaki, J., Maruyama, H., and Aoyagi, Y. (2006) Attenuation of mouse acute colitis by naked hepatocyte growth factor gene transfer into the liver. J Gene Med 8, 623-635.

Helwig, U., Gionchetti, P., Rizzello, F., Lammers, K., Kuhbacher, T., Schreiber, S., Baggiolini, M., Uguccioni, M, and Campieri, M. (2004) CXC and CC chemokine expression in inflamed and noninflamed pelvic ileal pouch tissue. Int J Colorectal Dis *19*, 165-170.

Hoogewerf, A.J., Kuschert, G.S.V., Proudfoot, A.E.I., Borlat, F., Clark-Lewis, I., Power, C.A., and Wells, T.N.C. (1997) Glycosaminoglycans mediate cell surface oligomerization of chemokines. Biochemistry 36, 13570-13578.

Hyun, J.G., Lee, G., Brown, J.B., Grimm, G.R., Tang, Y., Mittal, N., Dirisina, R., Zhang, Z., Fryer, J.P., Weinstock, J.V., Luster, A.D., and Barrett, T.A. (2005) Anti-interferon-inducible chemokine, CXCL10, reduces colitis by impairing T helper-1 induction and recruitment in mice. Inflamm Bowel Dis *11*, 799-805.

Inatomi, O., Andoh, A., Kitamura, K., Yasui, H., Zhang, Z., and Fujiyama, Y. (2005) Butyrate blocks interferon-g-inducible protein-10 release in human intestinal subepithelial myofibroblasts. J Gastroenterol 40, 483-489.

Izcue, A., Coombes, J.L., and Powrie, F. (2006) Regulatory T cells suppress systemic and mucosal immune activation to control intestinal inflammation. Immunol Rev *212*, 256-271.

Jolicoeur, P. (1991) Murine acquired immunodeficiency syndrome (MAIDS): An animal model to study the AIDS pathogenesis. FASEB J 5, 2398-2405.

Kaser, A., Zeissig, S., Blumberg, R.S. (2010) Inflammatory Bowel Disease. Annu Rev Immunol *28*, 573-621.

Kawauchi, Y., Suzuki, K., Watanabe, S., Yamagiwa, S., Yoneyama, H., Han, G.D., Palaniyandi, S.S., Veeraveedu, P.T., Watanabe, K., Kawachi, H., Okada, Y., Shimizu, F., Asakura, H., Aoyagi, Y., and Narumi, S. (2006) Role of IP-10/CXCL10 in the progression of pancreatitis-like injury in mice after murine retroviral infection. Am J Physiol Gastrointest Liver Physiol *291*, G345-G354.

Khan, I.A., MacLean, J.A., Lee, F.S., Casciotti, L., DeHaan, E., Schwartzman, J.D., Luster, A.D. (2000) IP-10 is critical for effector T cell trafficking and host survival in *Toxoplasma gondii* infection. Immunity *12*, 483-494.

Kuhn, R., Lohler, J., Rennick, D., Rajewsky, K., and Muller, W. (1993) Interleukin-10-deficient mice develop chronic enterocolitis. Cell 75, 263-274.

Loetscher, M., Gerber, B., Loetscher, P., Jones, S.A., Piali, L.Clark-Lewis, I., Baggiolini, M., and Moser, B. (1996) Chemokine receptor specific for IP10 and Mig:structure, function, and expression in activated T-lymphocytes. J Exp Med 184, 963-969.

Luster, A.D.,Unkeless, J.C., Ravetch, J.V. (1985) g-Interferon transcriptionally regulates an early-response gene containing homology to platelet proteins. Nature 315, 672-676.

Luster, A. (1998) Chemokines-chemotactic cytokines that mediate inflammation. New Engl J Med 338, 436-445.

Luster, A.D.,Greenberg, S.M., and Leder, P. (1995) The IP-10 chemokine binds to a specific cell surface heparan sulfate site shared with platelet factor 4 and inhibits endothelial cell proliferation. J Exp Med 182, 21-231.

MacDermott, R.P., Sanderson, I.R., and Reinnecker, HC. (1998) The central role of chemokines (chemotactic cytokines) in the immunopathogenesis of ulcerative colitis and Crohn's disease. Inflammatory Bowel Dis 4, 54-67.

MacDermott, R.P. (1999) Chemokines in the inflammatory bowel diseases. J Clin Immunol 19, 266-272.

Mackay, C.R. (2001). Chemokines: immunology's high impact factors. Nat Immunol 2, 95-101.

Mosier, D.E., Yetter, R.A., and Morse, H.C.III. (1985) Retroviral induction of acute lymphoproliferative disease and profound immunosuppression in adult C57BL/6 mice. J Exp Med 161, 766-784.

Mantovani, A. (1999) The chemokine system: redunduncy for robust outputs. Immunol Today 20, 254-57.

Narumi, S., Tominaga, Y., Tamaru, M. (1998) Expression of IFN-inducible protein 10 in chronic hepatitis.J Immunol 158, 5536-44.

Neville, L.F., Mathiak, G., and Bagasra, O. (1997) The immunobiology of interferon-gamma inducible protein 10 kD (IP-10): a novel, pleiotropic member of the C-X-C chemokine superfamily. Cytokine & Growth Factor Reviews 8, 207-219.

Nishimura, M., Kuboi, Y., Muramoto, K., Kawano, T., and Imai, T. (2009) Chemokines as novel therapeutic targets for inflammatory bowel disease. Ann NY Acad Sci 1173, 350-356.

Noguchi, A., Watanabe, K., Narumi, S., Yamagami, H., Fujiwara, Y., Higuchi, K., Oshitani, N., and Arakawa, T. (2007) The production of interferon-g-inducible protein 10 by granulocytes and monocytes is associated with ulcerative colitis disease activity. J Gastroenterol 42, 947-956.

Ogawa, N., Ping, L., Zhenjun, L., Takada, Y., and Sugai, S. (2002) Involvement of the interferon-g-inducible 10-kd protein (CXCL10) and monokine induced by interferon-g (CXCL9), in the salivary gland lesions of patients with Sjogren's syndrome. Arthritis Rheum 46, 2730-41.

Okayasu, I., Hatakeyama, S., Yamada, M., Ohkusa, T., Inagaki, Y., and Nakya, R. (1990) A novel method in the induction of reliable experimental acute and chronic ulerative colitis in mice. Gastroenterol 98, 694-702.

Ouyang, W., Kolls, J.K., and Zheng, Y. (2008) The biological function of T helper 17 cell effector cytokines in inflammation. Immunity 28, 454-467.

Papadakis, K.A., Prehn, J., Zhu, J.P., Landers, C., Gaiennie, j., Fleshner, P.R., and Targan, S.R. (2004) Expression and regulation of the chemokine receptor CXCR3 on lymphocytes from normal and inflammatory bowel disease mucosa. Inflamm Bowel Dis 6, 778-788.

Podolsky, D.K. (1999) Innate mechanisms of mucosal defense and repair: the best offense is a good defense. Am J Physiol 277, G495-499.

Rossi, D., Zlotnik, A. (2000) The biology of chemokines and their receptors. Ann Rev Immunol 18, 217-242.

Sasaki, S., Yoneyama, H., Suzuki, K., Suriki, H., Aiba, T., Watanabe, S., Kawauchi, Y., Kawachi, H., Shimizu, F., Matsushima, K., Asakura, H., and Narumi, S. (2002) Blockade of CXCL10 protects mice from acute colitis and enhances crypt cell survival. Eur J Immunol 32, 3197-3205.

Schall, T.J., and Proudfoot, A.E.I. (2011) Overcoming hurdles in developing successful drugs targeting chemokine receptors. Nat Rev Immunol 11, 355-363.

Shibahara, T., Wilcox, J.N., Couse, T., and Madara, J.L. (2001) Characterization of epithelial chemoattractants for human intestinal intraepithelial lymphocytes. Gastroenterol 120, 60-70.

Singh, U.P., Singh, S., Taub, D.D., and Lillard, Jr., J.W. (2003) Inhibition of IFN-g-inducible protein-10 abrogates colitis in IL-10$^{-/-}$ mice. J Immunol 171, 1401-1406.

Singh, U.P., Vekataraman, C., Singh, R., and Lillard, Jr., J.W. (2007) CXCR3 axis: role in inflammatory bowel disese and therapeutic implication. Endoc, Metab & Imm Dis-Drug Targets 7, 111-123.

Sorensen, T.L., Trebst, C., Kivisakk, P., Klaege, K.L., Majmudar, A., Ravid, R., Lassmann, H., Olsen, D.B., Striter, R.M., Rasohoff, R.M, and Sellebjerg, F. (2002) Multiple sclerosis: a study of CXCL10 and CXCR3 co-localization in the inflamed central nervous system. J Neuroimmunol 127, 59-68.

Stewenius, J., Adnerhill, I., Ekelund, G.R., Floren, C.H., Fork, F.T., Jenzon, I., Lindstrom, C., and Ogren, M. (1996) Operations in unselected patients with ulcerative colitis and indeterminate colitis: A long term follow-up study. Eur J Surg 162, 131-137.

Strober, W., and Fuss, I.J. (2011) Proinflammatory cytokines in the pathogenesis of inflammatory bowel diseases. Gastroenterol 140, 1756-1767.

Suriki, H., Suzuki, K., Baba, Y., Hasegawa, K., Narisawa, R., Okada, Y., Mizuochi, T., Kawachi, H., Shimizu, F., and Asakura, H. (2000) Analysis of cytokine production in the colon of nude mice with experimental colitis induced by adoptive transfer of imunocompetent cells from mice infected with a murine retrovirus. Clin Immunol 97, 33-42.

Suzuki, K, Kawauchi, Y., Palaniyandi, S.S., Veeraveedu, P.T., Fujii, M., Yamagiwa, S., Yoneyama, H., Han, G.D., Kawachi, H., Okada, Y., Ajioka, Y., Watanabe, K., Hosono, M., Asakura, H., Aoyagi, Y., and Narumi, S. (2007) Blockade of interferon-g-inducible protein-10 attenuates chronic experimental colitis by blocking cellular trafficking and protecting intestinal epithelial cells. Pathol Int 57, 413-420.

Suzuki, K., Narita, T., Yui, R., Ohtsuka, K., Inada, S., Kimura, T., Okada, Y., Makino, M., Mizuochi, T., Asakura, H., and Fujiwara, M. (1997) Induction of intestinal lesions in nu/nu mice induced by transfer of lymphocytes from syngeneic mice infected with murine retrovirus. Gut 41, 221-228.

Suzuki, K., Makino, M., Okada, Y., Kinoshita, J., Yui, R., Kanazawa, H., Asakura, H., Fujiwara, M., Mizuochi, T., and Komuro, K. (1993) Exocrinopathy resembling Sjogren's syndrome induced by a murine retrovirus. Lab Invest 69, 430-435.

Swaminathan, G.J., Holloway, D.E., Colvin, R.A., Campanella, G.K., Papageorgiou, A.C., Luster, A.D., and Acharya, K.R. (2003) Crystal structures of oligomeric forms of the IP-10/CXCL10 chemokine. Structure 11, 521-532.

Tanaka, Y., Adams, D.H., Hubscher, S., Hirano, H., Siebenlist, U., and Shaw S. (1993) T-cell adhesion induced by proteoglycan-immobilized cytokine MIP-1b. Nature 361, 79-82.

Taub, D.D., Lloyd, A.R., Conlon, K., Wang, J.M., Ortaldo, J.R., Harada, A., Matsushima, K., Kelvin, D.J., and Oppenheim, J.J. (1993) Recombinant human interferon-inducible protein 10 is a chemoattractant for human monocytes and T lymphocytes and promotes T cell adhesion to endothelial cells. J Exp Med 177, 1809-1814.

Uguccioni, M., Gionchetti, P., Robbiani, D.F., Rizzello, F., Peruzzo, S., Campieri, M., and Baggiolini, M. (1999) Increased expression of IP-10, IL-8, MCP-1, and MCP-3 in ulcerative colitis. Am J Pathol 155, 331-336.

Viola, A., and Luster, A.D. (2008) Chemokines and their receptors: drug targets in immunity and inflammation. Annu Rev Pharmacol Toxicol 48, 171-97.

Watanabe, S., Suzuki, K., Kawauchi, Y., Yamagiwa, S., Yoneyama, H., Kawachi, H., Okada, Y., Shimizu, F., Asakura, H., and Aoyagi, Y. (2003) Kinetic analysis of the development of pancreatic lesions in mice infected with a murine retrovirus. Clin Immunol 109, 212-223.

Xavier, R. J., and Podolsky, D. K. (2007). Unravelling the pathogenesis of inflammatory bowel disease. Nature 448, 427-434.

Part 3

Complications

9

Ulcerative Proctitis

Gino Caselli Morgado and George Pinedo Mancilla
Unit of Colorectal Surgery, Department of Digestive Surgery,
Pontifical Catholic University of Chile, Santiago
Chile

1. Introduction

Ulcerative colitis (UC) is a chronic inflammatory disease of digestive tract of unknown cause. This disease is characterized by a chronic course with alternating periods of activity and clinical remission. The incidence of UC in America has a range extending from 2.2 to 14.3 per 100,000 population per year [1]. The continuous involvement from the rectum to proximal presents an extension that is variable among patients and in the course of the disease [2]. The extension of the compromise determines its clinical presentation, the treatment and prognosis of UC [2]. Depending on the size, it is classified as proctitis or ulcerative proctitis (UP) when it affects the rectum; left or distal colitis when inflammation is distal to the splenic flexure and extended colitis when the inflammation reaches the transverse colon, right or has an involvement the entire colon [2]. Several studies have attempted to establish the factors that determine the extension of the involvement. Among the factors associated with rectal compromise are middle age patients, absence of serious bleeding and absence of extraintestinal manifestations [3]. However, these factors have not been replicated, so even today there are no factors strongly related to PU [1,4]. The mayority of the new cases are diagnosed in adults as a PU or distal colitis [1,5]. Although initial reports indicated that PU had a low frequency [6], recent studies reported that incidence has been increasing up to 48% and 60% [4,7], whereas the incidence of colitis has been decreasing in most geographic areas [8]. Some authors have suggested that PU represents a completely different clinical entity from the CU [8-9]. However, most authors agree that the PU is an initial form of CU with the potential to extend into the proximal segments of the colon [10-12]. Ulcerative proctitis, unlike other forms of more extensive presentation of CU, is clinically characterized by bleeding and or rectal pushing, without systemic symptoms or abnormal physical examination or laboratory tests and can be treated solely with topical rectal therapies [7].

The 5-aminosalicylates (5-ASA) and corticosteroids are available for topical use as a local anti-inflammatory agents [7]. These drugs can get straight to the site of inflammation, which decreases systemic absorption and minimize potential side effects [7,13]. The oral 5-ASA is also an alternative prior to the use of corticosteroids, as these have a number of risks and limitations in short and long term use, reserving for very severe active PU [14]. When refractory to previous treatment, drugs that can be used to induce and maintain remission are immunomodulators such as azathioprine [15], 6-mercaptopurine [16] and/or Infliximab therapy [17-18].

Mortality and cancer risk associated is no greater than the general population [2], as the PU is usually considered a mild form of UC. However, about 23% of PU patients can reach a colectomy [19] and from 41 to 54% of patients will increase proximally its compromise after 10 years of disease [2-11], indicating that the PU is not always a mild disease.

2. 5-ASA preparations

Topical treatment have been used for a long time and have offered the advantage of delivering a high dose of the compound directly to the site of inflammation, minimizing absorption and therefore limiting the frequency of systemic adverse events [20]. Rectal preparations of 5-ASA are the treatment of choice for distal UC and mild to moderate PU. Various forms of this compound have been tested in different trials, including suppositories, enemas, foams and gels. Mesalazine suppositories 1 g per day administered dose, preferably at night, should be considered as the treatment of choice for active PU, being superior to oral 5-ASA with 91% versus 41% as a induction of the remission [5,11,21,22,23,24]. Scintigraphic studies have shown that this drug consistently reaches the rectum and distal sigmoid to a length of 18-20 cms. from the anal verge [25], being as effective as enemas, but better tolerated and preferred by patients [26]. The dosage of 5-ASA enemas is 4 g in 60 ml with a dosage of 1-2 times daily for 4 weeks. Although equally effective as the enema, foams and gel might offer the advantage of longer intraluminal retention, more homogeneous distribution in the inflamed mucosa and better tolerance by the patients [26,28]. Maintenance treatment is indicated for all cases and the minimum is a one-year treatment [29-30]. A small percentage of patients who could completely stop the therapy, because the relapse is up to 86% to the completion of a twelve months treatment [31]. The algorithm of management of active PU and remission is shown on Fig.1.

3. 5-ASA oral administration

When the patient refuses the use of topical agents or if after 2-4 weeks of treatment with 5-ASA rectally there is no response, the oral 5-ASA (mesalazine or sulfasalazine) should be considered as an alternative. Randomized clinical trials have shown benefits of adding oral 5-ASA compounds (mesalazine) with a dose greater than 3 g per day in active distal UC [32]. No studies demonstrate the efficacy of these compounds as oral monotherapy for PU, although had been proven effective for more extensive UC. It has been postulated that it would be especially useful to prevent proximal extension of disease in the maintenance phase of treatment [32-33]. The administration might be associated with allergic phenomenon and headache among other side effects [13].

4. Steroids in the treatment of PU

For those patients in whom there is no response after 2-4 weeks of topical treatment with aminosalicylates is considering the use of corticosteroids. Several steroids have been effectively administered rectally (suppositories, enemas, foams), including hydrocortisone (100 to 200 mg in 60 to 200 ml), betamethasone, prednisolone phosphate [34] and recently the budesonide, included as a therapeutic agent [35]. Hydrocortisone enemas were significantly superior to placebo with 55% versus 10% induction of remission [36] and have comparable efficacy to systemic corticosteroids and less inhibition of the hypothalamic-pituitary-adrenal axis, as there is direct absorption through the superior and middle rectal veins into the systemic circulation, without passing through the hepatic portal system [35]. Budesonide has been extensively studied during the last decade, when compared with mesalazine and other corticoids. One study compared the response of budesonide foam and hydrocortisone foam in patients who failed to mesalazine, achieving a 52% response in the budesonide group and 37% remission in the group using hydrocortisone foam [36]. Remission with budesonide foam was achieved by 19% of the patients with a minimum dosage of 2 mg per 100 ml for a period of at least 6 weeks, but doses of 8 mg in 100 ml achieved remission in a higher percentage of 27% 4% versus placebo [35-37]. No studies support the use of steroids for maintenance of remission of PU [1]. Despite the benefits delivered by 5-ASA compounds and steroids for rectal administration, some patients fail to achieve remission and require additional therapy. The failure of the administration of drugs is considered the most important factor of refractoriness of the PU, so that by reintroducing the therapy, it could achieve a good response. Patients should also be evaluated for hypersensitivity to aminosalicylates, characterized by an allergic colitis, abdominal pain and diarrhea [1] and by examination or endoscopy to rule out a secondary infection by Clostridium difficile or cytomegalovirus, an extension of the disease to proximal segments the colon or the presence of Crohn's disease. Infection should also be excluded in refractory patients. Patients not responding to therapy, rectal and/or oral (5-ASA and steroids) are in a serious problem, and the options include azathioprine (AZA), 6-mercaptopurine (6-MP), immunomodulators, infliximab, antibiotics and even surgery [1].

5. Antibiotics

Unlike Crohn Disease (CD), the effectiveness of antibiotics in ulcerative colitis has not been proven [1]. Both ciprofloxacin, tobramycin and metronidazole have been studied, despite a clear trend toward improvement, showed no superiority in terms of the induction or maintenance of remission in UC [38]. Although in some studies there was a clinical/endoscopic response about 80%, sustained remission was not obtained, and recurrence was similar to placebo [39]. There are no studies showing the effect of the antibiotics in PU.

6. Azathioprine and 6-mercaptopurine in PU

The AZA and 6-MP are a key part in the therapy of IBD [40], mainly in steroid-dependent and resistant cases. Strong scientific evidence available on the role of AZA and 6-MP in UC is more limited than in CD [41], has been released placebo-controlled studies evaluating the efficacy of these drugs in the induction of remission in patients with active UC, in which it is established that AZA had no effect in achieving remission, but decreases the proportion of relapse [42-43]. Nor has largely been assessed for the maintenance of remission of UC. There are no studies evaluating exclusively the effectiveness of these compounds in PU or distal colitis, but it is considered as a valid alternative in the treatment [32].

7. Cyclosporine

Several studies show that cyclosporine is effective in inducing remission in severe UC [44]. The relatively fast response makes the use of cyclosporine potentially attractive, but long-term benefit are unclear, especially when life-threatening side effects can occur such as nephrotoxicity and opportunistic infections. There are no randomized trials showing the effectiveness of immunosuppression for refractory PU and studies are only anecdotal [45-46].

8. PU and biological therapy

Biologic therapies attempt to restore the balance between pro-inflammatory and anti-inflammatory effects observed in IBD. Infliximab is a chimeric monoclonal antibody (IgG) derived from recombinant DNA, consisting of genes of human and murine origin. These bonds and neutralizes tumoral necrosis factor alpha (TNFα), thus interrupting the sequential cascade of activation of inflammatory pathways mediated by this cytokine. Infliximab was reviewed in controlled randomized studies ACT 1 and ACT 2, demonstrating its benefit in patients with moderately to severely active UC, as well as refractory UC [47]. However, these tests excluded patients with only PU. Among the advantages of this drug include a rapid onset of action and the possibility of achieving endoscopic and histological normalization of the mucosa. It showed a 30% remission and 60% improvement in patients and close to 70% of the patients refractory to 5-ASA, corticosteroids or AZA/6-MP respond to Infliximab [48]. However, the use of infliximab in this condition is poor [1]. The algorithm for management of refractory PU is shown on Fig.2.

9. Other investigational therapies

Transdermal patches and nicotine enemas [47], low molecular weight heparins [50], light chain fatty acids rectal administration [45] and probiotics [51] have been dismissed for handling the left CU or PU, given the low level of evidence and its low efficacy in inducing remission in active crisis.

10. Surgery in ulcerative proctitis

Although PU can be sometimes refractory to all therapies available, it is rare surgery being considered as a treatment option. Surgery has being used between 2-9% at 5 years [52-53] to 23% at 20 years [54]. For those patients who do require surgery, proctocolectomy with end ileostomy or the confection of an ileal reservoir-anal anastomosis are the options [1]. We emphasize that no published studies that demonstrate short or long term results of surgery in refractory PU.

11. What is the future treatment for the PU?

Protocols of therapeutic strategies based on the best scientific evidence has improved significantly the prognosis of patients with PU in recent years. The availability of biological therapies and the advances in colorectal surgery opens up new prospects for evaluating the usefulness of these alternatives in the refractory PU to conventional treatment. This has been associated with the development of new drugs which would yield an improvement in symptoms with fewer side effects, which are not yet available.

The use of epidermal growth factor (EGF) enemas has delivered good results and it is an effective treatment for ulcerative left colitis and mild to moderate PU associated with oral mesalamine [55]. This compound stimulates the migration, proliferation and repair the injuries of the gastric, intestinal and colonic mucosa. Studies shows a 83% of remission in the EGF-enema group vs 8% of placebo group after 2 weeks of treatment. Despite reducing the activity and inducing clinical remission, clinical studies should be conducted to compare EGF versus high doses of mesalamine or corticosteroids [55]. Rebamipide is an aminoacid 2(1H)-quinolinone derivate, used for the protection of gastric and duodenal mucosa. It acts through the suppression of neutrophil functions, stimulation of epithelial cell regeneration and increased the expression of epidermal growth factor (EGF) and its receptor. Through a prospective study was found that Rebamipide enema in distal colitis and active PU local topical therapy could be effective in the treatment of mild to moderate active disease [56]. There were no adverse effects related to the Rebamipide in the 16 patients included in the study [57]. Tacrolimus is an immunosuppressive drug produced that has been used mainly in transplantation and autoimmune diseases. The mechanism is similar to cyclosporine, but is better tolerated and is a hundred times more potent than this. Acts directly on T-lymphocytes, inhibiting the transcription of IL-2, decreasing lymphocytic response to antigens [58] and inhibiting the release of inflammatory mediators from mast cells and basophils. Lawrence et al [58] achieved complete remission after 8 weeks of treatment with rectal tacrolimus in 75% of the patients studied, all resistant to conventional therapy. The patients who did not responded, presented proximal proggresion of the disease, where the compound did not reach topically. Randomized clinical trials are needed to evaluate its effectiveness versus placebo.

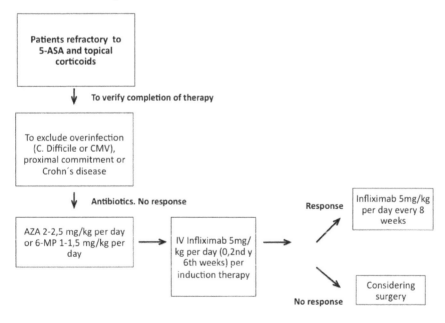

*Adapted from Clinical Guidelines. Inflamm Bowel Dis. 2006;12:972-978 Regueiro et al.

Fig. 1. Algorithm of management of active PU

In summary, topical administration of 5-ASA suppositories, enema or foam is the preferred treatment for most patients with PU. The local administration of 5-ASA is more effective than oral 5-ASA, but the combination of oral and topical should be considered for those without an adequate response to any of these therapies separately. Topical corticosteroids are the second-line treatment either as monotherapy or in combination with topical 5-ASA. Maintenance treatment is indicated in all cases and corresponds to the preferential use of topical 5-ASA, with the oral formulation is also an alternative. Refractory patients or intolerant to 5-ASA may require immunomodulators or biological therapy. Systemic steroids or surgery should be used in very special cases.

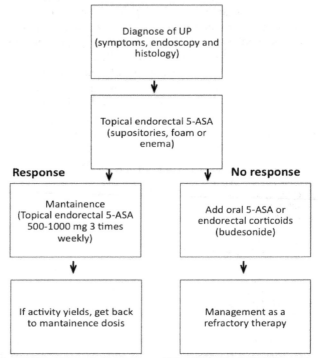

*Adapted from Clinical Guidelines. Inflamm Bowel Dis. 2006;12:972-978 Regueiro et al.

Fig. 2. Algorithm for management of refractory PU

12. References

[1] Regueiro M, Loftus E, Steinhart H, Cohen R. Clinical Guidelines for the medical management of left-sided ulcerative colitis and ulcerative proctitis: Summary statement. Inflamm Bowel Dis 2006;12:972-978.

[2] Silverberg M, Satsangi J, Ahmad T, Arnott I, Bernstein C, Brant S et al. Toward an integrated clinical, molecular and serological classification of inflammatory bowel disease: Report of a Working Party of the 2005 Montreal World Congress of Gastroenterology. Canadian Journal of Gastroenterology 2005; 19 Suppl A:5-36.

[3] Farmer R, Easley K, Rankin G. Clinical patterns, natural history, and progression of ulcerative colitis. A long-term follow-up of 1116 patients. Dig Dis Sci 1993; 38:1137-1146.

[4] Langholz E, Munkholm P, Davidsen M, Bonder V. Course of ulcerative colitis: analysis of changes in disease activity over years. Gastroenterology 1994;107:3-11.

[5] Loftus E. Clinical epidemiology of inflammatory bowel disease: incidence, prevalence and environmental influences. Gastroenterology 2004;126:1504-1517.

[6] Powell-Tuck J, Ritchie J, Lennard-Jones J. The prognosis of idiopathic proctitis. Scand J Gastroenterol 1977;12:727–732.

[7] Pica R, Paoluzi O, Iacopini F, Marcheggiano A, Crispino P, Rivera M et al. Oral mesalazine (5-ASA) treatment may protect against proximal extention of mucosal inflammation in ulcerative proctitis. Inflamm Bowel Dis 2004;10:731-736.

[8] Russel M, Stockbrugger R. Epidemiology of inflammatory bowel disease: An update. Scand J Gastroenterol 1996;31:417-427.

[9] Farmer R. Nonspecific ulcerative proctitis. Gastroenterol Clin North Am 1987;16:157-174.

[10] Ekbom A, Helmick C, Zack M, Adami H. Ulcerative proctitis in central Sweden 1965-1983: A population-based epidemiological study. Dig Dis Sci 1991;36:97-102.

[11] Campieri M, De Franchis R, Bianchi Porro G, Ranzi T, Brunetti G, Barbara L. Mesalazine (5-Aminosalicylic acid) suppositories in the treatment of ulcerative proctitis or distal proctosigmoiditis: A randomized controlled trial. Scandinavian Journal of Gastroenterology 1990;25:663-668.

[12] Breschi G, Parisi G, Gambardella L, Banti S, Bertoni M, Rindi G et al. Evaluation of clinical patterns in ulcerative colitis: a long-term follow-up. Int J Clin Pharmacol Res.1997;17:17-22.

[13] Loftus E Jr, Kane S, Bjorkman D. Systematic review: short-term adverse effects of 5-aminosalicylic acid agents in the treatment of ulcerative colitis. Aliment Pharmacol Ther 2004;19:179-189.

[14] Truelove S, Jewell D. Intensive intravenous regimen for severe attacks of ulcerative colitis. Lancet 1974;1:1041-1048.

[15] Hawthorne A, Logan R, Hawkey C, Foster P, Axon A, Swarbrick E. et al. Randomized controlled trial of azathioprine withdrawal in ulcerative colitis. BMJ 1992;305:20-22.

[16] George J, Present DH, Pou R Bodian C, Rubin P. The long-term outcome of ulcerative colitis treated with 6-mercaptopurine. Am J Gastroenterol 1996;91:1711-1714

[17] Eaden J, Abrams K, Mayberry J. The risk of colorrectal cancer in ulcerative colitis: a meta-analysis. Gut 2001;48:526-535.

[18] Rutgeerts P, Sandborn W, Feagan B, Reinisch W, Olson A, Johanns J et al. Infliximab for induction and maintenance therapy for ulcerative colitis. N Engl J Med 2005; 353:2462-2476

[19] Mir-Madjlessi S, Michener W, Farmer R. Course and prognosis of idiopathic ulcerative proctosigmoiditis in young patients. J Pediatr Gastroenterol Nutr 1986;5:571-575.

[20] Gionchetti P, Rizzello F, Morselli C, Campieri M. Review article: Problematic proctitis and distal colitis. Aliment Pharmacol Ther 2004;20 (Suppl.4):93S-96S.

[21] Gionchetti P, Rizzello F, Belluzzi A. 5-Aminosalicylic acid as enemas or suppositories in distal ulcerative colitis. J Clin Gastroenterol 1988;10:406-409.

[22] Gionchetti P, Rizzello F, Venturi A, Ferretti M, Brignola C, Miglioli M et al. Comparison of oral with rectal mesalazine in the treatment of ulcerative proctitis. Dis Colon Rectum 1998;41:93-97.

[23] NgoyY, Gelinet J, Ivanovic A, Kag J, Schenowitz G, Vilotte J, Rambaud J. Efficacy of a daily application of mesalazine (Pentasa) suppository with progressive release, in the treatment of ulcerative proctitis. A double-blind versus placebo randomized trial. Gastroenterol Clin Biol 1992;16:782-786.

[24] Campieri M, Gionchetti P, Belluzzi A, Brignola C, Tampieri M, Iannone P et al. Optimum dosage of 5-aminosalicylic acid as rectal enemas in patients with active ulcerative colitis. Gut 1991;32: 929-931.

[25] Williams C, Haber G, Aquino J. Double blind, placebo-controlled evaluation of 5-ASA suppositories in active proctitis and measurement of extent of spreads using 99m-Tc labelled 5-ASA suppositories. Dig Dis Sci 1987;32:71S-75S.

[26] Van Bodegraven A, Boer B, Lourens J, Tuynmn H, Sindram J. Distribution of mesalazine enemas in active and quiescent ulcerative colitis. Aliment Pharmacol Ther 1996;10:327-332.

[27] Campieri M, Paoluzi P, D'Albasio G, Brunetti G, Pera A, Barbara L. Better quality of therapy with 5-ASA colonic foam in patients with ulcerative colitis. Aliment Pharmacol Ther 1997;11:679-684.

[28] Marteau P, Crand J, Foucault M, Rambaud J. Use of mesalazine slow release suppositories 1 g three times per week to maintain remission of ulcerative proctitis: a randomised double blind placebo controlled multicentre study. Gut 1998;42:195-199.

[29] Mantzaris G, Hatzis A, Petraki K, Spiliadi C, Triantaphyllou G. Intermittent therapy with high-dose 5-aminosalicylic acid enemas maintains remission in ulcerative proctitis and proctosigmoiditis. Dis Colon Rectum 1994;37:58-62.

[30] Banerjee S, Peppercorn M. Inflammatory bowel disease: medical therapy for specific clinical presentations. Gastroenterol Clin N Am. 2002;31:185-202.

[31] Regueiro M, Loftus E, Steinhart H, Cohen R. Medical management of left-sided ulcerative colitis and ulcerative proctitis: Clinical Evaluation of Therapeutic Trials. Inflamm Bowel Dis 2006;12:979-994

[32] Lakatos P, Lakatos L. Ulcerative proctitis: a review of pharmacotherapy and management. Expert Opin Pharmacother 2008;9:741-749.

[33] Marshall J, Irvine E. Rectal corticosteroids versus alternative treatment in ulcerative colitis: a meta-analysis. Gut 1997;40:775-781.

[34] Truelove S, Hambling M. Treatment of ulcerative colitis with local hydrocortisone hemisuccinate sodium; a report on a controlled therapeutic trial. Br Med J 1958;2:1072-1077.

[35] Hanauer S, Robinson M, PruitT R, Lazenby A, Persson T, Nilsson L et al. Budesonide enema for treatment of active, distal ulcerative colitis and proctitis. A dose ranking study. U.S. Budesonide enema study group. Gastroenterology 1998;115:525-532.

[36] Bar-Meir S, Fidder H, Faszczyk M, Bianchi G, Stuirnolo G, Mickisch O et al. Budesonide foam vs. Hidrocortisone acetate foam in the treatment of active ulcerative proctosgmoiditis. Dis Colon Rectum 2003;46:929-936.

[37] Lobo A, Burke D, Sobala G, Axon A. Oral Tobramycin in ulcerative colitis: effect on maintenance of remission. Aliment Pharmacol Ther 1993;7:155-158.

[38] Turunen U, Frakkila M, Hakala K, Seppala K, Sivonen A, Ogren M. et al . Long-term treatment of ulcerative colitis with ciprofloxacin: a prospective double-blind, placebo-controlled study. Gastroenterology 1998;115:1072-1078.

[39] Ejderhamm J, Browaldh L, Oldaeus G, Saalman R, Stenhammar L. Treatment with glucocorticosteroid enemas in children with ulcerative colitis; a randomized single-blind multicenter comparison between budesonide and prednisolone. Gut 1999;45(Suppl V):A170.

[40] Gisbert J, Gomollon F, Mate J, Pajares J. Preguntas y respuestas sobre el papel de la azatioprina y la 6-mercaptopurina en el tratamiento de la enfermedad inflamatoria intestinal. Gastroenterol Hepatol 2002;25:401-415.

[41] Jewell D, Truelove S. Azathioprine in ulcerative colitis: final report on controlled therapeutic trial. Br Med J 1974;4:627-630.

[42] Caprilli R, Carratu R, Babbini M. A double-blind comparison of the effectiveness of azathioprine and sulfasalzine in idiopathic proctocolitis. Preliminary report. Dig Dis 1975;20:115-120.

[43] Sood A, Midha V, Sood N, Kaushal V. Role of azathioprine in severe ulcerative colitis: one-year, placebo- controlled, randomized trial. Indian J Gastroenterol 2000;19:14-16.

[44] Shibolet O, Regushevskaya E, Mayer Brezis, Soares-Weiser K, Cyclosporine A for induction of remission in severe ulcerative colitis (Review). Cochrane Database of Syst Rev 2005;1:1-16.

[45] Breuer R, Soergel K, Lashner B, Christ M. Hanauer S, Vanaguna A et al. Short-chain fatty acid rectal irrigation for left-sided ulcerative colitis: a randomised, placebo controlled trial. Gut 1997;40:485-491.

[46] Hyams J, Davis P, Lerer T, Colletti R, Bousvaros A, Leichter A et al. Clinical outcome of ulcerative proctitis in children. J Pediatr Gastroenterol Nutr 1997;25:149-152.

[47] Hanauer S, Feagan B, Lichtenstein G, Mayer L, Schreiber S, Colombel J et al. Mantainance infliximab for Crohn´s disease: the ACCENT I randomized trial. Lancet 2002;359:1541-1549.

[48] Van Der Hagen S, Baeten C, Soeters P, Russel M, Beets-Tan R, Van Gemert W. Anti-TNF-alpha (Infliximab) used as induction treatment in case of active proctitis in a multistep strategy followed by definitive surgery of complex anal fistulas in Crohn´s disease: a preliminar report. Dis Colon Rectum 2005;48:758-467.

[49] Sandborn W, Tremaine W, Leighton J, Lawson G, Zins B, Compton R et al. Nicotine tartrate liquid enemas for midly and moderately active left-sided ulcerative colitis unresponsive to first-line therapy: a pilot study. Aliment Pharmacol Ther 1997;11:661-671.

[50] Bloom S, Kiilerich S, Lassen M, Forbes A, Leiper K, Langholz E et al. Low molecular weight heparin (Tinziparin) vs. placebo in the treatment of mild to moderately active ulcerative colitis. Aliment Pharmacol Ther 2004;19:871-878.

[51] Biblioni R, Fedorak R, Tannock G, Madsen K, Gionchetti P, Campieri M et al. VSL#3 probiotic-mixture induces remission in patients with active ulcerative colitis. Am J Gastroenterol 2005;100:1539-1546.

[52] Moum B, Ekbom A, Vatn M, Aadland E, Sauar J, Lygren I et al. Clinical course during the 1st year after diagnosis in ulcerative colitis and Crohn´s disease. Results of a

large, prospective population-based study in Southeastern Norway, 1990-93. Scand J Gastroenterol. 1997;32:1005-1012.

[53] Ritchie J, Powell-Tuck J, Lennard-Jones J. Clinical outcome of the first ten years of ulcerative colitis and proctitis. Lancet 1978;1:1140-1143.

[54] Gionchetti P, Ardizzone S, Benvenuti M, Bianchi-Porro G, Biasco G, Cesari P et al. A new mesalazine gel enema in the treatment of left-sided ulcerative colitis: a randomized controlled trial. Aliment Pharmacol Ther 1999;13:381-388.

[55] Sinha A, Nightingale J, West K, Berlanga-Acosta J, Playford R. Epidermal growth factor enemas with oral mesalamine for mild-to-moderate left-sided ulcerative colitis or proctitis. N Engl J Med 2003;349:350-357.

[56] Mariyama K, Takeshima F, Hamamoto T. Efficacy of Rebamipide enemas in active distal ulcertive colitis and proctitis: A prospective study report. Dig Dig Sci 2005;50:2323-2329.

[57] Arakawa T, Kobayashi F, Yoshieaka T, Tarnawski A. Rebamipide: overview of its mechanism of action and efficacy in mucosal protection and ulcer healing. Dig Dis Sci 1998;43(Suppl 9):5S-13S.

[58] Lawrence I, Copeland T. Rectal Tacrolimus in the treatment of resistant ulcerative proctitis. Alimen Pharmacol Ther 2008;28:1214-1220.

Extraintestinal Manifestations of Ulcerative Colitis

Brian Huang, Lola Y. Kwan and David Q. Shih
Cedars Sinai Medical Center, Inflammatory Bowel and Immunobiology Institute (IB)
USA

1. Introduction

Inflammatory bowel disease (IBD) consists predominantly of ulcerative colitis (UC) and Crohn's disease (CD), which are clinically distinguished by intestinal localization, local features of inflammation, a profile of complications, and familial aggregation. UC is characterized by recurring episodes of continuous inflammation limited to the mucosal layer of the colon and rectum, and approximately 42% of UC patients have extraintestinal complications (Ozdil et al., 2004). This chapter highlights key features of each involved organ system including association, diagnosis, and treatment options.

2. Extraintestinal manifestations of Ulcerative Colitis

The extraintestinal manifestations (EIMs) of UC can affect any organ system ranging from more common ones including the skin and hepatobiliary systems, to less common ones including the cardiovascular and renal systems (Das, 1999). Studies have shown that the development of one EIM can increase the risk of developing additional complications (Monsen et al., 1990).

2.1 Skin and mucocutaneous complications

The skin is one of the most commonly affected organ systems in IBD patients. The two most common skin disorders associated with UC, erythema nodosum (EN) and pyoderma gangrenosum (PG), are reactive due to an immunologic response to UC. Non immunologic causes can also occur secondary to nutritional deficiencies and medication side effects. (Das, 1999; Timani & Mutasim, 2008). Skin disorders seen in UC caused by malnutrition include diseases such as pellagra and cheilitis. Aphthae are the most common complication of the oral mucosa, while fissures and fistulae are most common in the perianal mucosa. [FIGURES 1 AND 2] (Areias & Garcia E Silva, 1987). Standard medications used to treat UC include steroids and immunosuppressants which can cause skin disorders such as cushingoid features and drug eruptions (Timani & Mutasim, 2008). Other disorders, such as Sweet's syndrome and psoriasis have been associated with UC (Timani & Mutasim, 2008).

2.1.1 Erythema Nodosum

EN affects about 3% of patients with UC (Areias & Garcia E Silva, 1987; Evans & Pardi, 2007; Mir-Madjlessi et al., 1985; Timani & Mutasim, 2008). Lesions affect females with UC more

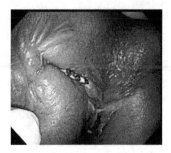

Fig. 1. Fistula with a seton

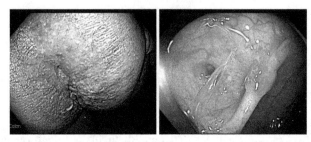

Fig. 2. UC patient with peri-anal fistula (left). Endoscopic view of fistula (right)

frequently than men and EN rarely precedes the initial diagnosis of UC (Trost & Mcdonnell, 2005; Weinstein et al., 2005). Typical EN lesions present as painful, raised subcutaneous lesions located on extensor surfaces of the extremities (Evans & Pardi, 2007; Timani & Mutasim, 2008). However, UC patients almost always have EN lesions on the anterior surface of the legs [FIGURE 3] (Mir-Madjlessi, Taylor et al., 1985). The skin nodules are non-ulcerating and resemble a bruise on the skin (Timani & Mutasim, 2008). Unlike PG, EN lesions mirror UC disease activity and worsen with colonic flares (Timani & Mutasim, 2008). The average lag time between initial UC diagnosis and appearance of EN is 5 years (Mir-Madjlessi, Taylor et al., 1985).

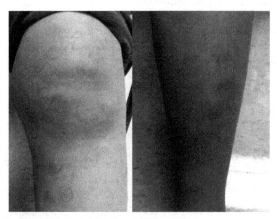

Fig. 3. EN affecting the lower extremities in a UC patient

As EN lesions and UC disease activity usually parallel each other, treatment of the underlying UC usually controls the EN lesions. Most lesions are self-limiting, thus a conservative approach to therapy is often practiced, such as leg elevation, rest, non-steroidal anti-inflammatory drugs (NSAIDs), and potassium iodide (Horio et al., 1981; Marshall & Irvine, 1997; Schulz & Whiting, 1976). In situations where lesions occur during quiescent phases of UC, treatment with oral steroids is effective. Studies have shown that time to remission in patients with EN is approximately 5 weeks which is significantly shorter than that seen in PG (Timani & Mutasim, 2008; Tromm et al., 2001).

2.1.2 Pyoderma Gangrenosum

The incidence of PG in patients with UC varies between 1.4 and 5% (Areias & Garcia E Silva, 1987; Mccallum & Kinmont, 1968). PG is more commonly seen in patients with UC as opposed to CD, and as with EN, there is a slight female predilection (Bernstein et al., 2001b; Greenstein et al., 1976). PG was initially described in 1930 as necrotic ulcers with expanding borders of erythema (Newell & Malkinson, 1982). The onset of noninfectious pustules and nodules eventually expand outwards to develop painful shallow and deep ulcers (Callen, 1998; Farhi & Wallach, 2008). PG usually occurs on the legs, but can also appear anywhere on the skin [FIGURE 4]. Pathergy, a phenomenon in which skin lesions develop secondary to local trauma, has been reported in approximately 30% of cases of PG (Blitz & Rudikoff, 2001; Callen, 1998). The average lag time between initial UC diagnosis and appearance of PG is 10 years (Mir-Madjlessi, Taylor et al., 1985). Diagnosis of PG is usually clinical, but skin biopsy may be necessary for confirmation. PG is classified as a type of neutrophilic dermatosis in which the inflammatory infiltrate seen on microscopic examination shows dense dermal neutrophilic infiltrates without any evidence of infection (Cohen, 2009; Timani & Mutasim, 2008). Unlike EN, there is no temporal relationship between onset of UC flares and the course of PG lesions (Thornton et al., 1980).

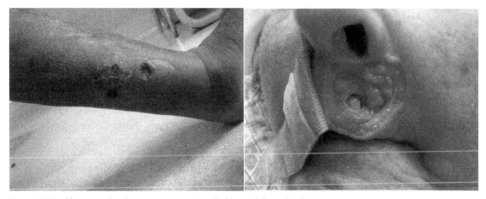

Fig. 4. PG affecting the lower extremity (left) and face (right)

In general, the PG lesions are more severe and refractory to therapy than EN. Treatment of the underlying UC activity does not always resolve the PG lesions and about 30% of patients require additional treatment (Mir-Madjlessi, Taylor et al., 1985). The mainstay of treating PG has been a combination of topical, intralesional, and systemic medications, but no specific therapy has proven to be universally effective (Cohen, 2009; Timani & Mutasim, 2008). Treatments with the best clinical evidence include systemic corticosteroids and cyclosporine as maintenance therapy (Wollina, 2002), assuming there is no concurrent infection. Initial doses of oral prednisone have ranged from 0.5 to 2 mg/kg/day and initial cyclosporine doses have ranged from 2 to 5 mg/kg/day (Timani & Mutasim, 2008; Wollina, 2002). Maintaining target trough serum levels of 150-350 ng/ml for cyclosporine has shown to be effective in improving PG lesions (Cohen, 2009; Curley et al., 1985; Matis et al., 1992; Turner et al., 2010). In small lesions, intralesional steroid injections can be considered (Timani & Mutasim, 2008). Other agents including azathioprine, cyclophosphamide, methotrexate, high dose intravenous immunoglobulin, mycophenolate mofetil, minocycline, plasmapheresis, and hyperbaric oxygen treatment have been employed with variable efficacy (Cohen, 2009; Timani & Mutasim, 2008; Tutrone et al., 2007; Wasserteil et al., 1992). Biologics including infliximab and adalimumab have also been reported to improve PG lesions (Alkhouri et al., 2009; Brooklyn et al., 2006). Additionally, optical treatments such as steroids, tacrolimus, benzoyl peroxide, and hydrogen peroxide have shown positive results (Callen & Jackson, 2007). To avoid pathergy, unnecessary surgical interventions should be avoided. However, surgery can be considered if medical therapies are not successful. Proper timing of the surgery with immunosuppressants is essential for optimal long term wound stabilization (Rozen et al., 2001; Wittekindt et al., 2007; Wollina, 2002).

2.1.3 Sweet's syndrome

Sweet's syndrome (SS), also known as acute febrile neutrophilic dermatosis, has a female predilection and classically affects women between the ages of 30 and 50 years (Timani & Mutasim, 2008). Although the pathogenesis is unclear, Sweet's syndrome usually develops as a response to some type of underlying systemic disease, such as infection, malignancy, medications, or IBD (Vij et al., 2010) In fact, studies have shown that patients with SS have underlying disease in 50% of cases and an underlying malignancy in 20% of cases (Kemmett & Hunter, 1990; Souissi et al., 2007). UC and CD are the most common systemic diseases associated with SS (Timani & Mutasim, 2008). SS is characterized by an acute onset of fever, leukocytosis, and tender, erythematous plaques that can occur on the extremities, face, neck, and trunk (Burrall, 1999; Kemmett & Hunter, 1990; Souissi, Benmously et al., 2007). When these lesions occur on the lower extremities, they often resemble EN and skin biopsy may be necessary to differentiate the two disease processes (Guhl & Garcia-Diez, 2008). These lesions are burning-like and non-pruritic in quality. Other associated symptoms include, but are not limited to arthralgia, headache, fatigue, and other constitutional symptoms. Other organ systems such as the eye, kidney, liver, and pancreas can be involved as well (Cohen et al., 1988). As is also seen with PG, skin biopsy reveals neutrophilic infiltrates in the reticular dermis upon histopathological examination (Kemmett & Hunter, 1990; Timani & Mutasim, 2008). The onset of symptoms from SS usually occur after the initial diagnosis of UC (Darvay, 1996).

The mainstay of treatment for SS is steroids and multiple studies have shown dramatic improvement with a 6 week course of systemic corticosteroid therapy (Cohen, Talpaz et al., 1988; Souissi, Benmously et al., 2007). Topical or intralesional steroids are effective for localized disease (Timani & Mutasim, 2008). Recurrence is common and has been reported to affect approximately 1/3 of patients (Kemmett & Hunter, 1990). Untreated lesions have been reported to heal after variable periods of time, but can be associated with scarring (Kemmett & Hunter, 1990; Timani & Mutasim, 2008). Other alternative first line treatments include potassium iodide and colchicine. Second line agents including indomethacin and clofazimine have been used with successful results, but are not as effective as corticosteroids, potassium iodide, and colchicine (Cohen, 2009; Cohen & Kurzrock, 2002).

2.1.4 Mucocutaneous manifestations

Aphthous Stomatitis. About 4.3% of UC patients experience recurrent aphthous stomatitis and symptom onset often parallels UC disease activity (Areias & Garcia E Silva, 1987; Timani & Mutasim, 2008). Minor aphthous ulcers are small, round, painful, and heal within 2 weeks without scarring, while major recurrent ulcers are larger, can last for 6 weeks, and frequently scar [FIGURE 5] (Ship, 1996; Timani & Mutasim, 2008). A study showed that a majority of patients with multiple aphthous ulcers had underlying IBD (Letsinger et al., 2005). The pathogenesis of aphthous stomatitis and UC is still unclear; studies have not been successful in proving that these ulcers are secondary to vitamin deficiencies as the lesions did not improve with vitamin therapy (Basu & Asquith, 1980). Treatment options include treating the underlying UC, symptomatic relief with steroid elixirs, and systemic treatment with steroids and immunosuppressants (Basu & Asquith, 1980; Timani & Mutasim, 2008).

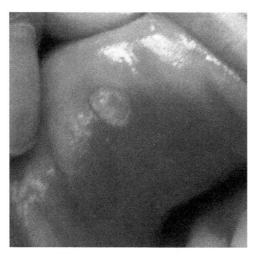

Fig. 5. Aphthous stomatitis in a UC patient

Pyostomatitis Vegetans. Pyostomatitis vegetans, a rare disorder of the oral mucosa, has been shown to be a specific marker for IBD, especially UC (Storwick et al., 1994; Timani & Mutasim, 2008). Lesions are hyperplastic folds of the mucosa with small abscesses and erosions and often manifest before the diagnosis of UC (Hansen et al., 1983).

Pyostomatitis vegetans is usually resistant to treatments such as topical steroids, antibiotic mouthwashes, or hydrogen peroxide. Systemic steroids and immunosuppressants have been employed with variable success, but were not always successful in maintaining remission (Timani & Mutasim, 2008). In one case report, topical fluocinonide gel resulted in temporary state of remission, but total colectomy was necessary to achieve complete remission (Calobrisi et al., 1995).

2.1.5 Miscellaneous skin disorders

Studies report an increased risk of psoriasis with UC. In one study, of 88 patients with UC, 5.7% had psoriasis, compared to 1.5% in the control group, suggesting some type of genetic relationship between the two (Yates et al., 1982). Another study found an association between UC and hidradenitis suppurativa [FIGURE 6].

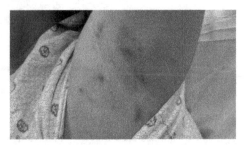

Fig. 6. UC patient with hidradenitis suppurativa

2.2 Hepatopancreatobiliary complications

There are multiple types of hepatic, biliary, and pancreatic complications associated with UC. Pancreatic complications are less common than hepatobiliary complications, but will be discussed in this section as well given its anatomic location.

2.2.1 Primary Sclerosing Cholangitis (PSC)

PSC is a chronic cholestatic liver disease that is caused by progressive inflammatory destruction of intra- and extra-hepatic bile ducts, which leads to multifocal biliary strictures, resulting in liver cirrhosis and failure. PSC is believed to be the result of a combination of genetic and immunological factors, resulting in immune dysfunction and improper targeting of the biliary system by lymphocytes and autoantibodies (Bergquist et al., 2008; Karlsen et al., 2007; Saarinen et al., 2000). Multiple autoantibodies including ANA, RF and atypical p-ANCA have been described in UC and PSC patients (Chapman et al., 2010; Terjung & Spengler, 2009). Atypical p-ANCA is detected by indirect immunofluorescence staining on ethanol fixed neutrophils in a perinuclear or nuclear pattern whereas classical ANCA targets myeloperoxidase and proteinase 3 in a perinuclear pattern (Terjung et al., 1998). Atypical p-ANCA is detectable in approximately 70% of PSC patients with or without UC and is also described in autoimmune hepatitis in patients with IBD (Duerr et al., 1991; Saxon et al., 1990; Terjung & Spengler, 2009). Atypical p-ANCA recognizes both beta isoform 5 in human neutrophils and bacterial cell division protein FtsZ, which is highly conserved across bacterial microflora in the gut (Terjung et al., 2010). This evidence supports the theory of a combined pathogenesis of PSC or autoimmune hepatitis in UC. It is proposed that an altered immune response to bacterial antigen in the gut lumen results in a "leaky gut" and stimulation of pattern recognition receptors (cross-recognition between bacterial antigen in the gut and host components, such as beta isoform 5 in neutrophils) which gives rise to autoimmunity phenomenon. (Terjung & Spengler, 2009).

PSC typically affects young to middle aged males (male to female ratio of 2:1) and while only 5% of patients with UC will develop PSC, about 70% to 80% of cases of PSC occur in patients with UC (Charatcharoenwitthaya & Lindor, 2006; Lundqvist & Broome, 1997). The onset of PSC can precede or follow the onset of UC, and may not be related to UC disease activity (Larsen et al., 2010). An isolated alkaline phosphatase level may be the only finding during the early stages of the disease, but PSC usually manifests with chronic intermittent obstructive jaundice. As the disease progresses, serum bilirubin will rise (Lee & Kaplan, 1995). In the latter course of the disease, the prothrombin time will be prolonged and serum albumin level will decrease, signaling progression to hepatic failure. Other symptoms such as right upper quadrant abdominal pain, pruritus, fatigue, fever, and weight loss are variably present. However, PSC should be suspected in asymptomatic patients with an isolated elevation of serum alkaline phosphatase (Larsen, Bendtzen et al., 2010). Symptomatic patients manifest with icterus, jaundice, hepatomegaly and splenomegaly (Chapman, Fevery et al., 2010; Farrant et al., 1991; Wiesner et al., 1989).

Pericholangitis, described by studies as PSC of the small bile ducts, is another complication of UC. A study of 107 patients with UC showed that 35% patients had "small duct" PSC compared to 17% with "large duct" PSC, but histologic examinations were indistinguishable from each other (Wee & Ludwig, 1985). These findings imply that rather than being separate disorders, PSC and pericholangitis merely affect different areas of the same disease process. Pericholangitis (or small-duct PSC) is now referred to patients with biochemical and histologic characteristics of PSC, but with normal appearing cholangiograms (Wee & Ludwig, 1985). Small-duct PSC is more often associated with Crohn's disease whereas large-duct PSC (classical PSC) is more often associated with UC (Bjornsson et al., 2008; Loftus, 1997; Rasmussen et al., 1997). Compared to large-duct PSC, small-duct PSC has a relatively favorable prognosis with longer transplant-free survival. Approximately 25% of patients with small-duct PSC progress to large-duct PSC, but usually does not develop into cholangiocarcinoma unless it progresses to large-duct PSC (Bjornsson, Olsson et al., 2008).

The gold standard for diagnosis is endoscopic retrograde cholangiopancreatography (ERCP) and typical radiographic findings include multifocal strictures and dilatation of the intra- and/or extra-hepatic biliary tracts, producing a "beaded pattern" (Lee & Kaplan, 1995; Maccarty et al., 1983). Recently, magnetic resonance cholangiopancreatography (MRCP) has emerged as a non-invasive alternative in diagnosing suspected PSC (Chapman, Fevery et al., 2010). ERCP may be more preferable over MRCP in diagnosing early stage PSC having a specificity and sensitivity near 100% (Angulo et al., 2000; Berstad et al., 2006; Moff et al., 2006). However, ERCP does carry potential for significant risks and complications (Larsen, Bendtzen et al., 2010). Hence, there has been an increased use of MRCP as an initial diagnostic tool, followed by ERCP as needed. If the diagnosis is in doubt, liver biopsy can assist in the confirmation of diagnosis as well as staging of disease (Charatcharoenwitthaya & Lindor, 2006). However, the classic pathognomonic finding of "onion-skin lesions" or periductal concentric fibrosis is rarely seen (Chapman, Fevery et al., 2010). Liver biopsy can be essential in the diagnosis of small-duct PSC, but is not required for the diagnosis of large-duct PSC (Burak et al., 2003; Chapman, Fevery et al., 2010).

Multiple studies show that using ursodeoxycholic acid (UDCA) at moderate to high dosages has been shown to improve liver histology and liver biochemistry (Smith & Befeler, 2007). Even though UDCA has not been demonstrated to improve either symptoms or mortality, it has been shown to reduce the incidence of colonic dysplasia, colorectal carcinoma and cholangiocarcinoma (Pardi et al., 2003). Focus should be on starting these patients early enough to delay progression to cirrhosis, cholangiocarcinoma, and death. This is especially important as UDCA is not as effective in patients with end stage PSC. During treatment with UDCA, stenosis of bile ducts may occur and endoscopic intervention with dilatation has been showed to be effective (Stiehl, 2004). At the present time, liver transplantation is the only effective treatment especially for end-stage PSC or PSC with cholangiocarcinoma (Chapman, Fevery et al., 2010; Navaneethan & Shen, 2010). Orthotopic liver transplantation is the established treatment in PSC with 85% to 90% of 5-year survival rate (Gow & Chapman, 2000). However, 20 to 25% of transplanted patients develop recurrent PSC 5 to 10 years after transplant (Alabraba et al., 2009; Campsen et al., 2008; Graziadei et al., 1999; Navaneethan & Shen, 2010).

2.2.2 Malignancies

PSC has been shown to be complicated by malignancies including cholangiocarcinoma (CCA), bile duct carcinoma, gall bladder carcinoma, and hepatocellular carcinoma. Studies have shown that patients with UC and PSC are more prone to develop cholangiocarcinoma, colorectal cancer, gallbladder cancer and hepatocellular carcinoma (Broome et al., 1995; Florin et al., 2004; Kitiyakara & Chapman, 2008). Typically CCA presents as an intraductal tumor, and at times can be quite difficult to differentiate from a benign PSC stricture [FIGURE 7]. Evidence supporting diagnosis of CCA include high levels of CA 19-9, cross sectional liver imaging with long, confluent strictures and ERCP with brush biopsy of strictures, in addition to overall clinical presentation (Chapman, Fevery et al., 2010; Charatcharoenwitthaya et al., 2008; Levy et al., 2005). The relative risk of bile duct carcinoma in UC patients is 31.3 compared to the general population and the prognosis is quite poor with a mean survival of less than one year. PSC and pericholangitis are common pre-existing lesions in UC patients with bile duct carcinoma (Mir-Madjlessi et al., 1987). A case report recommended that in patients with UC and PSC with abnormal gallbladders, liver biopsy and cholecystectomy should be performed (Dorudi et al., 1991). Another case report documented an association between fibrolamellar hepatocellular carcinoma and UC complicated by PSC (Snook et al., 1989).

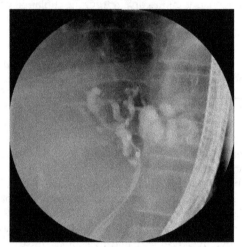

Fig. 7. ERCP of a UC patient with PSC showing high grade strictures within the right and left hepatic ducts with secondary pronounced intrahepatic ductal dilatation

2.2.3 Primary Biliary Cirrhosis (PBC)

PBC is autoimmune in nature with the unique presence of anti-mitochondrial antibodies (AMA) on laboratory testing. Studies have reported that in patients with UC, there is a 30 fold risk of primary biliary cirrhosis compared to the general population (Koulentaki et al., 1999). UC patients with PBC, as compared to patients without UC, are younger and more likely to be male. The mainstay treatment of PBC includes cholestyramine to relieve itching by reducing the amount of bile acid in the blood, UDCA to increase bile flow to reduce inflammation in bile ducts, fat soluble vitamins for nutritional supplementation, and ERCP for bile drainage. Ultimately, advanced PBC with liver failure and portal hypertension requires liver transplantation.

2.2.4 Autoimmune Hepatitis (AIH)

Autoimmune chronic active hepatitis (CAH) has been observed in UC patients with and without PSC (Rabinovitz et al., 1992; Snook, Kelly et al., 1989). In addition to laboratory tests showing the presence of autoantibodies, such ANA and anti-smooth muscle muscle antibody (ASMA) and abnormal liver function tests, liver biopsy may be necessary to confirm the diagnosis (Alvarez et al., 1999). In patients with both UC and autoimmune hepatitis, up to 42% have abnormal cholangiographic findings indicating the coexistence or overlap of PSC (Perdigoto et al., 1992). UC patients with both AIH and PSC respond relatively poorly to immunosuppression and progress more rapidly to cirrhosis. Autoimmune CAH responds to steroids, but in the presence of PSC, dual therapy with steroids and azathioprine is indicated (Perdigoto, Carpenter et al., 1992; Rabinovitz, Demetris et al., 1992). Thus, in patients with UC complicated by autoimmune CAH, cholangiography is necessary to rule out PSC to dictate further therapy.

2.2.5 Other hepatic complications

Fatty liver or hepatic steatosis can be observed in UC patients and appears to correlate with disease severity or duration and may contribute to abnormal liver function tests (Riegler et al., 1998). The ultrasound findings of fatty liver show hepatomegaly and a dysechogenic pattern (De Fazio et al., 1992). Causes of fatty liver include malnutrition, protein loss, and steroid use. Patients are usually asymptomatic and treatment is geared towards treatment of the underlying UC and improving nutritional status (Navaneethan & Shen, 2010).

Hepatic amyloidosis is an extremely rare complication of UC (0.07% vs. 0.9% in CD) and control of gut inflammation can reduce amyloid deposition severity (Greenstein et al., 1992; Navaneethan & Shen, 2010; Wester et al., 2001). Because of the rarity and asymptomatic nature of this complication, the need for liver biopsy remains unclear and should be made on a case-by-case basis.

Hepatic and/or splenic abscesses are rare complications of IBD and even more rare in UC. They are diagnosed by ultrasound or CT scan showing non-enhancing hypodense lesions in the liver and/or spleen. Clinical suspicion of hepatosplenic abscesses should be considered in febrile patients with IBD whose presentations are inconsistent with IBD exacerbation. The treatments of hepatosplenic abscesses include drainage, broad-spectrum antibiotics, and treatment of underlying IBD with sulfasalazine and/or steroids. The pathogenesis of hepatosplenic abscess in UC is unclear at this time with possible mechanisms including infectious and immunologic etiologies (Navaneethan & Shen, 2010).

2.2.6 Portal vein thrombosis

Portal vein thrombosis is considered an EIM of UC and is thought to be secondary to coagulation abnormalities caused by chronic bowel inflammation. Ulceration of the mucosa barrier can increase the chance of gut microbial translocation and thus portal vein thrombosis (Navaneethan & Shen, 2010). Portal vein thrombosis has also been observed in UC patients who were status post proctocolectomy (Navaneethan & Shen, 2010).

2.2.7 Pancreatic complications

Patients with UC have increased chances of developing both acute and chronic pancreatitis (Keljo & Sugerman, 1997). Causes include idiopathic, gallstones, PSC, and medication side effects from drugs such as 5-ASA, mesalamine, corticosteroids, azathioprine, and 6-mercaptopurine. Medication induced pancreatitis does not lead to chronic pancreatitis and treatment involves cessation of the insulting drug (Bank & Wright, 1984). On the other hand, the etiology of chronic pancreatitis is unknown. Chronic pancreatitis with UC is usually painless, but is associated with pancreatic duct strictures and severe pancreatic exocrine insufficiency (Pena et al., 2000).

Autoimmune pancreatitis (AIP) is a less common complication of UC compared to drug-induced or gallstone pancreatitis (Navaneethan & Shen, 2010). It affects elderly individuals and can present with obstructive jaundice. Steroids have become the standard treatment of AIP for obstructive jaundice, abdominal pain, and prevention of future episodes of pancreatitis (Finkelberg et al., 2006; Kamisawa et al., 2009). Failure to respond to steroids raises the possibility of pancreatic cancer and warrants further work up for malignancy.

2.3 Musculoskeletal complications

Musculoskeletal complications are quite common and affect approximately 25% of all IBD patients (Bourikas & Papadakis, 2009; Danese et al., 2005). The musculoskeletal involvement of UC patients can be divided into the following categories:

1. Arthritis: peripheral arthritis, axial arthritis including ankylosing spondylitis (AS) and sacroiliitis
2. Periarticular inflammation: enthesitis, tendonitis, dactylitis, clubbing, periostitis, myositis, fibromyalgia, and granulomatous lesions of the joint and bone
3. Metabolic bone disorders: osteoporosis, osteopenia, osteonecrosis
4. Localized myopathy: orbital myositis, gastrocnemius myalgia syndrome, polymyositis, dermatomyositis
5. Impaired growth: seen in children and adolescents

2.3.1 Arthritis

Peripheral Arthritis: Arthritis, located peripherally or axially, can precede, occur concurrently, or follow the diagnosis of UC (Bourikas & Papadakis, 2009). The type of articular involvement in UC is inflammatory and is associated with pain, heat, swelling, and decreased joint mobility. Similar to rheumatoid arthritis (RA), the pain and stiffness of arthritis in UC is worse in the morning and improves with physical activity. However, unlike RA arthritis, UC arthritis is typically seronegative, non-deforming, and non-erosive. The peripheral arthropathy seen with UC can be classified into two types: Type 1 and Type 2 (Atzeni et al., 2009; Bourikas & Papadakis, 2009; Brakenhoff et al., 2010; Jose & Heyman, 2008).

Type 1 is pauci-articular, asymmetrical in distribution, and typically affects less than 5 large joints, such as the knees, elbows, and ankles. The risk of developing peripheral arthritis is higher in UC patients and increases with colonic involvement (Bourikas & Papadakis, 2009; Jose & Heyman, 2008). The risk of developing type 1 peripheral arthritis is also increased with the presence of other EIMs, such as EN, PG, abscesses, stomatitis, and uveitis (Jose & Heyman, 2008). With the exception of small joints or type 2 polyarticular arthritis, the arthritis usually correlates with UC disease activity (Atzeni, Ardizzone et al., 2009). This type of arthritis is sometimes referred to as colitic arthritis, affects up to 20% of UC patients, and usually presents as an acute self-limiting episode that lasts less than 10 weeks with a median of 5 weeks (Bourikas & Papadakis, 2009; Das, 1999; Jose & Heyman, 2008). However, about 20% to 40% will experience recurrent episodes of arthritis.

Type 2 arthropathy is typically polyarticular, involving 5 or more joints including the small joints of the hands, and most commonly affects the MCP joints of the hands. This type of polyarticular arthritis with IBD is associated with uveitis, but not with other EIMs of IBD.

Unlike type 1 arthritis, symptoms of type 2 arthritis are independent of bowel disease activity and can persist for months to years with a median of 3 years (Bourikas & Papadakis, 2009; Jose & Heyman, 2008). Genetic factors implicated in the association between peripheral arthritis and UC include: HLA-B27, HLA-B35, HLA-DR, and HLA-B44 (Brakenhoff, Van Der Heijde et al., 2010).

Axial Arthritis: Axial arthritis, referred as type 3 arthritis, includes both AS and isolated sacroiliitis. This axial type of arthropathy occurs less frequently than peripheral arthritis, and as with type 2 arthropathy, does not parallel the underlying IBD in clinical course (Bourikas & Papadakis, 2009; Brakenhoff, Van Der Heijde et al., 2010; Jose & Heyman, 2008). In fact, studies have shown that axial arthropathy often precedes UC diagnosis by several years (Bourikas & Papadakis, 2009). In fact, studies have shown that AS occurs in approximately 5% to 10% of patients with IBD and patients are typically young and HLA-B27 positive [FIGURES 8 AND 9]. Presentation involves a severe onset of back pain with morning stiffness that is exacerbated by activity. Spondyloarthritis commonly coincides with periarticular involvement including synovitis, dactylitis, enthesitis, plantar fasciitis, and chest wall pain (Bourikas & Papadakis, 2009). Sacroiliitis seen with UC is often asymptomatic, but can manifest as pelvic pain that improves with movement and sacroiliac joint pain worsened with pelvic brim pressure [FIGURE 10] (Atzeni, Ardizzone et al., 2009).

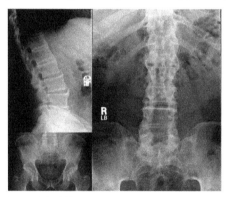

Fig. 8. X-Rays of a UC patient with AS

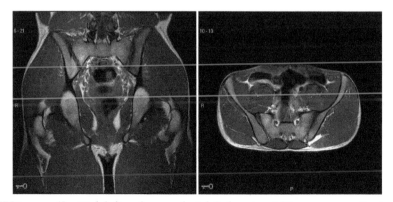

Fig. 9. MRI images (Sagittal, left and coronal, right) showing AS in a young patient with UC

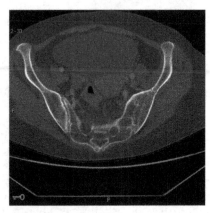

Fig. 10. MRI showing right sided SI and fused left sided joint space

Treatment: The treatment of UC-associated arthropathies is extrapolated from other forms of arthritis (Atzeni, Ardizzone et al., 2009). As with other types of UC EIMs, treatment of the underlying disorder with medical and/or surgical interventions can improve the peripheral arthritis seen with UC (Danese, Semeraro et al., 2005; Jose & Heyman, 2008). Symptomatic treatments include rest, physical therapy, and intra-articular steroid treatments. A short course of celecoxib (COX-2 inhibitor) for 2 weeks has been safely used to treat arthritis in UC (Sandborn et al., 2006). Patients failing to improve should be considered for second-line therapy, including sulfasalazine and immunomodulators (Danese, Semeraro et al., 2005). In patients with active colonic inflammation and peripheral arthritis, biologic agents such as infliximab should be considered (Atzeni, Ardizzone et al., 2009).

In contrast to peripheral arthritis which generally responds to treatment of the colitis, medical and surgical therapy of the underlying bowel disease does not affect the disease course of axial arthropathy. Traditionally, mainstay treatments of AS included intensive physical therapy plus disease-modifying drugs such as sulfasalazine and methotrexate (Atzeni, Ardizzone et al., 2009). However, recent studies have shown that TNF-alpha inhibitor agents such as infliximab are effective in treating AS, IBD, and IBD-associated peripheral and axial arthritis (Atzeni, Ardizzone et al., 2009; Bourikas & Papadakis, 2009; Danese, Semeraro et al., 2005).

2.3.2 Periarticular Inflammation
Periarticular inflammation including enthesitis, tendonitis, clubbing, dactylitis, periostitis, fibromyalgia, and granulomatous lesions of the joints and bones, have been described in UC patients in the presence and absence of arthritis (Bourikas & Papadakis, 2009; Salvarani et al., 2000). These types of periarticular involvement usually do not alter inflammatory markers, but can severely compromise quality of life.

2.3.3 Metabolic bone disorders
Bone disorders such as osteoporosis, osteopenia, and osteonecrosis are associated with UC and this relationship is intensified with concomitant steroid use (Jose & Heyman, 2008). Some studies have shown that in IBD patients, the prevalence rate of osteoporosis can range from 2% to 30% and as high as 40% to 50% for osteopenia (Danese, Semeraro et al., 2005). However, there is still controversy on the exact relationship between UC and osteoporosis.

While one study found approximately 25% of UC patients to have decreased bone mineral density (BMD), another group in Norway found that unlike CD patients, UC patients had relatively normal body compositions without significantly decreased body mass index (BMI) or BMD (Jahnsen et al., 1997; Jahnsen et al., 2003; Vestergaard, 2004). The exact pathogenesis between UC and metabolic bone disorders is not entirely clear, but suggested causes include nutritional deficiency, malabsorption of calcium and vitamin D, steroid use, immobility, and elevated inflammatory cytokines (Danese, Semeraro et al., 2005). Consequently, calcium and vitamin D levels should be checked in UC patients taking steroids. Attempts to minimize steroid dosage and/or duration, substituting steroids with steroid-sparing immunomodulators, or supplementation with bisphosphonates or calcitonin can prevent bone loss and reduce morbidity in these patients (Jose & Heyman, 2008).

Osteonecrosis, also known as aseptic or avascular necrosis, is characterized by bone tissue death secondary to poor vascular supply. Believed to be the result of ischemia of the juxta-articular bone, osteonecrosis has been described in both children and adults with IBD with a prevalence of <1% of all IBD patients and up to 4% of patients taking steroids (Jose & Heyman, 2008; Madsen & Andersen, 1994). Osteonecrosis is a serious complication of UC that should be diagnosed early by magnetic resonance imaging and/or bone scan to prevent serious complications (Madsen & Andersen, 1994). Treatment includes medical management with calcium, vitamin D, bisphosphonates, hydrochlorothiazide, or anti-hypertensive to reduce bone edema. Surgical options include core-decompression biopsy, arthroplasty, or joint replacement (Jose & Heyman, 2008).

2.3.4 Localized myopathy

Muscle involvement is a rare EIM and UC patients are less affected than CD (Bourikas & Papadakis, 2009). The myopathy seen in UC patients can be a direct result of the underlying autoimmune disorder or a side effect of the IBD therapy. In most patients, diagnosis of IBD usually precedes the development of myopathy symptoms. Myopathy disorders that have been associated with UC include orbital myositis, gastrocnemius myalgia syndrome, polymyositis, and dermatomyositis (Bourikas & Papadakis, 2009). Orbital myositis in UC patients is rare and only a handful of cases have been reported (Macarez et al., 2005). It presents as acute orbital pain, diplopia, eyelid swelling, exophthalmos, and conjunctival injection. Diagnosis is made by CT or MRI that can show proptosis and extra-ocular muscle swelling. A case report documented successful results with a short course of systemic steroids and long-term mesalamine therapy (Macarez, Bazin et al., 2005). Gastrocnemius myalgia syndrome usually presents as calf tenderness and is less commonly reported in UC compared to CD. Polymyositis and dermatomyositis in UC patients usually present with proximal muscle weakness (Bourikas & Papadakis, 2009). Diagnostic work up should include CPK, ESR, muscle/skin biopsy, and EMG. Mainstay treatment of the various types of myositis should always include glucocorticoids. TNF-alpha blockers may be required for orbital myositis and azathioprine for polymyositis and dermatomyositis (Bourikas & Papadakis, 2009). A case report of an elderly woman with UC and polymyositis who was treated with corticosteroids and 5-ASA had marked improvement of her muscle weakness (Chugh et al., 1993).

2.3.5 Impaired growth

About 33% of patients with IBD develop symptoms during childhood and adolescence (Ballinger et al., 2001). Of this young population, approximately 28% of UC patients have evidence of growth impairment and delay with onset of bowel symptoms (Berger et al., 1975; Stawarski et al., 2006). The underlying UC causes of this chronic under-nutrition include poor oral intake from fear of colitis exacerbation, malabsorption from inflammation, and hypoalbuminemia secondary to protein-losing enteropathies (Jose & Heyman, 2008). There is evidence that inflammatory cytokines such as IL-6 and TNF-alpha account for the chronic inflammation that impairs linear growth and thus development (Ballinger, Camacho-Hubner et al., 2001). Studies have also shown that high dose daily steroid therapy is associated with diminished type 1 collagen production, which is also important for linear growth. Interestingly, low dose and alternate-day steroid regimens have less dramatic impacts on growth velocity and should be considered as treatment regimens for UC (Berger, Gribetz et al., 1975). Height, weight, puberty staging, and bone age should be regularly checked in young UC patients to prevent poor development. Optimal management of these young patients involves a balance between selecting an appropriate regimen that adequately treats the UC while minimally compromising normal growth and development. Ideally, keeping the underlying bowel disease in remission, especially during puberty, can improve the chance of reaching full growth potential. Calorie supplementation and enteral nutrition should be utilized to meet individualized nutritional goals. (Ballinger, Camacho-Hubner et al., 2001). Surgical interventions eradicating medically refractory disease activity have had more success in reversing growth retardation than high dose steroids, assuming that there was not a significant preexisting delay (Berger, Gribetz et al., 1975).

2.4 Ocular complications

Ocular complications associated with UC were first described in 1925 in two patients with corneal inflammation and conjunctivitis (Crohn, 1925). A large study of 465 UC patients showed that 17 patients (3.6%) had ocular involvement. Of these 17 patients, 7 patients had episcleritis and 5 had iritis or anterior uveitis (Billson et al., 1967). Two patients had blepharo-keratitis and there were single cases of interstitial keratitis, choroiditis, and dacryocystitis reported in this study. Episcleritis, uveitis and conjunctivitis are the most frequent eye manifestations of IBD. Females are affected more frequently than males and eye manifestations were found to be well correlated with UC flares (Billson, De Dombal et al., 1967). Another study reported a higher incidence with 10 out of 78 UC patients (12.8%) having ocular complications (Ozdemir et al., 2000).

2.4.1 Episcleritis

The episclera is the connective tissue between the conjunctiva and sclera. Episcleritis is thus defined as an inflammation of the episclera and its adjacent tissues. The inflammation is usually segmental and bilateral in distribution and associated with eye discomfort, irritation, redness, and tearing [FIGURE 11]. However, there is usually no visual impairment or purulent discharge. Episcleritis responds well to topical steroids (Billson, De Dombal et al., 1967).

2.4.2 Uveitis

The uvea is the middle layer of the eye and is situated between the retina and sclera. It includes the iris, ciliary body, and the choroid of the eye. Uveitis refers to an inflammation of the uvea. Multiple studies and case reports have demonstrated that UC can be associated not only with anterior uveitis, but also posterior, peripheral, or even pan-uveitis (Ozdemir et al., 2000). Symptoms of uveitis include photophobia, blurred vision, pain, and conjunctival injection. Anterior uveitis or iritis is distinguished from other causes of red eye by slit lamp examination and leukocytes seen in the anterior chamber is diagnostic of anterior uveitis. Posterior uveitis can be diagnosed by one of two ways: either by direct visualization of the active chorioretinal inflammation and/or by detecting leukocytes in the vitreous humor by slit lamp or indirect ophthalmoscope. Uveitis usually responds to topical steroid treatment. Severe cases of iritis should be treated with mydriatics to dilate pupils to prevent synechia, in which there is adhesion of the iris to the cornea or lens. It has been speculated that primary treatment of the UC with systemic steroids could account for the relatively low incidence of uveitis in patients with UC (Billson, De Dombal et al., 1967).

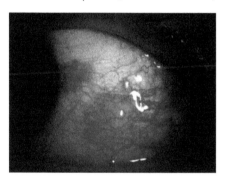

Fig. 11. UC Patient with episcleritis

2.4.3 Scleritis
UC has been associated with different types of anterior scleritis: diffuse, nodular, and posterior scleritis (Ozdemir et al., 2000). Symptoms of scleritis include deep eye pain with radiation to eyebrows, cheeks and temples, eye redness, tearing, photophobia and blurred vision. Severe cases can ultimately lead to blindness. Initial treatments include NSAIDs; oral steroids or immunosuppressants may be necessary for advanced disease. Necrotizing scleritis, the most severe form of scleritis, causes severe inflammation and pain in part of or the entire sclera. This serious disorder is associated with RA, but has also been reported in UC (Lyne & Pitkeathley, 1968). A case report documented a case of severe necrotizing scleritis in a patient with UC that was surgically treated with an amniotic membrane graft and successfully preserved the patient's vision (Lazzaro, 2010).

2.4.4 Optic neuritis
Optic neuritis is inflammation of optic nerve and studies have shown that optic neuritis can be the sole ocular manifestation of UC (Sedwick et al., 1984). Patients with UC who develop rapid and progressive reduction in vision should be suspected to have optic neuritis. Untreated optic neuritis can lead to permanent loss of vision and treatment of optic neuritis typically includes systemic steroid (Nakamura et al., 2005).

One of the key inflammatory mediators of UC includes the cytokine tumor necrosis-alpha (TNF-α). As such, anti-TNF-α therapies are often used to treat patients with UC and are generally well tolerated (Rutgeerts et al., 2005). However, there have been reports of the development of demyelinating disease such as optic neuritis in patients receiving anti-TNF-α therapy (Nash & Florin, 2005). A study of 15 patients who presented with optic neuritis following TNF-α antagonist therapy showed that 9 of these patients experienced full recovery, 2 had partial resolution, and 4 patients continued to be symptomatic (Simsek et al., 2007). It is recommended that patients on anti-TNF-α therapy should be monitored for signs and symptoms of optic neuritis and if symptomatic, should have the medication discontinued.

2.4.5 Other ocular complications

Other ocular complications include marginal keratitis and corneal ulcers, cataracts, recurrent conjunctivitis, blepharitis, retinal vasculitis, retinal vein occlusion, and neuroretinitis (Billson, De Dombal et al., 1967).

In summary, routine eye examinations are recommended for UC patients. Early diagnosis and treatment of ocular involvement can prevent serious and potentially irreversible complications of UC.

2.5 Hematologic and vascular complications

Hematological complications that are associated with UC include (Gomollon & Gisbert, 2009; Imagawa, 1999; Wilson et al., 2004):

1. Anemia of various causes: iron deficiency anemia (IDA), anemia of chronic disease (ACD), folic acid or B12 deficiency, megaloblastic anemia, autoimmune hemolytic anemia, or anemia secondary to marrow-suppressing medications.
2. Granulocytopenia, thrombocytopenia
3. Idiopathic thrombocytopenic purpura
4. Neoplastic (rare): myelodysplastic syndrome, acute or chronic leukemia

In IBD, the prevalence of anemia ranges from 8.8% to 73.7% and the major types of anemia are IDA and ACD (Giannini & Martes, 2006).

2.5.1 Iron deficiency anemia

In addition to biochemical values (serum iron, total iron binding capacity, transferrin, ferritin), new indices of iron metabolism (for example soluble transferrin receptors or sTfR, sTfR-ferritin index, hepcidin, ferritin: transferrin receptor ratio, reticulocyte hemoglobin content or percentage of hypochromic red blood cells) may help with the assessment of IDA and ACD in IBD (Stein et al., 2010; Zhu et al., 2010). Traditionally, IDA is treated with oral iron supplementation. However in patients with UC, not only can oral iron cause more GI side effects, but it is also poorly absorbed in the gut secondary to mucosal inflammation and altered distribution. As a result, the strong oxidizing properties of the unabsorbed iron inside the gut lumen can exacerbate the UC (Zhu, Kaneshiro et al., 2010). Hence, parenteral iron therapy and erythropoietin have been advocated in the treatment of IDA in UC patients (Gomollon & Gisbert, 2009; Stein, Hartmann et al., 2010; Wilson, Reyes et al., 2004; Zhu, Kaneshiro et al., 2010).

2.5.2 Anemia of Chronic Disease

ACD, seen in patients with acute or chronic inflammation, is the second most common anemia in both the general and IBD population (Weiss & Goodnough, 2005). The pathogenesis of ACD is immune driven by cytokines and cells of the reticuloendothelial system. Erythropoiesis is decreased secondary to the chronic inflammation and corresponding anti-inflammatory treatments for IBD (Zhu, Kaneshiro et al., 2010). In UC, recombinant human erythropoietin is recommended for ACD and IDA if parenteral iron therapy is ineffective (Stein, Hartmann et al., 2010; Weiss & Goodnough, 2005; Zhu, Kaneshiro et al., 2010).

2.5.3 Autoimmune Hemolytic Anemia

The association of autoimmune hemolytic anemia (AIHA) with UC is rare, occurring in less than 1% of cases. However, AIHA should be suspected in patients with anemia, painless jaundice, and unconjugated hyperbilirubinemia (Gumaste et al., 1989; Valderrama Rojas et al., 2003). The diagnosis of AIHA includes a positive direct Coombs test that detects IgG or complement absorbed onto red blood cells. However, studies have shown that approximately 1.82% of UC patients without signs of hemolysis can have a positive direct Coombs test (Valderrama Rojas, Rodriguez Gorostiza et al., 2003). Systemic steroids are the first line of therapy, produce remission in 21% to 50% of cases, and should be continued for 3 weeks before being considered ineffective (Gumaste, Greenstein et al., 1989; Veloso et al., 1991). For cases unresponsive to steroids, immunosuppressive therapy with agents such as cyclophosphamide or azathioprine and surgical intervention including splenectomy should be considered. A case report describes a patient with UC and AIHA in which immunosuppression with steroids and azathioprine was not successful in achieving remission. Ultimately, splenectomy was performed and the patient went into remission allowing her immunosuppressants to be discontinued (Wodzinski & Lawrence, 1985). If the hemolysis is not responding to the aforementioned treatments, colectomy or total proctocolectomy are advisable and effective (Gumaste, Greenstein et al., 1989)(Sharma 2002). Thrombocytopenia with AIHA is known as Evan's syndrome. A case report describes an association of Evan's syndrome with UC that responded to immunosuppressive therapy (Ucci et al., 2003).

2.5.4 Other hematologic complications

Agranulocytosis and thrombocytopenia have been reported to be associated with UC. This can be secondary to medication side effects: for example, sulfasalazine has been shown to cause agranulocytosis and mesalamine has been showed to cause thrombocytopenia (Farrell et al., 1999; Roddie et al., 1995). Immune-mediated neutropenia and thrombocytopenia have also been reported in UC (Kim et al., 1995). Idiopathic thrombocytopenic purpura (ITP), documented by various case reports to occur in patients with UC, is autoimmune in nature and treatment is similar to that of AIHA with steroids, splenectomy, and if necessary, colectomy (Mizuta et al., 2003; Yoshida et al., 1996).

Various hematologic malignancies have been reported as UC complications and include: acute promyelocytic leukemia, acute myelogenous leukemia, chronic granulocytic leukemia, and myelodysplastic syndrome (Braverman & Bogoch, 1978; Fabry et al., 1980; Hebbar et al., 1997; Rosen & Teplitz, 1965). However, the pathogenesis of the association remains unclear (Fabry, Sachar et al., 1980; Hebbar, Kozlowski et al., 1997; Rosen & Teplitz, 1965; Suzuki et al., 1995).

2.5.5 Vascular complications

Venous thromboembolism (VTE) such as deep vein thrombosis (DVT) and pulmonary embolism (PE) are known complications of UC (Braverman & Bogoch, 1978). This is attributable to the hypercoagulable state associated with UC with patients often having active disease at time of VTE (Koutroubakis, 2005). Treatment is similar to that of patients without IBD. Arterial thrombosis is a rare complication of UC and sites of thrombosis involving radial, brachial and common carotid arterial thrombosis have been reported (Braverman & Bogoch, 1978; Mikroulis et al., 1999; Nogami et al., 2007). The pathogenesis of arterial thrombosis is related to increased fibrinogen levels, increased platelet counts, and decreased anti-thrombin III levels (Mikroulis, Antypas et al., 1999). Treatment with antithrombotic therapy can often worsen the UC and in patients who fail antithrombotic or anticoagulation therapies, colectomy is often necessary (Mikroulis, Antypas et al., 1999; Nogami, Iiai et al., 2007).

UC has been reported to be associated with several vasculitides including: Takayasu's arteritis and giant cell arteritis (Jacob et al., 1990; Kawashima et al., 1999; Shibata et al., 2002). Takayasu's arteritis is a granulomatous arteritis involving the aorta and its branches. Involvement of the common carotid artery will show typical tenderness of carotid artery, an early but pathognomonic symptom of Takayasu's arteritis. MRI is helpful for the early diagnosis of Takayasu's arteritis (Kawashima, Koike et al., 1999). Giant cell arteritis is granulomatous arteritis involving medium and large-sized arteries. Giant cell arteritis, also known as temporal arteritis and cranial arteritis, usually presents with headache, blurred vision, and sometimes sensorineural deafness (Jacob, Ledingham et al., 1990). Biopsy of temporal artery is needed for definitive diagnosis of temporal arteritis. Both Takayasu's arteritis and Giant cell arteritis respond to steroids (Jacob, Ledingham et al., 1990; Kawashima, Koike et al., 1999; Shibata, Funayama et al., 2002). Early diagnosis is important as delayed treatment can lead to permanent loss of vision.

2.6 Renal and genitourinary tract complications

A significant number of UC patients can develop complications involving the kidney and genitourinary tract. These complications include urolithiasis, chronic renal disease, ureteral obstruction, fistulas, and renal cell carcinoma.

2.6.1 Urolithiasis

Kidney stones, usually composed of either calcium oxalate or uric acid, are more prevalent in UC patients than in the general population (Caudarella et al., 1993). UC patients, especially those who have undergone surgery, have been shown to have decreased urinary volume, pH, magnesium, and excretion of citrate, all of which are significant risk factors for renal stone formation. Dehydration from diarrhea during UC flares further increases one's chance of developing nephrolithiasis.

2.6.2 Chronic renal disease

A statistically significant increased risk for renal disease is found in UC but not in CD patients (Bernstein et al., 2005). Reported chronic renal diseases associated with UC include: glomerulonephritis, immunoglobulin A nephropathy, nephrotic syndrome, idiopathic interstitial nephritis, drug-induced nephritis by mesalamine, NSAID induced nephropathy, type AA renal amyloidosis, or secondary amyloidosis (Basili et al., 2002; Skhiri et al., 1998; rStokke et al., 1976; Tokuyama et al., 2010). Kidney biopsy is indicated in order to confirm the diagnosis.

Nephrotic syndrome as a complication of UC has been reported to be related to an underlying complement and immune disorder and usually responds favorably to steroid treatment. A case report documents rapid improvement in renal function after colectomy (Stokke, Teisberg et al., 1976). UC patients found to have micro- or macro-hematuria should receive a renal biopsy for possible immunoglobulin A nephropathy (Trimarchi et al., 2001). Many of these diagnoses can end in renal failure and may ultimately require hemodialysis.

2.6.3 Ureteral obstruction

Ureteral involvement has been reported to occur in 3-6% of IBD cases (Ruffolo et al., 2004).

Ureteral obstruction in UC can be caused by kidney stone or retroperitoneal inflammation and fibrosis. Intravenous pyelography (IVP) is used to diagnose non-calculous ureteral obstruction and is found in 14% of UC patients (Fleckenstein et al., 1977). These patients are initially asymptomatic, but chronic obstruction and lead to pyelonephritis, hydronephrosis, hypertension, and eventual loss of kidney function. Because occult ureteral stenosis without gastrointestinal symptoms may be present, the possibility of IBD should be raised in patients who present with isolated ureteral stenosis (Kruglik et al., 1977). Initial management focuses on medical treatment of UC, but nephrostomy tubes or ureteral stents are indicated to relieve any obstructions.

2.6.4 Renal Cell Carcinoma
Renal cell carcinoma (RCC), although relatively uncommon, has been documented to occur in UC patients. While the association is unclear, possible etiologies include genetic predisposition or immunosuppression from medications. Treatment usually requires surgical intervention including nephrectomy (Satsangi et al., 1996).

2.7 Neurological complications
Both central and peripheral neurological disorders have been reported to occur in patients with UC. These include strokes, cerebral sinus thrombosis, cerebral vasculitis, acute disseminated encephalomyelitis, multiple sclerosis, peripheral neuropathies, and many other disorders (Jose & Heyman, 2008). Neurological complications of UC can be differentiated into three major categories: cerebrovascular disease, cerebral vasculitis, and immune mediated neuropathy. (Pandian et al., 2004)

2.7.1 Cerebrovascular disease
Compared to venous thrombotic events such as DVT and pulmonary emboli, thrombotic events occurring in the CNS are relatively rare occurring in up to 7.5% of cases (Nudelman et al., 2010). Cerebral sinus thrombosis typically presents with headache, convulsions, hemiparesis, and/or other neurologic signs and diagnosis is made by MRI angiogram (Tsujikawa et al., 2000). Because untreated cerebral sinus thrombosis can result in fatal cerebral edema and herniation, rapid diagnosis and treatment aimed to reduce intracranial pressure with a combination of steroids, diuretics, anticoagulants, and antithrombotic therapy is essential (Nudelman, Rosen et al., 2010; Tsujikawa, Urabe et al., 2000).
Cerebral arterial thrombosis is also a rare complication of UC, but has been described in young patients without any other significant risk factors of cerebral vascular accidents such as hyperlipidemia, cardiac arrhythmia, or carotid artery disease (Katsanos & Tsianos, 2002). Unfortunately, due to the rarity of cases, there are no official guidelines on the treatment of strokes in patients with IBD. Case reports have documented that arterial thrombotic events in UC patients is often associated with severe pan-colonic disease and generally carries a poor prognosis (Novotny et al., 1992). Colectomy may be necessary in these patients.

2.7.2 Cerebral vasculitis
Cerebral vasculitis is another complication of UC and can manifest as seizures and severe headaches (Masaki et al., 1997; Nomoto et al., 2006). Diagnosis is typically made with MRI

digital subtraction angiogram that shows a "beaded" appearance with multiple areas of irregularities of the intracerebral arteries. Treatment is similar to that of systemic vasculitis and usually involves steroids and/or immunosuppressants (Nelson et al., 1986; Nomoto, Nagao et al., 2006).

2.7.3 Immune mediated neuropathy

An association between UC and multiple sclerosis (MS) has been found both within families and within individuals (Hoffmann & Kruis, 2004). MS affects UC more than CD patients and the prevalence of MS in IBD patients is about 3.7 times more than seen in the average (Kimura et al., 2000). There are clearly common factors between IBD and MS, but more research is necessary to establish specific relationships between the two disorders (Pandian, Pawar et al., 2004). Management of these patients including diagnosis and treatment is generally similar to patients without UC (Pandian, Pawar et al., 2004).

Other rare neurological complications of UC that have been reported include: acute disseminated encephalomyelitis, optic neuritis, sensorineural hearing loss, myelopathy, peripheral polyneuropathy, Guillain-Barre syndrome, and myasthenia gravis (Gondim et al., 2005; Kanra et al., 2002; Krystallis et al., 2010; Lossos et al., 1995; Scheid & Teich, 2007; Tan, 1974; Yesilova et al., 2006). Many of these complications are autoimmune in nature and respond to steroids and/or immunosuppressive therapy.

2.8 Pulmonary complications

A variety of pulmonary complications associated with UC have been well documented and reported in medical and scientific literature. Virtually any part of the respiratory system can be involved and the pulmonary complications can be classified into airway, parenchymal, vascular, thromboembolic, and pleural disease.

2.8.1 Airway disease

Almost any part of the airway ranging from the trachea to the bronchi and bronchioles, can be associated with UC with the most common complications involving the bronchi (Higenbottam et al., 1980). Bronchial involvement may present as a chronic persistent cough with mucopurulent production suggesting chronic bronchitis or bronchiectasis (Gibb et al., 1987). In general, these symptoms do not respond to antibiotics, but do respond to inhaled steroids (Higenbottam, Cochrane et al., 1980). Studies have shown that in UC patients, colonic and pulmonary flares often parallel each other, suggesting a common embryonic origin of the colonic and pulmonary epithelium (Higenbottam, Cochrane et al., 1980; Wilcox et al., 1987). Furthermore, the histopathology of sclerosing cholangitis, another EIM of UC, has been shown to be quite similar to that of the airway inflammation associated with UC (Janssen et al., 2006).

Tracheal involvement can present as cough, hoarseness, dyspnea or even stridor due to inflammation and stenosis in subglottic or upper tracheal area. Depending on the severity of the inflammation and degree of respiratory compromise, systemic steroids and sometimes endotracheal intubation may be indicated (Janssen, Bierig et al., 2006; Rickli et al., 1994).

Less frequently seen in UC patients is bronchiole and small airways inflammation manifested as constrictive bronchiolitis or bronchiolitis obliterans with organizing pneumonia (BOOP) (Ward et al., 1999). Constrictive bronchiolitis is defined as concentric fibrosis in the bronchiolar submucosal layer with continuous external circular scarring

(Epler, 2007). BOOP is an inflammatory disease involving the terminal bronchiole and alveoli (lung parenchyma), and has been reported to be associated with UC. Symptoms seen with small airway involvement include cough, sputum production, wheezing, dyspnea, fever, flu-like symptoms, and pleuritic chest pain. These symptoms can manifest acutely or in chronic fashion and systemic steroids are indicated in the treatment of small airway inflammation.

Diagnosis

1. Routine laboratory tests: Sputum culture can rule out a respiratory infection. Observing peripheral eosinophilia on complete blood count can help differentiate inflammation from infection. Chest X-ray may show diffuse narrowing of the trachea in tracheal stenosis, thickening of the bronchial wall in bronchiectasis, or ground glass opacities in BOOP (Epler, 2001; Gibb, Dhillon et al., 1987; Janssen, Bierig et al., 2006).

2. Pulmonary function tests: An obstructive pattern is usually seen in large airway inflammation while a restrictive pattern is usually seen in small airway or parenchymal inflammation. Patients with inflammation affecting various parts of the airway and parenchyma can have mixed patterns on pulmonary function tests (Gibb, Dhillon et al., 1987). In patients with upper airway obstruction, flow-volume loops will show showing flattening of the inspiratory and expiratory limbs (Janssen, Bierig et al., 2006). A low lung diffusing capacity for carbon monoxide (DLco) can help to diagnose small airway inflammation such as BOOP or parenchymal disease such as interstitial lung disease.

3. CT scan: CT scans, especially High Resolution CT (HRCT) scans are more sensitive than plain chest films in differentiating between the pulmonary complications of UC. Irregular narrowing of the trachea or main bronchi can be seen in large airway involvement, thickened bronchial walls and dilated airways with mucoid impaction can be seen with bronchial involvement, and bilateral consolidation and peripheral (pleural-based) ground glass opacities are observed in BOOP (Epler, 2001; Garg et al., 1993; Spira et al., 1998; Wilcox, Miller et al., 1987).

4. Bronchoscopy: Bronchial epithelial biopsy can help diagnose tracheal stenosis with extensive inflammation with granulation tissue, basal reserve cell hyperplasia, thickening of the basement membrane, and submucosal inflammation (Gibb, Dhillon et al., 1987; Janssen, Bierig et al., 2006).

5. Surgery: Open lung biopsy or video-assisted thoracoscopic (VATS) procedure with biopsy may be needed to establish a diagnosis of BOOP or interstitial lung disease (Epler, 2001).

2.8.2 Lung parenchymal disease

BOOP, a disorder with both airway and parenchymal involvement, has been discussed under the airway disease section. Interstitial lung disease as a pulmonary complication of UC is extremely rare and is usually steroid-responsive, but cases of mortality have been reported (Marten et al., 2005). In a case report, a patient with UC was described to present with dyspnea and fatigue, but unlike BOOP, cough or fever was absent. Physical examination revealed inspiratory crackles and chest x-ray revealed reticular densities in the mid- to lower lung field bilaterally. CT scan revealed honeycombing and ground glass opacification with traction bronchiectasis and bronchiolectasis in similar lung field. Pulmonary function test revealed restriction pattern with reduced DLco and the patient ultimately developed respiratory failure requiring mechanical ventilation and passed away from acute right ventricular failure (Marten, Fend et al., 2005). Pulmonary infiltrates with eosinophilia (PIE syndrome) is a recognized pulmonary complication of UC and has been documented to occur in patients receiving and not receiving sulfasalazine/mesalamine therapy (Camus et al., 1993; Saltzman et al., 2001). Typical chest x-ray appearance of PIE is peripheral homogenous nonsegmental air-space infiltrate or a "reverse pulmonary edema" pattern (Saltzman, Rossoff et al., 2001). The patient presents with dry cough, wheezing, fever, night sweat, and malaise. Peripheral blood and bronchoalveolar lavage can demonstrate eosinophilia. Systemic steroid treatment causes prompt and sustained resolution of clinical and radiographic abnormalities (Saltzman, Rossoff et al., 2001).

Necrobiotic nodules (sterile abscesses) are rare pulmonary complications of UC. Patients usually present with high fever and constitutional symptoms. The lesions show PMNs and fibrin with necrosis, a similar pattern seen in PG, a dematologic complication of IBD (Camus, Piard et al., 1993; Warwick et al., 2009). Chest X-ray can show multiple cavitary and non-cavitary nodules. In 2 case reports, therapy with steroids with or without cyclophosphamide successfully produced remission without relapse (Camus, Piard et al., 1993).

2.8.3 Vascular disease

Pulmonary vasculitis is a rare complication of UC (Black et al., 2007; Forrest & Shearman, 1975; Hilling et al., 1994; Isenberg et al., 1968). Patients can present with fever, dyspnea, or cough with blood-tinged sputum (Forrest & Shearman, 1975; Hilling, Robertson et al., 1994). Other vascular diseases associated with UC include Wegener granulomatosis, Churg-Strauss syndrome, and microscopic polyangiitis(Black, Mendoza et al., 2007). Nodular lung lesions can be seen in pulmonary vasculitis and Wegener's granulomatosis and are usually responsive to systemic steroids (Black, Mendoza et al., 2007; Forrest & Shearman, 1975; Hilling, Robertson et al., 1994; Isenberg, Goldstein et al., 1968; Stebbing et al., 1999).

2.8.4 Vascular thromboembolic disease

The incidence of VTE is about 3 to 4 times higher for patients with IBD in comparison with controlled age-matched groups (Bernstein et al., 2001a; Miehsler et al., 2004; Stebbing, Askin et al., 1999). The age-adjusted incidence ratios of UC compared to age-matched population was 2.8 for DVT and 3.6 for pulmonary embolism (PE) (Bernstein, Blanchard et al., 2001). IBD patients have increased risk factors for thromboembolism secondary to the underlying disease process or its associated complications including dehydration, inactivity, hospitalization, surgery, and central venous catheterization. However, up to 1/3 of VTE events occur in patients while the underlying disease process is quiescent, suggesting that there are additional risk factors unrelated to disease activity or accompanying therapies (Stebbing, Askin et al., 1999; Tsiolakidou & Koutroubakis, 2008). The following genetic factors have been suggested to increase the incidence of VTE in IBD patients: factor V Leiden, factor II (prothrombin, G20210A), methylenetetrahydrofolate reductase gene mutation (MTHFR, 6777T), plasminogen activator inhibitor type 1 (PAI-1) gene mutation and factor XIII (val34leu) (Tsiolakidou & Koutroubakis, 2008). The symptoms, diagnosis and treatment of DVT and PE in UC are similar to patients without IBD.

2.8.5 Pleural disease

Pleural and pericardial complications of IBD in the form of serositis, pleural effusions, pleuritis, pericarditis, pleuro-pericarditis or myo-pericarditis are uncommon (Tsiolakidou &

Koutroubakis, 2008). When they do occur, they are usually diagnosed in young male patients with UC (Camus, Piard et al., 1993; Stebbing, Askin et al., 1999). The pleural effusion is almost always unilateral and exudative in nature. The symptoms and diagnosis of serositis are similar to other patients without UC and the treatment of serositis includes steroid and NSAIDs such as aspirin and Indocin (Stebbing, Askin et al., 1999).

2.9 Cardiac complications

In general, cardiovascular involvement with UC is uncommon, but complications such as intracavitary thrombosis, endocarditis, myocarditis, pericarditis, coronary artery disease, arrhythmias, and heart failure have been described in case reports (Katsanos & Tsianos, 2002).

2.9.1 Thrombosis

Intracavitary thrombosis, diagnosed by echocardiogram, has been reported to occur in the right atrium and left ventricle of UC patients (Saleh, 2010; Sasvary et al., 1996). Early diagnosis and treatment is essential as RA thrombus can lead to PE and LV thrombus can lead to systemic embolism.

2.9.2 Endocarditis

In UC patients, endocarditis can occur as a result of bacteremia, prolonged total parenteral nutrition (TPN) usage, or immunosuppression (Katsanos & Tsianos, 2002). Responsible organisms include streptococcus bovis, enterococcus faecium, and candida albicans (Christakis et al., 2007; Moshkowitz et al., 1992). Other complications that have been reported of endocarditis in UC patients include cerebral infarction and mitral valve leaflet aneurysm for which surgical intervention is indicated (Katsanos & Tsianos, 2002; Tomomasa et al., 1993).

2.9.3 Myocardial Involvement

Although relatively rare, myocardial involvement in UC patients compared with the general population has an incidence ratio of 2.6 (Sorensen & Fonager, 1997). A majority of cases in UC patients with myocardial involvement is complicated by pericarditis or pleural effusion. Prolonged corticosteroid use has been implicated in the cause of hypertrophic cardiomyopathy and mesalamine has been reported to cause myocarditis and perimyocarditis (Katsanos & Tsianos, 2002).

Case reports of acute myocardial infarction have been documented to occur during flares (Efremidis et al., 1999). The pathogenesis behind this ischemia is presumed to be reversible vasoconstriction of varying severity decreasing blood flow to myocardial tissue (Katsanos & Tsianos, 2002).

2.9.4 Pericarditis

The most commonly reported cardiac complication of UC is pericarditis which can be caused by drugs (5-aminosalicylic acid, mesalamine, azathioprine), pericardio-colonic fistulas, or idiopathic mechanisms (Katsanos & Tsianos, 2002). Both acute and chronic pericarditis with and without cardiac tamponade have been reported (Cappell & Turkieh, 2008; Dubowitz & Gorard, 2001). Drug induced pericarditis typically resolves after omission of the offending drug and treatment with NSAIDs is effective. Cardiac tamponade is a rare, but life threatening complication of UC that can be diagnosed by echocardiogram or cardiac catheterization. Treatment includes emergent pericardiocentesis and pericardiectomy is indicated for recurrent pericardial effusion and chronic constrictive pericarditis (Cappell & Turkieh, 2008; Rezaie et al., 2010).

2.9.5 Valvular Involvement
Valvular involvement in UC is relatively common and can manifest as endocardium and aortic root involvement. Aortic and mitral valve involvement may require surgical replacement, but generally carries with good outcomes and prognosis (Katsanos & Tsianos, 2002).

2.9.6 Arrhythmias
Various types of cardiac arrhythmia have been reported to occur in UC, including Wenckebach, complete heart block, atrial fibrillation, supraventricular tachycardia, ventricular tachyarrhythmia, and mesalamine related sinus bradycardia (Katsanos & Tsianos, 2002). A permanent pacemaker is indicated for complete heart block (Maeder, 1996). Hypomagnesemia is frequently seen in UC due to ongoing fecal losses and this can lead to ventricular tachycardia. Treatment with magnesium infusion is effective (Levine et al., 1982). Interestingly, in patients with no prior cardiac history or electrolyte balance, QT intervals were found to be significantly higher in UC than CD, suggesting an increased risk of dangerous arrhythmias (Curione et al., 2010).

2.9.7 Heart failure
Heart failure in UC can be acute (acute myocardial infarction, myocarditis, cardiac tamponade, valvular deterioration) or chronic (myocardium or valvular involvement, heart muscle atrophy with TPN and prolonged steroid use) (Katsanos & Tsianos, 2002). Aortic valve insufficiency can cause heart failure and cardiogenic shock (Lidon & Ariza, 1993). Sudden cardiac arrest in UC patients can be secondary to acute myocardial infarction, cardiogenic shock, or ventricular arrhythmias (Katsanos & Tsianos, 2002).

3. Conclusion

UC is a systemic disease, since its clinical manifestations can affect not only the bowel, but can also involve almost any organ including the skin, eyes, liver, musculoskeletal cardiovascular, hematologic, and renal systems (Table 1). These EIM can influence both morbidity and mortality. Most of the patients with IBD associated EIMs have extensive colitis and family history of the disease. With the exception of PSC, AS, PG, and type 2 arthritis, extraintestinal complications tend to follow the clinical course of IBD. Awareness and understanding of the disease manifestations extrinsic to the gastrointestinal tract are essential in the management of IBD patients.

4. Acknowledgment

The authors thank Cindy Ting for critical reading of this manuscript. Dr. Jamil Laith (Cedars-Sinai Medical Center) for providing Figure 7. Drs. Dmitry Karayev and Thomas J. Learch for providing Figures 8-10. Gary Holland and Yen Tran (Jules Stein Eye Institute, UCLA) for providing Figure 11.

Common Manifestations

Organ System	Features	CD or UC	IBD Activity Correlation	Therapy
Dermatologic				
Erythema nodosum	Painful, raised subcutaneous lesions on extensor surfaces	Both	Yes	Conservative therapies: leg elevation, rest, NSAIDS, potassium iodide Treatment of the underlying IBD
Pyoderma gangrenosum	Early: noninfectious pustules and nodules Late: Painful ulcers that can be shallow or deep	Both	No	Corticosteroids Cyclosporine Biologics Hyperbaric oxygen therapy Surgery Glucocorticoids
Aphthous stomatitis	Small, round, painful ulcers in oral mucosa	Both	Yes	Immunosuppressants Treatment of the underlying IBD
Pyostomatitis vegetans	Hyperplastic folds of oral mucosa with small abscesses and erosions	Both, but especially UC	Yes, occurs prior to flares	Glucocorticoids and immunosuppressants with variable success Colectomy may be required for complete remission
Hepatopancreatobiliary				
Primary Sclerosing Cholangitis	Progressive inflammatory destruction of bile ducts Chronic intermittent obstructive jaundice Abdominal pain, pruritus, fatigue, fever, weight loss	Both, but more common in UC	No	Ursodeoxycholic Acid (UDCA) Endoscopic Intervention with bile duct stent placement Liver transplantation
Primary Biliary Cirrhosis	Progressive cholestatic liver disease Pruritus, jaundice, skin pigmentation, fatigue, abominal pain	Both	Chronic disease progression	Cholestyramine Ursodeoxycholic Acid (UDCA) ERCP for bile drainage

Common Manifestations

Organ System	Features	CD or UC	IBD Activity Correlation	Therapy
Autoimmune Hepatitis	Acute/chronic hepatitis or cirrhosis Fever, right upper quadrant pain, jaundice	Both	No	Glucocorticoids Azathioprine Liver transplantation
Pancreatitis	Abdominal pain, nausea/vomiting Acute and chronic: idiopathic, gallstones, PSC, medication induced Autoimmune: obstructive jaundice	Both	Controversial	Treatment of underlying process Autoimmune: steroids
Musculoskeletal	Basic Features: Clinical or Histologic Pain, heat, swelling, decreased mobility in affected joint.			
Peripheral arthritis	Non-deforming, non-erosive Worse in AM, improves with activity Type 1: acute, pauci-articular (<5 joints), asymmetrical, self-limiting Type 2: poly-articular (≥ 5 joints), migratory arthritis, chronic with relapsing/remitting course	Both, more common in CD	Type 1: Yes Type 2: No	Type 1: Treatment of underlying IBD Type 2: COX-2 inhibitors, sulfasalazine, immunomodulators, TNF-alpha inhibitors Both: Symptomatic: rest, physical therapy, intra-articular steroids
Axial Arthritis (Sacroiliitis and Ankylosing Spondylitis)	Back pain Back stiffness in morning or after rest	Both	No	Intense physical therapy Glucocorticoids, sulfasalazine, methotrexate, TNF-alpha inhibitors
Osteoporosis	Bone pain Increased fracture risk	Both, more severe in CD than UC	Indirectly related to nutrition, absorption, and treatment	Symptomatic: Analgesics Medical: Calcium, Vitamin D, bisphosphonates Surgical: correction of fractures
Polymyositis/Dermatomyositis	Muscle pain/weakness Elevated serum CPK	Both	No	Glucocorticoids 5-ASA

Common Manifestations

Organ System	Features	CD or UC	IBD Activity Correlation	Therapy
Orbital Myositis	Sudden orbital pain Periorbital/eyelid edema Diplopia Exophthalmos Conjunctival injection	Rare in both	No	Glucocorticoids
Gastrocnemius Myalgia Syndrome	Calf tenderness	Both, more common in CD	No	Glucocorticoids
Ocular				
Episcleritis	Acute onset of injection, irritation of eye Vision typically not affected	Both	Yes	Topical steroids Treatment of underlying IBD
Uveitis	Photophobia, blurred vision, pain, conjuctival injection	Both	Unpredictable, but can parallel luminal IBD activity	Topical steroids Mydriatics Infliximab
Scleritis	Deep eye pain with radiation to eyebrows, cheeks, temples Eye redness, tearing, photophobia, blurred vision Blindness	Both	May precede or follow IBD diagnosis	Oral steroids NSAIDS Immunosuppressants Surgical repair

Less Common Manifestations

Organ System	Features	CD or UC	IBD Activity Correlation	Therapy
Hematologic				
Iron deficiency anemia	UC: more often secondary to blood loss CD: more often secondary to poor absorption	Both, more common in UC	Yes	Iron (parenteral therapy as first line therapy) Erythropoietin if iron alone ineffective
Anemia of chronic disease	Secondary to inflammatory cytokines and/or low erythropoietin	Both, more common in CD	Yes	Erythropoietin + iron supplementation
Megaloblastic anemia	From folic acid or B12 deficiency	Both, more common in CD (ileal disease/resection)	Yes	Intramuscular or intranasal Vitamin B12 Folic Acid supplementation
Autoimmune hemolytic anemia (AIHA)	Anemia, painless jaundice, unconjugated hyperbilirubinemia	Both, more common in UC	Controversial	Steroids Splenectomy Immunosuppressants Colectomy, proctocolectomy
Idiopathic Thrombocytopenic Purpura (ITP)	Petechiae, purpura, epistaxis	Both, more common in UC	No	Steroids Immunosuppressants Splenectomy Colectomy
Evan's Syndrome	ITP + AIHA Autoantibodies to platelets and RBCs	Both, more common in UC	No	Treatment similar as for ITP
Vascular				
Venous Thromboembolism	Deep vein thrombosis Pulmonary embolism	Both	Yes	Similar anticoagulation treatments as for patients without IBD

Less Common Manifestations

Organ System	Features	CD or UC	IBD Activity Correlation	Therapy
Arterial Thrombosis	Thrombosis of radial, brachial and common artery	Both	Yes	Antithrombotic/anticoagulation therapies Colectomy
Renal				
Urolithiasis	Sudden, severe, colicky pain in back, flank, or groin Nausea/vomiting	Both	No	Narcotics, hydration Lithotripsy Surgery
Chronic Renal Disease	Glomerulonephritis, immunoglobulin A nephropathy, nephrotic syndrome, interstitial nephritis, drug-induced nephritis, renal amyloidosis	UC	Variable	Hemodialysis for those that result in renal failure
Neurological				
Cerebrovascular Disease (Cerebral sinus/arterial thrombosis)	Headache, convulsions, hemiparesis, focal neurological signs	Both	No	Sinus thrombosis: Intracranial pressure reduction with steroids, diuretics, anticoagulants, antithrombotics Arterial thrombosis: no official guidelines, colectomy may be indicated
Cerebral Vasculitis	Seizures Severe headaches "Beaded" appearance of intracerebral arteries with MRI	Both	unclear	Steroids Immunosuppressants Anticoagulation
Immune Mediated Neuropathy (Multiple Sclerosis)	Diplopia, numbness, slurred speech, other neurological signs	Both	unclear	Steroids Immunosuppressants

Less Common Manifestations

Organ System	Features	CD or UC In general UC > CD	IBD Activity Correlation	Therapy
Pulmonary				
Upper Airway Disease (Epiglottitis, Laryngotracheitis, Subglottic, or Tracheal stenosis)	Cough, hoarseness, dysphonia, dyspnea, stridor	Both	No	Inhaled steroids Systemic steroids Laser ablation for refractory obstruction
Large Airway Disease (Chronic bronchitis, Bronchiectasis)	Cough, mucopurulent sputum production	Both	No	Inhaled steroids Low dose oral steroids
Small Airway Disease (Constrictive bronchiolitis)	Cough, sputum, dyspnea, wheezing, fever Concentric fibrosis in bronchiolar submucosal layers with continuous external circular scarring inflammation in terminal bronchiole	Both	No	Inhaled steroids Low dose oral steroids
Small Airway and Lung Parenchymal Disease (BOOP)	Dry cough, dyspnea, fever, wheezing, pleuritic chest pain, flu-like symptoms	Both, more common in UC	No	High dose oral steroids Systemic steroids
Interstitial Lung Disease	Dyspnea, fatigue	Both	No	Oral steroids with or without other immunomodulators
Pulmonary infiltrates with eosinophilia (PIE)	Dry cough, wheezing, fever, chest tightness, night sweats, malaise Eosinophilia in blood and bronchoalveolar lavage	Both	No	Oral steroids
Lung necrobiotic nodules (Sterile abscesses)	High fever, constitutional symptoms PMNs and fibrin with necrosis, absence of giant cells, vasculitis, or capillaritis	Both, more common in UC	No	Oral steroids with or without cyclophosphamide

Less Common Manifestations

Organ System	Features	CD or UC	IBD Activity Correlation	Therapy
Pulmonary Vasculitis	Fever, dyspnea, cough, blood-tinged sputum / Nodular density on lung biopsy	Both	No	Oral steroids
Pleural Effusion/Pleuritis	Dyspnea, pleuritic chest pain / Unilateral and exudative effusion	Both	No	Steroids / NSAIDs / Therapeutic thoracentesis
Cardiac				
Intracavitary Thrombosis	RA Thrombosis: pulmonary embolism / LV Thrombosis: cerebrovascular event	Both	No	Anticoagulation
Infectious endocarditis	Septicemia, related to TPN catheters and immunosuppressive therapy	Both, more common in CD	No	Antibiotics / Valvular replacement
Myocarditis (idiopathic, drug induced, selenium deficiency)	Asymptomatic / Chest pain, dyspnea	Both, more common in UC	No	Withdrawal of offending drugs / Treatment of underlying IBD / Selenium supplementation
Myocardial Infarction	Angina, chest pain, diaphoresis / Usual pathophysiologic mechanisms and risk factors / Ischemia secondary to reversible vasoconstriction	Both	Yes	Steroids / Treatment as per ACS protocol / Treatment of underlying IBD
Pericarditis	Pleuritic chest pain, fever, dyspnea, cough	Both	No	Omission of offending drug / NSAIDs / Pericardiocentesis for cardiac tamponade / Pericardiectomy for constrictive pericarditis

Less Common Manifestations

Organ System	Features	CD or UC	IBD Activity Correlation	Therapy
Valvular Involvement (from endocarditis or aortitis)	Aortic regurgitation, mitral regurgitation, tricuspid regurgitation, mitral valve aneurysm	Both	No	Treat underlying disease Valvular replacement for complicated cases
Cardiac Arrhythmia	Various types including Wenckebach, complete heart block, atrial fibrillation, SVT, etc.	Both	No	Treat the arrhythmia Magnesium supplementation Permanent pacemaker for complete heart block
Heart Failure	Acute: AMI, myocarditis, tamponade, valvular deterioration Chronic: myocardium or valvular involvement, myocardial atrophy due to prolonged TPN or steroid use	Both	No	Treat underlying disease
Cardiac Related Sudden Death	Sudden AMI, cardiogenic shock, cardiac tamponade, or arrhythmia	Both	No	Treat underlying disease

Table 1. Extraintestinal Manifestations of IBD

5. References

Alabraba, E., P. Nightingale, et al. (2009). A re-evaluation of the risk factors for the recurrence of primary sclerosing cholangitis in liver allografts. *Liver Transpl* 15(3): 330-340.

Alkhouri, N., V. Hupertz, et al. (2009). Adalimumab treatment for peristomal pyoderma gangrenosum associated with Crohn's disease. *Inflamm Bowel Dis* 15(6): 803-806.

Alvarez, F., P. A. Berg, et al. (1999). International Autoimmune Hepatitis Group Report: review of criteria for diagnosis of autoimmune hepatitis. *J Hepatol* 31(5): 929-938.

Angulo, P., D. H. Pearce, et al. (2000). Magnetic resonance cholangiography in patients with biliary disease: its role in primary sclerosing cholangitis. *J Hepatol* 33(4): 520-527.

Areias, E.&L. Garcia e Silva (1987). [Cutaneous manifestations of ulcerative colitis]. *Med Cutan Ibero Lat Am* 15(3): 185-197.

Atzeni, F., S. Ardizzone, et al. (2009). Combined therapeutic approach: inflammatory bowel diseases and peripheral or axial arthritis. *World J Gastroenterol* 15(20): 2469-2471.

Ballinger, A. B., C. Camacho-Hubner, et al. (2001). Growth failure and intestinal inflammation. *QJM* 94(3): 121-125.

Bank, L.&J. P. Wright (1984). 6-Mercaptopurine-related pancreatitis in 2 patients with inflammatory bowel disease. *Dig Dis Sci* 29(4): 357-359.

Basili, E., M. Cazo, et al. (2002). [Secondary amyloidosis complicating ulcerative colitis]. *Gastroenterol Clin Biol* 26(5): 529-531.

Basu, M. K.&P. Asquith (1980). Oral manifestations of inflammatory bowel disease. *Clin Gastroenterol* 9(2): 307-321.

Berger, M., D. Gribetz, et al. (1975). Growth retardation in children with ulcerative colitis: the effect of medical and surgical therapy. *Pediatrics* 55(4): 459-467.

Bergquist, A., S. M. Montgomery, et al. (2008). Increased risk of primary sclerosing cholangitis and ulcerative colitis in first-degree relatives of patients with primary sclerosing cholangitis. *Clin Gastroenterol Hepatol* 6(8): 939-943.

Bernstein, C. N., J. F. Blanchard, et al. (2001a). The incidence of deep venous thrombosis and pulmonary embolism among patients with inflammatory bowel disease: a population-based cohort study. *Thromb Haemost* 85(3): 430-434.

Bernstein, C. N., J. F. Blanchard, et al. (2001b). The prevalence of extraintestinal diseases in inflammatory bowel disease: a population-based study. *Am J Gastroenterol* 96(4): 1116-1122.

Bernstein, C. N., A. Wajda, et al. (2005). The clustering of other chronic inflammatory diseases in inflammatory bowel disease: a population-based study. *Gastroenterology* 129(3): 827-836.

Berstad, A. E., L. Aabakken, et al. (2006). Diagnostic accuracy of magnetic resonance and endoscopic retrograde cholangiography in primary sclerosing cholangitis. *Clin Gastroenterol Hepatol* 4(4): 514-520.

Billson, F. A., F. T. De Dombal, et al. (1967). Ocular complications of ulcerative colitis. *Gut* 8(2): 102-106.

Bjornsson, E., R. Olsson, et al. (2008). The natural history of small-duct primary sclerosing cholangitis. *Gastroenterology* 134(4): 975-980.

Black, H., M. Mendoza, et al. (2007). Thoracic manifestations of inflammatory bowel disease. *Chest* 131(2): 524-532.

Blitz, N. M.&D. Rudikoff (2001). Pyoderma gangrenosum. *Mt Sinai J Med* 68(4-5): 287-297.

Bourikas, L. A.&K. A. Papadakis (2009). Musculoskeletal manifestations of inflammatory bowel disease. *Inflamm Bowel Dis* 15(12): 1915-1924.

Brakenhoff, L. K., D. M. van der Heijde, et al. (2010). The joint-gut axis in inflammatory bowel diseases. *J Crohns Colitis* 4(3): 257-268.

Braverman, D.&A. Bogoch (1978). Arterial thrombosis in ulcerative colitis. *Am J Dig Dis* 23(12): 1148-1150.

Brooklyn, T. N., M. G. Dunnill, et al. (2006). Infliximab for the treatment of pyoderma gangrenosum: a randomised, double blind, placebo controlled trial. *Gut* 55(4): 505-509.

Broome, U., R. Lofberg, et al. (1995). Primary sclerosing cholangitis and ulcerative colitis: evidence for increased neoplastic potential. *Hepatology* 22(5): 1404-1408.

Burak, K. W., P. Angulo, et al. (2003). Is there a role for liver biopsy in primary sclerosing cholangitis? *Am J Gastroenterol* 98(5): 1155-1158.

Burrall, B. (1999). Sweet's syndrome (acute febrile neutrophilic dermatosis). *Dermatol Online J* 5(1): 8.

Callen, J. P. (1998). Pyoderma gangrenosum. *Lancet* 351(9102): 581-585.

Callen, J. P.&J. M. Jackson (2007). Pyoderma gangrenosum: an update. *Rheum Dis Clin North Am* 33(4): 787-802, vi.

Calobrisi, S. D., D. F. Mutasim, et al. (1995). Pyostomatitis vegetans associated with ulcerative colitis. Temporary clearance with fluocinonide gel and complete remission after colectomy. *Oral Surg Oral Med Oral Pathol Oral Radiol Endod* 79(4): 452-454.

Campsen, J., M. A. Zimmerman, et al. (2008). Clinically recurrent primary sclerosing cholangitis following liver transplantation: a time course. *Liver Transpl* 14(2): 181-185.

Camus, P., F. Piard, et al. (1993). The lung in inflammatory bowel disease. *Medicine (Baltimore)* 72(3): 151-183.

Cappell, M. S.&A. Turkieh (2008). Chronic pericarditis and pericardial tamponade associated with ulcerative colitis. *Dig Dis Sci* 53(1): 149-154.

Caudarella, R., E. Rizzoli, et al. (1993). Renal stone formation in patients with inflammatory bowel disease. *Scanning Microsc* 7(1): 371-379; discussion 379-380.

Chapman, R., J. Fevery, et al. (2010). Diagnosis and management of primary sclerosing cholangitis. *Hepatology* 51(2): 660-678.

Charatcharoenwitthaya, P., F. B. Enders, et al. (2008). Utility of serum tumor markers, imaging, and biliary cytology for detecting cholangiocarcinoma in primary sclerosing cholangitis. *Hepatology* 48(4): 1106-1117.

Charatcharoenwitthaya, P.&K. D. Lindor (2006). Primary sclerosing cholangitis: diagnosis and management. *Curr Gastroenterol Rep* 8(1): 75-82.

Christakis, G. B., S. P. Perlorentzou, et al. (2007). Bacteremia caused by Pantoea agglomerans and Enterococcus faecalis in a patient with colon cancer. *J BUON* 12(2): 287-290.

Chugh, S., J. B. Dilawari, et al. (1993). Polymyositis associated with ulcerative colitis. *Gut* 34(4): 567-569.

Cohen, P. R. (2009). Neutrophilic dermatoses: a review of current treatment options. *Am J Clin Dermatol* 10(5): 301-312.

Cohen, P. R.&R. Kurzrock (2002). Sweet's syndrome: a review of current treatment options. *Am J Clin Dermatol* 3(2): 117-131.

Cohen, P. R., M. Talpaz, et al. (1988). Malignancy-associated Sweet's syndrome: review of the world literature. *J Clin Oncol* 6(12): 1887-1897.

Curione, M., A. Aratari, et al. (2010). A study on QT interval in patients affected with inflammatory bowel disease without cardiac involvement. *Intern Emerg Med* 5(4): 307-310.

Curley, R. K., A. W. Macfarlane, et al. (1985). Pyoderma gangrenosum treated with cyclosporin A. *Br J Dermatol* 113(5): 601-604.

Danese, S., S. Semeraro, et al. (2005). Extraintestinal manifestations in inflammatory bowel disease. *World J Gastroenterol* 11(46): 7227-7236.

Darvay, A. (1996). Sweet's syndrome preceding inflammatory bowel disease. *Clin Exp Dermatol* 21(2): 175.

Das, K. M. (1999). Relationship of extraintestinal involvements in inflammatory bowel disease: new insights into autoimmune pathogenesis. *Dig Dis Sci* 44(1): 1-13.

de Fazio, C., G. Torgano, et al. (1992). Detection of liver involvement in inflammatory bowel disease by abdominal ultrasound scan. *Int J Clin Lab Res* 21(4): 314-317.

Dorudi, S., R. W. Chapman, et al. (1991). Carcinoma of the gallbladder in ulcerative colitis and primary sclerosing cholangitis. Report of two cases. *Dis Colon Rectum* 34(9): 827-828.

Dubowitz, M.&D. A. Gorard (2001). Cardiomyopathy and pericardial tamponade in ulcerative colitis. *Eur J Gastroenterol Hepatol* 13(10): 1255-1258.

Duerr, R. H., S. R. Targan, et al. (1991). Anti-neutrophil cytoplasmic antibodies in ulcerative colitis. Comparison with other colitides/diarrheal illnesses. *Gastroenterology* 100(6): 1590-1596.

Efremidis, M., E. Prappa, et al. (1999). Acute myocardial infarction in a young patient during an exacerbation of ulcerative colitis. *Int J Cardiol* 70(2): 211-212.

Epler, G. R. (2001). Bronchiolitis obliterans organizing pneumonia. *Arch Intern Med* 161(2): 158-164.

Epler, G. R. (2007). Constrictive bronchiolitis obliterans: the fibrotic airway disorder. *Expert Rev Respir Med* 1(1): 139-147.

Evans, P. E.&D. S. Pardi (2007). Extraintestinal manifestations of inflammatory bowel disease: focus on the musculoskeletal, dermatologic, and ocular manifestations. *MedGenMed* 9(1): 55.

Fabry, T. L., D. B. Sachar, et al. (1980). Acute myelogenous leukemia in patients with ulcerative colitis. *J Clin Gastroenterol* 2(3): 225-227.

Farhi, D.&D. Wallach (2008). The neutrophilic dermatoses. *Dermatol Nurs* 20(4): 274-276, 279-282.

Farrant, J. M., K. M. Hayllar, et al. (1991). Natural history and prognostic variables in primary sclerosing cholangitis. *Gastroenterology* 100(6): 1710-1717.

Farrell, R. J., M. A. Peppercorn, et al. (1999). Mesalamine-associated thrombocytopenia. *Am J Gastroenterol* 94(8): 2304-2306.

Finkelberg, D. L., D. Sahani, et al. (2006). Autoimmune pancreatitis. *N Engl J Med* 355(25): 2670-2676.

Fleckenstein, P., L. Knudsen, et al. (1977). Obstructive uropathy in chronic inflammatory bowel disease. *Scand J Gastroenterol* 12(5): 519-523.

Florin, T. H., N. Pandeya, et al. (2004). Epidemiology of appendicectomy in primary sclerosing cholangitis and ulcerative colitis: its influence on the clinical behaviour of these diseases. *Gut* 53(7): 973-979.

Forrest, J. A.&D. J. Shearman (1975). Pulmonary vasculitis and ulcerative colitis. *Am J Dig Dis* 20(5): 482-486.

Garg, K., D. A. Lynch, et al. (1993). Inflammatory airways disease in ulcerative colitis: CT and high-resolution CT features. *J Thorac Imaging* 8(2): 159-163.

Giannini, S.&C. Martes (2006). Anemia in inflammatory bowel disease. *Minerva Gastroenterol Dietol* 52(3): 275-291.

Gibb, W. R., D. P. Dhillon, et al. (1987). Bronchiectasis with ulcerative colitis and myelopathy. *Thorax* 42(2): 155-156.

Gomollon, F.&J. P. Gisbert (2009). Anemia and inflammatory bowel diseases. *World J Gastroenterol* 15(37): 4659-4665.

Gondim, F. A., T. H. Brannagan, 3rd, et al. (2005). Peripheral neuropathy in patients with inflammatory bowel disease. *Brain* 128(Pt 4): 867-879.

Gow, P. J.&R. W. Chapman (2000). Liver transplantation for primary sclerosing cholangitis. *Liver* 20(2): 97-103.

Graziadei, I. W., R. H. Wiesner, et al. (1999). Recurrence of primary sclerosing cholangitis following liver transplantation. *Hepatology* 29(4): 1050-1056.

Greenstein, A. J., H. D. Janowitz, et al. (1976). The extra-intestinal complications of Crohn's disease and ulcerative colitis: a study of 700 patients. *Medicine (Baltimore)* 55(5): 401-412.

Greenstein, A. J., D. B. Sachar, et al. (1992). Amyloidosis and inflammatory bowel disease. A 50-year experience with 25 patients. *Medicine (Baltimore)* 71(5): 261-270.

Guhl, G.&A. Garcia-Diez (2008). Subcutaneous sweet syndrome. *Dermatol Clin* 26(4): 541-551, viii-ix.

Gumaste, V., A. J. Greenstein, et al. (1989). Coombs-positive autoimmune hemolytic anemia in ulcerative colitis. *Dig Dis Sci* 34(9): 1457-1461.

Hansen, L. S., S. Silverman, Jr., et al. (1983). The differential diagnosis of pyostomatitis vegetans and its relation to bowel disease. *Oral Surg Oral Med Oral Pathol* 55(4): 363-373.

Hebbar, M., D. Kozlowski, et al. (1997). Association between myelodysplastic syndromes and inflammatory bowel diseases. Report of seven new cases and review of the literature. *Leukemia* 11(12): 2188-2191.

Higenbottam, T., G. M. Cochrane, et al. (1980). Bronchial disease in ulcerative colitis. *Thorax* 35(8): 581-585.

Hilling, G. A., D. A. Robertson, et al. (1994). Unusual pulmonary complication of ulcerative colitis with a rapid response to corticosteroids: case report. *Gut* 35(6): 847-848.

Hoffmann, R. M.&W. Kruis (2004). Rare extraintestinal manifestations of inflammatory bowel disease. *Inflamm Bowel Dis* 10(2): 140-147.

Horio, T., S. Imamura, et al. (1981). Potassium iodide in the treatment of erythema nodosum and nodular vasculitis. *Arch Dermatol* 117(1): 29-31.

Imagawa, M. (1999). [Extra-intestinal complications of ulcerative colitis: hematologic complication]. *Nippon Rinsho* 57(11): 2556-2561.

Isenberg, J. I., H. Goldstein, et al. (1968). Pulmonary vasculitis--an uncommon complication of ulcerative colitis. Report of a case. *N Engl J Med* 279(25): 1376-1377.

Jacob, A., J. G. Ledingham, et al. (1990). Ulcerative colitis and giant cell arteritis associated with sensorineural deafness. *J Laryngol Otol* 104(11): 889-890.

Jahnsen, J., J. A. Falch, et al. (1997). Bone mineral density is reduced in patients with Crohn's disease but not in patients with ulcerative colitis: a population based study. *Gut* 40(3): 313-319.

Jahnsen, J., J. A. Falch, et al. (2003). Body composition in patients with inflammatory bowel disease: a population-based study. *Am J Gastroenterol* 98(7): 1556-1562.

Janssen, W. J., L. N. Bierig, et al. (2006). Stridor in a 47-year-old man with inflammatory bowel disease. *Chest* 129(4): 1100-1106.

Jose, F. A.&M. B. Heyman (2008). Extraintestinal manifestations of inflammatory bowel disease. *J Pediatr Gastroenterol Nutr* 46(2): 124-133.

Kamisawa, T., T. Shimosegawa, et al. (2009). Standard steroid treatment for autoimmune pancreatitis. *Gut* 58(11): 1504-1507.

Kanra, G., A. Kara, et al. (2002). Sensorineural hearing loss as an extra-intestinal manifestation of ulcerative colitis in an adolescent girl with pyoderma gangrenosum. *Eur J Pediatr* 161(4): 216-218.

Karlsen, T. H., E. Schrumpf, et al. (2007). Genetic epidemiology of primary sclerosing cholangitis. *World J Gastroenterol* 13(41): 5421-5431.

katsanos, K. H.&E. V. Tsianos (2002). The heart in inflammatory bowel disease. *Annals of Gastroenterology* 15(2): 124-133.

Kawashima, M., R. Koike, et al. (1999). [A case of Takayasu's arteritis with ulcerative colitis diagnosed by carotodynia and MRI findings]. *Nihon Rinsho Meneki Gakkai Kaishi* 22(5): 317-323.

Keljo, D. J.&K. S. Sugerman (1997). Pancreatitis in patients with inflammatory bowel disease. *J Pediatr Gastroenterol Nutr* 25(1): 108-112.

Kemmett, D.&J. A. Hunter (1990). Sweet's syndrome: a clinicopathologic review of twenty-nine cases. *J Am Acad Dermatol* 23(3 Pt 1): 503-507.

Kimura, K., S. F. Hunter, et al. (2000). Concurrence of inflammatory bowel disease and multiple sclerosis. *Mayo Clin Proc* 75(8): 802-806.

Kitiyakara, T.&R. W. Chapman (2008). Chemoprevention and screening in primary sclerosing cholangitis. *Postgrad Med J* 84(991): 228-237.

Koulentaki, M., I. E. Koutroubakis, et al. (1999). Ulcerative colitis associated with primary biliary cirrhosis. *Dig Dis Sci* 44(10): 1953-1956.

Koutroubakis, I. E. (2005). Therapy insight: Vascular complications in patients with inflammatory bowel disease. *Nat Clin Pract Gastroenterol Hepatol* 2(6): 266-272.

Kruglik, G. D., H. L. Neiman, et al. (1977). Urological complications of regional enteritis. *Gastrointest Radiol* 1(4): 375-378.

Krystallis, C. S., D. K. Kamberoglou, et al. (2010). Guillain-Barre syndrome during a relapse of ulcerative colitis: a case report. *Inflamm Bowel Dis* 16(4): 555-556.

Larsen, S., K. Bendtzen, et al. (2010). Extraintestinal manifestations of inflammatory bowel disease: epidemiology, diagnosis, and management. *Ann Med* 42(2): 97-114.

Lazzaro, D. R. (2010). Repair of necrotizing scleritis in ulcerative colitis with processed pericardium and a Prokera amniotic membrane graft. *Eye Contact Lens* 36(1): 60-61.

Lee, Y. M.&M. M. Kaplan (1995). Primary sclerosing cholangitis. *N Engl J Med* 332(14): 924-933.

Letsinger, J. A., M. A. McCarty, et al. (2005). Complex aphthosis: a large case series with evaluation algorithm and therapeutic ladder from topicals to thalidomide. *J Am Acad Dermatol* 52(3 Pt 1): 500-508.

Levine, S. R., T. J. Crowley, et al. (1982). Hypomagnesemia and ventricular tachycardia: a complication of ulcerative colitis and parenteral hyperalimentation in a nondigitalized noncardiac patient. *Chest* 81(2): 244-247.

Levy, C., J. Lymp, et al. (2005). The value of serum CA 19-9 in predicting cholangiocarcinomas in patients with primary sclerosing cholangitis. *Dig Dis Sci* 50(9): 1734-1740.

Lidon, R. M.&A. Ariza (1993). [Heart failure, changes in heart rhythm, and cardiogenic shock in a 46-year-old patient]. *Med Clin (Barc)* 101(20): 789-794.

Loftus, E. V., Sandborn WJ, Lindor KD, et al. (1997). Interactions between chronic liver disease and inflammatory bowel disease. *Inflamm Bowel Dis* 3: 288-302.

Lossos, A., Y. River, et al. (1995). Neurologic aspects of inflammatory bowel disease. *Neurology* 45(3 Pt 1): 416-421.

Lundqvist, K.&U. Broome (1997). Differences in colonic disease activity in patients with ulcerative colitis with and without primary sclerosing cholangitis: a case control study. *Dis Colon Rectum* 40(4): 451-456.

Lyne, A. J.&D. A. Pitkeathley (1968). Episcleritis and scleritis. Association with connective tissue disease. *Arch Ophthalmol* 80(2): 171-176.

Macarez, R., S. Bazin, et al. (2005). [Orbital myositis associated with ulcerative colitis]. *J Fr Ophtalmol* 28(6): 610-613.

MacCarty, R. L., N. F. LaRusso, et al. (1983). Primary sclerosing cholangitis: findings on cholangiography and pancreatography. *Radiology* 149(1): 39-44.

Madsen, P. V.&G. Andersen (1994). Multifocal osteonecrosis related to steroid treatment in a patient with ulcerative colitis. *Gut* 35(1): 132-134.

Maeder, H. U. (1996). The complete heart-block--an extraintestinal manifestation of ulcerative colitis. *Z Gastroenterol* 34(1): 27-29.

Marshall, J. K.&E. J. Irvine (1997). Successful therapy of refractory erythema nodosum associated with Crohn's disease using potassium iodide. *Can J Gastroenterol* 11(6): 501-502.

Marten, K., F. Fend, et al. (2005). Case report: Fatal acute exacerbation of usual interstitial pneumonia in ulcerative colitis. *Br J Radiol* 78(932): 762-766.

Masaki, T., T. Muto, et al. (1997). Unusual cerebral complication associated with ulcerative colitis. *J Gastroenterol* 32(2): 251-254.

Matis, W. L., C. N. Ellis, et al. (1992). Treatment of pyoderma gangrenosum with cyclosporine. *Arch Dermatol* 128(8): 1060-1064.

McCallum, D. I.&P. D. Kinmont (1968). Dermatological manifestations of crohn's disease. *Br J Dermatol* 80(1): 1-8.

Miehsler, W., W. Reinisch, et al. (2004). Is inflammatory bowel disease an independent and disease specific risk factor for thromboembolism? *Gut* 53(4): 542-548.

Mikroulis, D. A., G. D. Antypas, et al. (1999). Arterial Thrombosis in Ulcerative Colitis: Case Report. *Int J Angiol* 8(1): 62-64.

Mir-Madjlessi, S. H., R. G. Farmer, et al. (1987). Bile duct carcinoma in patients with ulcerative colitis. Relationship to sclerosing cholangitis: report of six cases and review of the literature. *Dig Dis Sci* 32(2): 145-154.

Mir-Madjlessi, S. H., J. S. Taylor, et al. (1985). Clinical course and evolution of erythema nodosum and pyoderma gangrenosum in chronic ulcerative colitis: a study of 42 patients. *Am J Gastroenterol* 80(8): 615-620.

Mizuta, Y., H. Isomoto, et al. (2003). Immune thrombocytopenic purpura in patients with ulcerative colitis. *J Gastroenterol* 38(9): 884-890.

Moff, S. L., I. R. Kamel, et al. (2006). Diagnosis of primary sclerosing cholangitis: a blinded comparative study using magnetic resonance cholangiography and endoscopic retrograde cholangiography. *Gastrointest Endosc* 64(2): 219-223.

Monsen, U., J. Sorstad, et al. (1990). Extracolonic diagnoses in ulcerative colitis: an epidemiological study. *Am J Gastroenterol* 85(6): 711-716.

Moshkowitz, M., N. Arber, et al. (1992). Streptococcus bovis endocarditis as a presenting manifestation of idiopathic ulcerative colitis. *Postgrad Med J* 68(805): 930-931.

Nakamura, M., A. Kanamori, et al. (2005). Alternate total ophthalmoplegia and optic neuropathy associated with ulcerative colitis. *Eye (Lond)* 19(2): 235-237.

Nash, P. T.&T. H. Florin (2005). Tumour necrosis factor inhibitors. *Med J Aust* 183(4): 205-208.

Navaneethan, U.&B. Shen (2010). Hepatopancreatobiliary manifestations and complications associated with inflammatory bowel disease. *Inflamm Bowel Dis* 16(9): 1598-1619.

Nelson, J., M. M. Barron, et al. (1986). Cerebral vasculitis and ulcerative colitis. *Neurology* 36(5): 719-721.

Newell, L. M.&F. D. Malkinson (1982). Pyoderma (ecthyma) gangrenosum by Brunsting, Goeckerman and O'Leary, October 1930. Commentary: Pyoderma gangrenosum. *Arch Dermatol* 118(10): 743-773.

Nogami, H., T. Iiai, et al. (2007). Common carotid arterial thrombosis associated with ulcerative colitis. *World J Gastroenterol* 13(11): 1755-1757.

Nomoto, T., T. Nagao, et al. (2006). Cerebral arteriopathy with extracranial artery involvement in a patient with ulcerative colitis. *J Neurol Sci* 243(1-2): 87-89.

Novotny, D. A., R. J. Rubin, et al. (1992). Arterial thromboembolic complications of inflammatory bowel disease. Report of three cases. *Dis Colon Rectum* 35(2): 193-196.

Nudelman, R. J., D. G. Rosen, et al. (2010). Cerebral sinus thrombosis: a fatal neurological complication of ulcerative colitis. *Patholog Res Int* 2010: 132754.

Ozdil, S., F. Akyuz, et al. (2004). Ulcerative colitis: analyses of 116 cases (do extraintestinal manifestations effect the time to catch remission?). *Hepatogastroenterology* 51(57): 768-770.

Pandian, J. D., G. Pawar, et al. (2004). Multiple sclerosis in a patient with chronic ulcerative colitis. *Neurol India* 52(2): 282-283.

Pardi, D. S., E. V. Loftus, Jr., et al. (2003). Ursodeoxycholic acid as a chemopreventive agent in patients with ulcerative colitis and primary sclerosing cholangitis. *Gastroenterology* 124(4): 889-893.

Pena, E., V. F. Moreira, et al. (2000). [Idiopathic chronic pancreatitis (with diffuse stenosis of Wirsung's duct) in ulcerative colitis]. *Gastroenterol Hepatol* 23(8): 389-391.

Perdigoto, R., H. A. Carpenter, et al. (1992). Frequency and significance of chronic ulcerative colitis in severe corticosteroid-treated autoimmune hepatitis. *J Hepatol* 14(2-3): 325-331.

Rabinovitz, M., A. J. Demetris, et al. (1992). Simultaneous occurrence of primary sclerosing cholangitis and autoimmune chronic active hepatitis in a patient with ulcerative colitis. *Dig Dis Sci* 37(10): 1606-1611.

Rasmussen, H. H., J. F. Fallingborg, et al. (1997). Hepatobiliary dysfunction and primary sclerosing cholangitis in patients with Crohn's disease. *Scand J Gastroenterol* 32(6): 604-610.

Rezaie, A., K. Wong, et al. (2010). Pericardial tamponade in a patient with inactive ulcerative colitis. *Case Report Med* 2010: 352417.

Rickli, H., C. Fretz, et al. (1994). Severe inflammatory upper airway stenosis in ulcerative colitis. *Eur Respir J* 7(10): 1899-1902.

Riegler, G., R. D'Inca, et al. (1998). Hepatobiliary alterations in patients with inflammatory bowel disease: a multicenter study. Caprilli & Gruppo Italiano Studio Colon-Retto. *Scand J Gastroenterol* 33(1): 93-98.

Roddie, P., H. Dorrance, et al. (1995). Treatment of sulphasalazine-induced agranulocytosis with granulocyte macrophage-colony stimulating factor. *Aliment Pharmacol Ther* 9(6): 711-712.

Rosen, R. B.&R. L. Teplitz (1965). Chronic Granulocytic Leukemia Complicated by Ulcerative Colitis: Elevated Leukocyte Alkaline Phosphatase and Possible Modifier Gene Deletion. *Blood* 26: 148-156.

Rozen, S. M., M. Y. Nahabedian, et al. (2001). Management strategies for pyoderma gangrenosum: case studies and review of literature. *Ann Plast Surg* 47(3): 310-315.

Ruffolo, C., I. Angriman, et al. (2004). Minimally invasive management of Crohn's disease complicated by ureteral stenosis. *Surg Laparosc Endosc Percutan Tech* 14(5): 292-294.

Rutgeerts, P., W. J. Sandborn, et al. (2005). Infliximab for induction and maintenance therapy for ulcerative colitis. *N Engl J Med* 353(23): 2462-2476.

Saarinen, S., O. Olerup, et al. (2000). Increased frequency of autoimmune diseases in patients with primary sclerosing cholangitis. *Am J Gastroenterol* 95(11): 3195-3199.

Saleh, T. (2010). Left Ventricular Thrombosis in Ulcerative Colitis. *Case Rep Gastroenterol* 4(2): 220-223.

Saltzman, K., L. J. Rossoff, et al. (2001). Mesalamine-induced unilateral eosinophilic pneumonia. *AJR Am J Roentgenol* 177(1): 257.

Salvarani, C., G. Fornaciari, et al. (2000). Musculoskeletal manifestations in inflammatory bowel disease. *Eur J Intern Med* 11(4): 210-214.

Sandborn, W. J., W. F. Stenson, et al. (2006). Safety of celecoxib in patients with ulcerative colitis in remission: a randomized, placebo-controlled, pilot study. *Clin Gastroenterol Hepatol* 4(2): 203-211.

Sasvary, F., J. Murin, et al. (1996). [Intracavitary thrombosis--unusual complications in ulcerative colitis]. *Bratisl Lek Listy* 97(11): 669-672.

Satsangi, J., J. Marshall, et al. (1996). Ulcerative colitis complicated by renal cell carcinoma: a series of three patients. *Gut* 38(1): 148-150.

Saxon, A., F. Shanahan, et al. (1990). A distinct subset of antineutrophil cytoplasmic antibodies is associated with inflammatory bowel disease. *J Allergy Clin Immunol* 86(2): 202-210.

Scheid, R.&N. Teich (2007). Neurologic manifestations of ulcerative colitis. *Eur J Neurol* 14(5): 483-493.

Schulz, E. J.&D. A. Whiting (1976). Treatment of erythema nodosum and nodular vasculitis with potassium iodide. *Br J Dermatol* 94(1): 75-78.

Sedwick, L. A., T. G. Klingele, et al. (1984). Optic neuritis in inflammatory bowel disease. *J Clin Neuroophthalmol* 4(1): 3-6.

Shibata, C., Y. Funayama, et al. (2002). Takayasu's arteritis after total proctocolectomy for ulcerative colitis: report of a case. *Dis Colon Rectum* 45(3): 422-424.

Ship, J. A. (1996). Recurrent aphthous stomatitis. An update. *Oral Surg Oral Med Oral Pathol Oral Radiol Endod* 81(2): 141-147.

Simsek, I., H. Erdem, et al. (2007). Optic neuritis occurring with anti-tumour necrosis factor alpha therapy. *Ann Rheum Dis* 66(9): 1255-1258.

Skhiri, H., B. Knebelmann, et al. (1998). Nephrotic syndrome associated with inflammatory bowel disease treated by mesalazine. *Nephron* 79(2): 236.

Smith, T.&A. S. Befeler (2007). High-dose ursodeoxycholic acid for the treatment of primary sclerosing cholangitis. *Curr Gastroenterol Rep* 9(1): 54-59.

Snook, J. A., P. Kelly, et al. (1989). Fibrolamellar hepatocellular carcinoma complicating ulcerative colitis with primary sclerosing cholangitis. *Gut* 30(2): 243-245.

Sorensen, H. T.&K. M. Fonager (1997). Myocarditis and inflammatory bowel disease. A 16-year Danish nationwide cohort study. *Dan Med Bull* 44(4): 442-444.

Souissi, A., R. Benmously, et al. (2007). [Sweet's syndrome: a propos of 8 cases]. *Tunis Med* 85(1): 49-53.

Spira, A., R. Grossman, et al. (1998). Large airway disease associated with inflammatory bowel disease. *Chest* 113(6): 1723-1726.

Stawarski, A., B. Iwanczak, et al. (2006). [Intestinal complications and extraintestinal manifestations in children with inflammatory bowel disease]. *Pol Merkur Lekarski* 20(115): 22-25.

Stebbing, J., F. Askin, et al. (1999). Pulmonary manifestations of ulcerative colitis mimicking Wegener's granulomatosis. *J Rheumatol* 26(7): 1617-1621.

Stein, J., F. Hartmann, et al. (2010). Diagnosis and management of iron deficiency anemia in patients with IBD. *Nat Rev Gastroenterol Hepatol* 7(11): 599-610.

Stiehl, A. (2004). [Primary sclerosing cholangitis]. *Internist (Berl)* 45(1): 27-32.

Stokke, K. T., P. A. Teisberg, et al. (1976). Nephrotic syndrome in ulcerative colitis. *Scand J Gastroenterol* 11(6): 571-576.

Storwick, G. S., M. B. Prihoda, et al. (1994). Pyodermatitis-pyostomatitis vegetans: a specific marker for inflammatory bowel disease. *J Am Acad Dermatol* 31(2 Pt 2): 336-341.

Suzuki, Y., K. Nakase, et al. (1995). [Acute promyelocytic leukemia following ulcerative colitis]. *Rinsho Ketsueki* 36(7): 707-709.

Tan, R. S. (1974). Ulcerative colitis, myasthenia gravis, atypical lichen planus, alopecia areata, vitiligo. *Proc R Soc Med* 67(3): 195-196.

Terjung, B., V. Herzog, et al. (1998). Atypical antineutrophil cytoplasmic antibodies with perinuclear fluorescence in chronic inflammatory bowel diseases and hepatobiliary disorders colocalize with nuclear lamina proteins. *Hepatology* 28(2): 332-340.

Terjung, B., J. Sohne, et al. (2010). p-ANCAs in autoimmune liver disorders recognise human beta-tubulin isotype 5 and cross-react with microbial protein FtsZ. *Gut* 59(6): 808-816.

Terjung, B.&U. Spengler (2009). Atypical p-ANCA in PSC and AIH: a hint toward a leaky gut ? *Clin Rev Allergy Immunol* 36(1): 40-51.

Thornton, J. R., R. H. Teague, et al. (1980). Pyoderma gangrenosum and ulcerative colitis. *Gut* 21(3): 247-248.

Timani, S.&D. F. Mutasim (2008). Skin manifestations of inflammatory bowel disease. *Clin Dermatol* 26(3): 265-273.

Tokuyama, H., S. Wakino, et al. (2010). Acute interstitial nephritis associated with ulcerative colitis. *Clin Exp Nephrol* 14(5): 483-486.

Tomomasa, T., K. Itoh, et al. (1993). An infant with ulcerative colitis complicated by endocarditis and cerebral infarction. *J Pediatr Gastroenterol Nutr* 17(3): 323-325.

Trimarchi, H. M., A. Iotti, et al. (2001). Immunoglobulin A nephropathy and ulcerative colitis. A focus on their pathogenesis. *Am J Nephrol* 21(5): 400-405.

Tromm, A., D. May, et al. (2001). Cutaneous manifestations in inflammatory bowel disease. *Z Gastroenterol* 39(2): 137-144.

Trost, L. B.&J. K. McDonnell (2005). Important cutaneous manifestations of inflammatory bowel disease. *Postgrad Med J* 81(959): 580-585.

Tsiolakidou, G.&I. E. Koutroubakis (2008). Thrombosis and inflammatory bowel disease-the role of genetic risk factors. *World J Gastroenterol* 14(28): 4440-4444.

Tsujikawa, T., M. Urabe, et al. (2000). Haemorrhagic cerebral sinus thrombosis associated with ulcerative colitis: a case report of successful treatment by anticoagulant therapy. *J Gastroenterol Hepatol* 15(6): 688-692.

Turner, R. B., J. J. Emer, et al. (2010). Rapid resolution of pyoderma gangrenosum after treatment with intravenous cyclosporine. *J Am Acad Dermatol* 63(3): e72-74.

Tutrone, W. D., K. Green, et al. (2007). Pyoderma gangrenosum: dermatologic application of hyperbaric oxygen therapy. *J Drugs Dermatol* 6(12): 1214-1219.

Ucci, G., P. Ferrando, et al. (2003). A case of Evans' syndrome in a patient with ulcerative colitis. *Dig Liver Dis* 35(6): 439-441.

Valderrama Rojas, M., F. J. Rodriguez Gorostiza, et al. (2003). [Autoimmune hemolytic anemia: a rare complication of ulcerative colitis]. *An Med Interna* 20(2): 78-80.

Veloso, F. T., J. Fraga, et al. (1991). Autoimmune hemolytic anemia in ulcerative colitis. A case report with review of the literature. *J Clin Gastroenterol* 13(4): 445-447.

Vestergaard, P. (2004). Prevalence and pathogenesis of osteoporosis in patients with inflammatory bowel disease. *Minerva Med* 95(6): 469-480.

Vij, A., G. M. Modi, et al. (2010). Chronic, recurrent neutrophilic dermatosis: a case report. *Dermatol Online J* 16(10): 1.

Ward, H., K. L. Fisher, et al. (1999). Constrictive bronchiolitis and ulcerative colitis. *Can Respir J* 6(2): 197-200.

Warwick, G., T. Leecy, et al. (2009). Pulmonary necrobiotic nodules: a rare extraintestinal manifestation of Crohn's disease. *Eur Respir Rev* 18(111): 47-50.

Wasserteil, V., S. Bruce, et al. (1992). Pyoderma gangrenosum treated with hyperbaric oxygen therapy. *Int J Dermatol* 31(8): 594-596.

Wee, A.&J. Ludwig (1985). Pericholangitis in chronic ulcerative colitis: primary sclerosing cholangitis of the small bile ducts? *Ann Intern Med* 102(5): 581-587.

Weinstein, M., D. Turner, et al. (2005). Erythema nodosum as a presentation of inflammatory bowel disease. *CMAJ* 173(2): 145-146.

Weiss, G.&L. T. Goodnough (2005). Anemia of chronic disease. *N Engl J Med* 352(10): 1011-1023.

Wester, A. L., M. H. Vatn, et al. (2001). Secondary amyloidosis in inflammatory bowel disease: a study of 18 patients admitted to Rikshospitalet University Hospital, Oslo, from 1962 to 1998. *Inflamm Bowel Dis* 7(4): 295-300.

Wiesner, R. H., P. M. Grambsch, et al. (1989). Primary sclerosing cholangitis: natural history, prognostic factors and survival analysis. *Hepatology* 10(4): 430-436.

Wilcox, P., R. Miller, et al. (1987). Airway involvement in ulcerative colitis. *Chest* 92(1): 18-22.

Wilson, A., E. Reyes, et al. (2004). Prevalence and outcomes of anemia in inflammatory bowel disease: a systematic review of the literature. *Am J Med* 116 Suppl 7A: 44S-49S.

Wittekindt, C., J. C. Luers, et al. (2007). Pyoderma gangrenosum in the head and neck. *Arch Otolaryngol Head Neck Surg* 133(1): 83-85.

Wodzinski, M. A.&A. C. Lawrence (1985). Severe Coombs positive autoimmune haemolytic anaemia associated with ulcerative colitis. *Postgrad Med J* 61(713): 261-262.

Wollina, U. (2002). Clinical management of pyoderma gangrenosum. *Am J Clin Dermatol* 3(3): 149-158.

Yates, V. M., G. Watkinson, et al. (1982). Further evidence for an association between psoriasis, Crohn's disease and ulcerative colitis. *Br J Dermatol* 106(3): 323-330.

Yesilova, Z., I. Naharci, et al. (2006). Motor axonal polyneuropathy in the course of ulcerative colitis: a case report. *Turk J Gastroenterol* 17(1): 58-61.

Yoshida, E. M., H. Chaun, et al. (1996). Immune thrombocytopenic purpura in three patients with preexisting ulcerative colitis. *Am J Gastroenterol* 91(6): 1232-1235.

Zhu, A., M. Kaneshiro, et al. (2010). Evaluation and treatment of iron deficiency anemia: a gastroenterological perspective. *Dig Dis Sci* 55(3): 548-559.

11

Kallikrein – Kinin System and Coagulation System in Inflammatory Bowel Diseases

Antoni Stadnicki[1,2]
[1]Department of Basis Biomedical Sciences, Medical University of Silesia, Katowice,
[2]Section of Gastroenterology, District Hospital, Jaworzno
Poland

1. Introduction

Inflammatory bowel diseases (IBD), including Crohn's disease and ulcerative colitis (UC), are complex disorders characterized by chronic, local and systemic inflammation and spontaneously relapsing course. The causes of these diseases are unknown, however they display genetic and environmental components and appear to be immunologically mediated in part by enteric microbiota (Baumgart & Carding, 2007).

There are convincing evidences that IBD are diseases of immunological hyperresponsiveness within the mucosa. Immunological reactions may be directed against luminal bacteria and their products normally present in the intestine (Sartor, 2006). Alternatively, mucosal inflammation in IBD might represent an immune response against unusual antigens such as environmental factors and/or epithelial HLA halotypes. The initiating events may be nonspecific and induce transient injury. The normal response is suppression of inflammation, but genetically susceptible host amplifies the inflammatory response. The activation of intestinal T helper cells (TH1, TH2 and TH17) play a pivotal role in experimental and human IBD because they modulate of the response to enteric microbiota and autoimmunity which is probably critical to IBD chronicity. Crohn's disease is TH1 and TH17 related disorder with local over-production of interleukin – 2 (IL-2), interpheron γ (INFγ), IL - 12, and IL-23, whereas in UC it is apparent activation of TH2 lymphocyte cytokine profile, mostly IL-4 and IL-10 as well as IL-13 by natural killer T cells. Interaction of activated T cells with effector cells (macrophages and neutrophils) leads to release of cytokines, eicosanoids and activation of complement cascade and coagulation and kallikrein - kinin systems which cause tissue injury. Many cytokines including interleukin 1 (IL-1), tumor necrosis factor (TNF) and IL-8 are increased in both active UC and Crohn's disease. The tissue levels of arachidonic acid metabolites; prostaglandins,leukotrienes and thromboxanes correlate with gross and histological evidence of intestinal inflammation in IBD. The activation of coagulation has been recognized as important component of the inflammatory response in both Crohn's disease and UC, and also is significant in progression and possibly pathogenesis of these entities (Danese et al., 2007). A significance the kallikrein – kinin system in human IBD is still uncertain although in animal IBD models kallikreins and kinins have been documented in part to mediate intestinal and systemic inflammation. There are two types of kallikreins, plasma and tissue; both serine protease enzymes may cleave kininogens to release kinins, a potent inflammatory mediators (Bhoola et al., 1992).

2. Plasma kallikrein-kininogen system

A single gene codes for plasma kallikrein, which is synthetized in the liver. The plasma kallikrein-kinin system is comprised of factor XII (Hageman factor) factor XI (initiator of intrinsic coagulation pathway), plasma prekallikrein, and high molecular weight kininogen (HK). Activation of the plasma kallikrein – kinin system (known also as the contact system) is initiated by autoactivation of factor XII yielding factor XIIa, which, in turn, activates prekallikrein to kallikrein. Kallikrein can cleave its own heavy chain (56 kDa) at Lys140-Ala141 to form two fragments of 28kDa and 18 kDa. Kallikrein can also react with C1-inhibitor (C1-INH) to form an inactive complex (Mr 190 kDa) (Campbell, 2001; Colman, 2006 c). Plasma kallikrein cleaves HK to release bradykinin, and enhances plasmin formation by activating prourokinase to urokinase (Ichinose et al., 1986). The major regulator of activation of the contact system is the plasma protease inhibitor, C1-INH, which inhibits activated factor XIIa, kallikrein, and factor XIa. In addition, alfa- 2 macroglobulin is an important inhibitor of kallikrein and a 1-antitrypsin for factor XIa. Plasma kallikrein exists as a zymogen, prekalliktein, 75% of which circulates in the blood in a noncovalent complex with HK. HK is multifunctional protein, β-globulin, with a plasma concentration about 80 µg/ml. HK is consisted of 6 domains divided into heavy chain (HK domains 1-3), and light chain (HK domains 5-6), linked by domain 4 which contains the sequence of bradykinin. Low molecular weight kininogen (LK) is present in plasma and various tissues. LK is β-globulin with a plasma concentration of 220 µg/ml, it has identical domain 1 through domain 4 of HK. However LK domain 5 is completely different from HK and domain 6 is lacking (Colman, 2006). Cleavage of HK by plasma kallikrein generates proinflammatory and proangiogenic bradykinin, and forming biologically active kininogen fragment HKa. Products of this pathway induce a variety of inflammatory events. Kallikrein is also implicated in neutrophil activation with release of lysosomal enzymes, such as elastase (Wachtfogelet al., 1983), as well as potentiation of superoxide formation (Schapira et al., 1982). In addition, plasma kallikrein and factor XII fragments may activate the alternative and classical complement pathways, respectively. Recent studies shown that HKa may stimulate in vitro secretion of cytokines; IL-1 β, IL-6, and TNF and chemokines from monocytes through signaling pathways by urokinase –type plasminogen receptor, integrin α-1 β2 (MAC-1) receptor, and complement protein C1q receptor (Khan et al., 2006). IL1- β release is localized to domain – 3 and domain -5 of HK. In addition HK and HKa have an-adhesive properties and HKa and domain 5 of HK inhibit angiogenesis (Colman 2006 b).

3. Tissue kallikreins and kinins

Tissue and plasma kallikreins differ in their molecular weight, isoelectric point, immunological properties, and substrate preference. Tissue kallikreins is a member of a multigene family that shows different patterns of tissue specific gene expression ((Clements et al., 1992). Under physiological conditions, tissue kallikrein is present in the highest concentration in exocrine glands, mostly in salivary glands and pancreas (Wolf et al., 1998). In salivary glands tissue kallikrein occurs in active form, while in pancreas is present as proenzym.Both active and precursor forms are present in excretory product such as urine and sweat. Kallikrein purified from both rat and human colon was found to be biochemically similar, if not identical, to tissue kallikrein for salivary gland and pancreas (Chen et al., 1995). Although HK is a better substrate for plasma kallikrein to release bradykinin and low molecular weight kininogen (LK) is better substrate for tissue kallikrein liberates kallidyn (Lys – bradykin), both are substrate for both plasma and tissue kallikreins. Kallistatin present in tissues and plasma is a main inhibitor of tissue kallikrein (Chao et al., 1996). Plasma kallikrein releases nonapeptide, bradykinin from HK, while tissue and glandular kallikreins liberates decapeptide, kallidyn (Lys–bradykinin) from LK. Kallidyn is rapidly converted to bradykinin by aminopeptidase. Bradykinin has short half life – 30 second in circulation. Kinins are rapidly destroyed by kininases, which are present in blood and in tissues. Removal of its C-terminal arginine by kininase I (carboxypeptidase N) forms an active metabolite des-Arg ^{9} bradykinin, which has a half life approximately 2 hours. Kininase II, known also as angiotensin converting enzyme (ACE) to remove the COOH – terminal peptides metabolizes kinins to their inactive forms (Bhoola et al., 1992). The final metabolite of bradyninin and des-Arg^9-bradykinin is bradykinin 1-5. T-kinins forming by

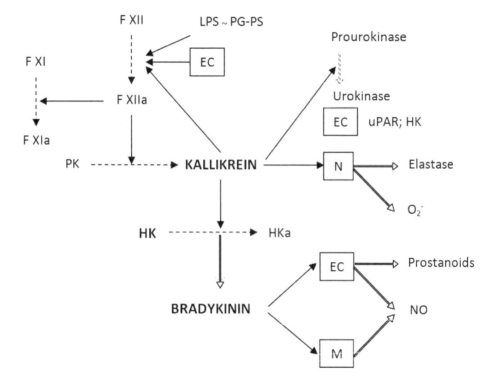

Fig. 1. Potential significance of plasma kallikrein- kinin system in inflammation.
PG-PS: peptidoglycan – polysaccharide; LPS: lipopolysaccharide; EC: endothelial cell; M: monocyte; N: neutrophil, HK: high molecular weight kininogen; TF: tissue factor; NO: nitric oxide, uPAR: urokinase plasminogen activated receptor. Solid arrows designate activation or cofactor amplification, dashed arrows designate conversion, and open arrows indicate release, expression, or synergistic properties

cleavage T – kininogen were exclusively identified   in rats (Okamoto et al., 1993). Bradykinin and kallidin and theirs active metabolite, des-Arg^9-bradykinin and Lys - des-Arg^9-bradykinin respectively bind to   two transmembran G protein - coupled receptors designated as bradykinin receptor - 2 (B2R) and bradykinin receptor – 1 (B1R). BR2 are constitutive mainly expressed in endothelial cells, stimulated by bradykinin to release nitric oxide and other negative regulators of smooth muscle tone and platelet function. However BR2 might also be upregulated in the acute phase of inflammation (Calixto et al., 2003; Moreau et al., 2005). B1R are inducible following tissue injury or after treatment with bacterial endotoxins or inflammatory cytokines such as interleukin -1 β (IL1- β) or tumor necrosis factor – α (TNF- α). Cytokine-induced B1R expression is mediated by nuclear factor – κ β (NF- κ β) and specific MAP – kinase pathways (mainly p38 and JNK) (Ni et al., 1998).

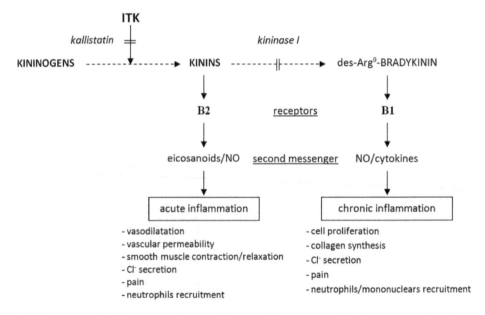

Fig. 2. Potential role of intestinal tissue kallikrein – kinin system in inflammatory bowel disease. Solid arrows designate activation, dashed arrows designate conversion, open arrows indicate induction, and interrupted lines indicate blockade. B2 and B1: kinin receptors; NO: nitric oxide; ITK: intestinal tissue kallikrein

4. Plasma kallikrein – kinin system in IBD

In the past two decades, the role of plasma kallikrein- kinin system in experimental and human sepsis (Pixley et al., 1995), and other acute inflammatory states including Rocky Mountains spotted fever (Rao et al., 1988), human experimental endotoxemia (DeLa Cadena et al., 1998), and acute pancreatitis has been well delineated . In 1990s we have developed experimental model of enterocolitis induced by bacterial cell wall polymer peptidoglycan – polysaccharide from group A streptococci (PG – APS) (Sartor at al., 1996). Female Lewis rats, the highest responders injected intramurally by PG-APS developed acute intestinal inflammation that peaks 1-2 days after PG – APS injection, gradually decreases over the next 10 days and spontaneously reactivates beginning on day 14, accompanied by peripheral erosive arthritis, granulomatous hepatitis, normochromic anemia and leukocytosis, with histological findings of intestinal fibrosis and granulomas. Acute intestinal inflammation developed in all rat strains investigated, but chronic, transmural, granulomatous reactivation only in genetically susceptible Lewis rats, but not in Buffalo or Fisher rats. This model has unique features resembling Crohn's disease. Inflammation induced by APG – PS, similar to human IBD is mediated by large number of inflammatory cascades and liberation of soluble mediators including cytokines, prostanoids and activation of the kallikrein-kinin system. We have developed a specific plasma kallikrein inhibitor (P8720) to evaluate a direct relationship between the plasma kallikrien- kinin activation and inflammatory changes. Treatment with the specific, oral plasma kallikrein inhibitor, P8720, in the acute and chronic granulomatous phase of enterocolitis in Lewis rat decreased the increase of gut gross and histological score and systemic inflammation, and prevented the decrease of plasma FXI and HK. (Stadnicki et al., 1996; Stadnicki et al., 1998 b). This activation is not specific for PG-APS since it has been demonstrated that it can also be induced in Lewis rats chronic enrerocolitis model- induced by indomethacin (Stadnicki et al., 1998 c). Looking for a functional mechanism involved in selective activation of the kallikrein- kinin system in genetically susceptible Lewis rats, we found that HK cleavage and yielding bradykinin by plasma kallikren was faster in Lewis rat plasma than in Buffalo rat plasma and Fisher rat plasma (Sartor at al., 1996). It has been found that a single point mutation at nucleotide 1586 translating from Ser511 (Buffalo and Fisher) to Asn511 (Lewis) is associated with N-glycolization indicating that this molecular alteration may be one contributing factor resulting in chronic reactive colitis in Lewis rats (Isordia Salas et al., 2003). Administration of PG – APS causes a similar biological response as triggered by endotoxins (LPS) which is detectable in plasma in most IBD patients during relapse (Gardiner et al 1995) indicating that both bacterial products act through similar the innate immunity activation, cytokines and mediators. Later it has been demonstrated that in patients with UC in active disease phase (but not in inactive UC) there was moderate activation of this system as significant decrease of plasma prekallikrein, HK and functional levels of C1 – inhibitor, and in some patients formation of kallikrein – inhibitor complexes on Western blot (Stadnicki et al., 1997). However in Crohn's disease study it not been found these chances in plasma of patients probably due the high plasma levels of C1 – inhibitor (Devani et al., 2002).

5. Intestinal tissue kallikrein – kinin system in IBD

5.1 Intestinal tissue kallikrein

The presence of kallikrein in gastrointestinal tract has been observed since 1960s (Schachter et al., 1986; Werle, 1960) but little has been done to evaluate its role in IBD. Long time ago only one study (Zeitlin & Smith, 1973) reported the presence of tissue kallikrein in normal human colon and a higher concentration in the inflamed colon of patients with UC. In rat model of PG – APS stimulated chronic inflammation we have shown that the normal location of ITK was the goblet cells and substantial amounts of ITK were present in the macrophages of the granulomas found in the submucosa indicating that ITK is present at the site of inflammation (Stadnicki et al., 1998 a). ITK concentrations were markedly reduced in the inflamed cecum as compared with the normal, but ITK protein concentration was associated with unchanged ITK mRNA levels, which indicated that its reduction was not due to suppression of its gene expression. Further evidence that inflamed intestinal tissue cells had secreted ITK to a greater extend that normal it has got from in vitro culture study showing marked IIK decrease in supernatant from in vitro cultures of inflamed intestine. In addition a potent tissue kallikrein inhibitor, kallikrein binding protein in the rat (whose human homolog is kallistatin) was decreased in rat plasma during inflammation suggesting release ITK into plasma. In human studies we have demonstrated that ITK was in goblet cells in normal and inflamed human colon which was in agreement with previous findings in rats (Stadnicki et al., 2003). Again ITK levels were significantly decreased in inflamed intestinal tissue from patients with IBD compared to normal controls consistent with its secretion in vivo. The kallistatin, a specific inhibitor, naturally occurring serine protein inhibitor (serpin) of human tissue kallikrein, was localized to epithelial cells. Kallistatin apparently colocalizes within ITK in the macrophages within the granulomas. It has been shown also decreased plasma levels of kallistatin in IBD patients similarly like kallikrein binding protein in rat enterocolitis which indicated that the secretion of ITK results in active form since kallistatin only steichometrically combines with enzymatically active tissue kallikrein (Xiong et al., 1992). Other study indicated that the goblet cells may have a more active role in the regulation of intestinal homeostasis and immunologic processes by interaction this other cells such as macrophages and lymphocytes (Lichtenstein, 2000). The factors which determine ITK secretion and activation are still not defined. It is known that inactive tissue prokallikrein can be activated by trypsin, plasmin, or even plasma kallikrein (Bhoola et al., 1992). Such enzymes could enter the intestinal space through several routes: by transudation of plasma or release from inflammatory cells. Interestingly a proinflammatory effect of ITK in the intestine are due to macrophage production and secretion. It has been demonstrated tissue kallikrein on human blood neutrophils, but did not detect the enzyme in monocytes (Figueroa et al., 1989). It is possible that tissue kallikrein is only expressed in stimulated monocytes or macrophages, as is the case for tissue factor (Gregory & Edgington, 1985). However, luminal ITK may enter the inflamed mucosa due to enhanced permeability, where it could hydrolyze growth factors and peptides which could act on the epithelial mucosa cells. In fact it has been demonstrated that ITK immunoreactivity was significantly weaker in gobled cells in both Crohn's disease and ulcerative colitis patients, but with strong reactivity in intestinal interstitium of IBD patients (Devani et al., 2005). ITK can cleave low kininogen which is present in intestine as well as both LK and HK, which are present in plasma and likely to be present in the protein – rich exudates of the inflamed intestine. Apart from its kininogenase activity, tissue kallikrein has been implicated in the processing of grow factors and peptide hormones. Tissue kallikrein hydrolyze vasoactive intestinal peptide and procollagenase in vitro (Techesche et al., 1983). If these reactions take place in IBD, ITK may influence intestinal motility, secretion and connective tissue metabolism. Moreover in experimental and human IBD the number of mast cells and mast cells tryptase expression are increased in the colonic mucosa and submucosa (He, 2004). In addition, activated basophils and mast cells contain and can release kallikrein as an additional local intestinal source of tissue kallikrein (Min & Paul, 2008).

5.2 Kinins and kinin receptors in IBD

Almost fifty years ago it has been demonstrated that bradykinin was able to evoke cardinal signs of inflammation (Lewis, 1964). In addition in chronic inflammation B1R seems to be important in neutrophil accumulation in inflamed tissue (McLean et al., 2000). Both B1R and B2R are involved in onset and maintenance of nociceptive alterations and inflammatory pain perceptions (Drey, 1997; Rupniak et al., 1997). Research on involvement of B2Rs in inflammatory states has progressed more quickly than that on B1Rs, and it was favored by the systematic development of selective peptidic B2R antagonists by the pharmaceutical companies, at this time. Thus we described B2Rs distribution in PG – APS induced model of granulomatous enterocolitis in intestinal layer showing B2R in epithelial cells, smooth muscle cells, and in serosa (Stadnicki et al., 1998 c). In this model a specific bradykinin BR2 antagonist (HOE – 140) attenuated arthritis but exhibited only minimal preventive effect on enterocolitis suggesting that kinin stimulation via B2R was a more important in arthritis than of enterocolitis (Stadnicki et al., 1999). In dextran sulfate (DDS) - induced colitis model in mice a selective B2R antagonist suppressed shortening of the large intestine (Arai et al., 1999), which was in agreement with future results indicated that intestinal contraction was regulated by B2R (Hara et al., 2007), however demonstrated only limited effect in intestinal inflammatory lesions. Later in human studies we demonstrated the increase in the ratio of B1R to B2R gene expression in relation to the degree of intestinal inflammation, and visualized both B1R and B2R in normal as well as inflammatory human colon and ileum (Stadnicki et al., 2005). B2R protein was normally present in the apices of enterocytes in the basal area and intracellularly in inflammatory tissue. In contrast, B1R protein was found in the basal area of enterocytes in normal intestine, but in the apical portion of enterocytes in inflamed tissue. B1R protein was significantly increased in both active UC and Crohn's disease intestines compared to controls. In addition B1R was observed in the nerve of the colonic submucosa. Importantly B1R but not B2 was present in macrophages inside granulomas of Crohn's intestine. The total level of B1R was significantly higher in enterocytes of patients with active phase of UC as well as in Crohn's disease as compared with controls. Recent studies have demonstrated that the B2R receptor may be recycled several times in the same enterocytes after internalization (Bachvarov et al., 2001; Souza et al., 2007). This process was supported by the appearance of B2R intracellularly in some enterocytes in UC intestine. In contrast B1R normally do not internalize following agonist stimulation, but they seem to translocate and aggregate after agonist binding, probably to facilitate the amplification of B1 receptor mediated responses (Sabourin et al., 2002). Taken together the results strongly indicated that the B1R receptor is a major structural background for kinins function in human IBD. Kinins are involved in intestinal glucose and electrolyte transport and local blood flow under normal conditions. However in intestine, kinins may be more important as pathophysiological mediators. It has been shown that bradykinin produces 2 – 4 – fold greater concentration of prostanoids in animals with experimental colitis than in normal controls, which may contribute to the increased intestinal secretion of chloride (Zipser et al. 1985). Bradykinin – induced chloride secretion by the guinea pig ileum occurs by direct binding of the ligand to its receptor (Maning et al., 1982). It has been shown that both inducible B1R and constitutive B2R mediate the ion transport in intestinal epithelium (Cuthbert, 2001). The secretion of chloride into the lumen is accompanied with natrium secretion and in turn water, thus leading to secretory diarrhea, and this effect of kinins is much prostaglandin-independent. In relation to IBD kinins may act on endothelial cells, smooth muscle cells, epithelial cells, and fibroblasts, which stimulate cell response through G proteins - coupled kinin receptors. By opening the tight junctions between endothelial cells, kinins can increase capillary permeability (Gaginella & Kachur, 1989). Kinins may stimulate though B2R inflammatory cell adhesion molecules, and white blood cells migration. Subsequently B1R stimulation promote more cell adhesion molecules, and cells influx mainly neutrophils into extravascular comparment(McLean et al., 2003;

Ulbrich et al., 2000). Kinins may act as mitogens to increase DNA synthesis, thereby promoting cell proliferation. The ability of kinins to stimulate fibroblast proliferation may contribute to fibrosis in chronic intestinal inflammation (Marceau et al., 1986). Kinins may stimulate macrophage release of IL-1 and TNF – α (Tiffany & Burch, 1989). This effect is probably mediated by stimulation of the RB1, since a specific RB1 antagonist block kinin-induced cytokine release. In human study it has been demonstrated a positive staining for TK, kallistatin and the B1R (but not the B2R) in macrophages forming granuloma and for B1R in plasmocytes in the border of granulomas which emphasizes the close relationship between the immune responses important in IBD and the inflammatory mediators including the ITK – kinins. Kinins may also evoke pain by stimulating sensory nerves to mechanical stimuli and other chemical mediators and, in turn, causes hyperalgesia (Drey, 1997). The role of B1R and its agonists in inflammatory pain has been shown in animals (Rupniak et al., 1997). In addition, bradykinin accelerates mucin discharge from goblet cells (Stanley & Philips, 1994). Although it is not know if ITK is co – secreted with mucin after bradykinin action, it raises the possibility of positive feedback loop between local ITK release and bradykinin generation. In addition, it has been demonstrated a B1R polymorphism in human IBD, but its clinical significance remains unknown (Bachvarov at al., 1998). The recent experimental study investigated the role of BR1s in TNBS - induced mouse model of colitis showing that that selective, orally active, non - peptide B1R antagonist SSR240612 markedly reduced TNBS – induced colitis e.g. intestinal tissue damage and neutrophil influx (Hara et al., 2008). Importantly this study clarified evidence that TNF – α may upregulate B1R expression in TNBS colitis model suggesting that anti- TNF- α monoclonal antibodies may in part modulate IBD by regulation of BR1 expression. It should be noted that kinins are implicated in the regulation of blood pressure, sodium homeostasis and the cardioprotective effect of preconditioning (Chao et al., 2004). Angiotensin- converting enzyme (kininase II) inhibition increase blood levels of bradykinin and kallidin peptides (Colman et al., 2006 c). Thus, the potentially salutary role of kinins in the circulation not encourage systemic administration of B1R antagonist. In fact commonly used ACE inhibitors are cardioprotective in part by elevating bradykinin, and thus increasing nitric oxide as well as decreasing angiotensin II formation (Colman et al., 2006c). Kinins have been demonstrated to stimulate synthesis of eicosanoids, nitric oxide and cytokines by white blood cells, endothelial cells and epithelial cells, and promote adhesion molecule – neutrophil cascade known to be important in IBD. A selective B1R receptor antagonist may have potential in therapeutic trial. It has been postulated that topical drug delivery to intestine as for 5 – ASA compounds to avoid side effect may be appropriate for the management of IBD (Marceau & Regoli, 2008). In fact the levels of kinin peptides in tissue were higher than in blood suggesting the primary tissue localization of the kallikrein – kinin system (Campbell, 2001). Nevertheless it seems that the contact system plays an important role in many inflammatory cascades by activation of the complement system, enhances liberation of prostanoids and cytokines, and specifically interacts with coagulation, fibrinolytic components and platelets.

6. Hemostatic alterations in IBD

The current model of coagulation in vivo emphasizes tissue factor as initiator of coagulation activation, underlines main role of thrombin in amplification of coagulation, and the interaction of coagulation factors with blood cells and endothelial cells (Hoffman & Monroe,

2007). Activated cells, especially platelets are critical in amplification and propagation phases providing a negatively – charged phosfolipid surface on which clotting reactions may take place. In IBD the coagulation system may be activated following cellular injury mainly through the extrinsic pathway. Tissue factor, a potent trigger of coagulation, functions as a monocyte and endothelia cell receptor which binds factor VII and facilitates activation of both factor IX and factor X. Activated factor X (FXa), Ca ++ , activated factor V (FVa), and platelet phospholipid form the prothrombinase complex that cleaves prothrombin, producing thrombin and liberating a prothrombin fragment, F1 + 2. Thrombin hydrolyzes fibrinogen forming fibrin, which is cross-linked by activated factor XIII. Cross-linked fibrin is then degraded by plasmin with the liberation of D-dimer and other degradation products. Factor XII converts the zymogen, factor XI, to an active enzyme, factor XIa, which, in turn, converts factor IX to factor IXa, thereby activating the intrinsic pathway of coagulation. (Clolman, 2006 a).

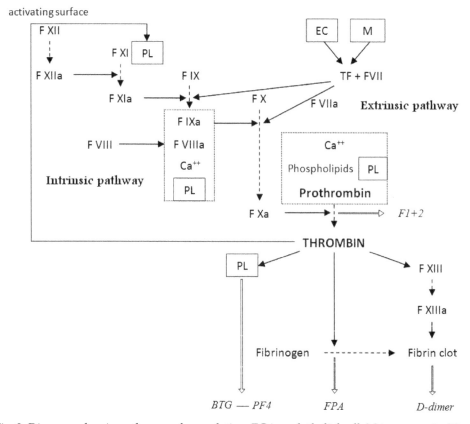

Fig. 3. Diagram of main pathways of coagulation. EC is endothelial cell, M is monocyte, PL is platelet, F1+2 is prothrombin fragment, FPA is fibrinopeptide A, βTG is β-thromboglobulin, TF is tissue factor. Solid arrows designate activation or cleavage, dashed arrows conversion, and open arrows indicate release, expression, or synergistic properties

6.1 Systemic coagulation changes

Early reports have presented hemostatic changes in IBD patients; elevation of plasma factor V, factor VIII, fibrinogen and thrombocytosis observed in the active IBD phase (Lam et al., 1975; Morowitz et al., 1968). Later reports have shown an acquired plasma antithrombin deficiency in active IBD patients, a feature which implies a real risk of thrombosis (Knot et al., 1985). Subsequent studies have shown the presence of increased markers of activate coagulation in both active and quiescent IBD (van Bodegraven et al., 2002; Hudson et al., 1992; Souto et al., 1995). In contrast other investigators did not found a significant increase of coagulation intermediates in IBD patients with an inactive stage (Edwards et al., 1987; Novacek et al., 1997; Stadnicki et al., 1997). It is assumed that the reaction with thrombin during the clotting activation causes consumption of plasma FXIIIa and, therefore, a fall in FXIII may be sign of clotting activation (Ichinose, 2001). In fact it has been found a decrease of FXIII subunit A, but not FXIII subunit B in both active UC (Stadnicki et al., 1991) and Crohn's disease (Hudson at al., 1993). Later other investigators shown reduced level of FXIII active subunit A (but not carries subunit B) in active IBD patients, but generally not in patients with quiescent disease suggesting its consumption as result of active coagulation and increased turnover during active inflammation (van Bodegraven et al., 1995; Hayat et al., 2002). In addition, elevated D-dimer was found almost exclusively in active IBD patients which provides evidence of fibrin formation and reactive fibrinolysis (Chiarantini et. al., 1996, Hudson et al.,1992, Stadnicki et al., 1997). Natural coagulation inhibitor, protein C plasma level has been shown to be unchanged or decreased in IBD (Larsen et al., 2002)), while decreased its cofactor, protein S plasma level was demonstrated in most studies (Aadland et al., 1994; Saibeni et al., 2001). In addition, an inhibitor of tissue factor, tissue factor protease – inhibitor (TFPI) plasma levels have been reported to be lower in IBD (Souto et al., 1995). Differences between ulcerative colitis and Crohn's diseases including disease location, histology, clinical course and complications although it is likely that both entities share similar immunoregulatory abnormalities and common pathways. The lower levels of coagulation intermediates or fragments in UC patients, as compared with Crohn's disease, may be simply due to more superficial distribution of intestinal inflammation always found in UC. In addition patients with Cronh's disease have higher tissue IL-1 β and plasma IL-6 levels (Mazlam & Hodgson, 1994). A role of intrinsic coagulation activation pathway, associated with the contact system, in IBD is unclear. FXI (an initiator of intrinsic pathway) is activated by thrombin (Olivier et al., 1999), or by the contact pathway initiated by autoactivation of FXII. Surprisingly in two large studies plasma factor XI functional level remained unchanged in active UC (Stadnicki et al., 1997) and Crohn's disease (Devani et al., 2002). In contrast other authors observed increased active plasma level of FXII and FXI among other signs of thrombin generation in active UC patients suggesting both extrinsic and intrinsic coagulation pathways activation in active UC stage (Kume et al., 2007; Kyriakou et al., 2002). However whether the plasma contact system is activated in intestinal circulation and if so, what is the role of HKa to maintain inflammation remains to be investigated.

6.2 Systemic fibrinolytic capacity

Disturbed fibrinolysis, which has been reported in general circulation and in colonic mucosa, has also been postulated to play a role in procoagulant potential in systemic circulation, however also in intestinal bleeding of IBD. It have been demonstrated the decrease of plasma t-PA with concomitant increase of its inhibitor, plasma PAI-1 indicated hypofibrinolytic capacity in general circulation of IBD patients (de Jong et al., 1989). T- PA is mainly released by vascular endothelium, thus its plasma decrease in IBD suggests endotheliopathy. This phenomenon is supported by data (Gris et al., 1991) indicating impaired fibrinolytic response to the venous occlusion test in patients with colitis. Systemic endothelial cell dysfunction has been reported in both UC and Crohn's disease. A serum von Willebrand factor concentration and thrombomodulin level, the markers of vascular injury have been shown to be increased in serum of IBD patients in relation with disease activity (Boehme MW et al., 1997; Wan der Wouwer et al., 2004). Recently discovered thrombin activatable fibrinolysis inhibitor (TAFI) provides link between coagulation and fibrinolysis (Bouma, 2004), and primarily its levels have been linked with thrombophilia in IBD. However TAFI plasma level in IBD is equivocal thus its significance is unclear (Koutroubakis et al., 2008; Saibeni et al., 2004). In addition, Italian group (Saibeni et al., 2006) has been demonstrated a prevalence of anti – t- PA antibodies in IBD patients which may reduce systemic fibrinolysis.

6.3 Intestinal coagulation and fibrinolytic disturbances

Nevertheless, those alterations occur in systemic circulation and, while reflecting the systemic inflammatory response, does not portray the actual events within the inflamed intestine. It has been indicated that regional vasculopathy leading to activation of coagulation cascade and local fibrin formation are pathogenic factors in Crohn's disease (Wakefield et al., 1989, 1991). Platelets thrombi linked with fibrin, and expression of tissue factor were also observed in Crohn's intestinal lesions (More et al., 1993; Wakefield et al., 1989). Similarly mucosal capillary thrombi have been identified in UC, but similar changes were also found in self – limited colitis, thus their pathogenic significance in UC is less appreciated (Dhillon et al., 1992). However a higher platelets aggregation has been found in mesenteric circulation in IBD, hence circulating platelets aggregates may contribute to ischemic damage, and platelets aggregates have been identified histologically in rectal biopsies from patients with UC (Collins et al., 1997). Latter data demonstrated that CD40L positive platelets adhere to mucosal endothelium in IBD, hence trigger proinflammatory reactions (Danese et al., 2003 a). Importantly, platelets may mediate leukocyte recruitment to the inflamed colon via CD40 – CD40L (Danese et al., 2003 a), and independently platelets taken from IBD patients release RANTES, a chemokine recruiting monocyte and T – memory cells (Fagerstam et al., 2000). In addition interaction of platelets expressed CD40 with CD40 expressed vascular component may increase influx of white blood cells to extravascular compartment. Activated protein C (APC) exert anti- inflammatory effect and directly maintain vascular barrier integrity. However protein C anticoagulant pathway has been found to be impaired in IBD, hence it may enhance thrombin generation. A reduced expression of endothelial protein C receptor (EPCR) in microvasculature endothelium has been shown in IBD patients (Faioni et al., 2004). It is still uncertain if the intestinal vascular alterations in IBD is the primum movens of the disease (Wakefield et al., 1989), or the consequence of inflammation (Binion et al., 1998). In the inflamed mucosa of IBD patients it has been presented a decrease of t-PA and increase of u-PA (de Bruin et al., 1988; de Jong et al., 1989). U-PA, in contrast to t-PA, is less fibrin dependent; thus plasmin generated due to u-PA may act as proinflammatory protease as well as enhance intestinal bleeding which is typical feature especially in UC. Interestingly u-PA is secreted as prourokinase which can be activated to urokinase by plasmin itself or in the cells surface by plasma kallikrein in the presence of high kininogen (Ichinose et al., 1986). Urokinase binds to its receptor, uPAR, on the endothelial – cell surface (Colman, 2006). Prekallikrein binds to HK, which associates with the same receptor hence the conversion of plasminogen to plasmin is efficient. Thus prekallikrein may be anti- thrombotic by virtue of its role in the fibrinolytic system. Although a moderate amount of FXIII has proved sufficient to secure hemostasis, its low level in the presence of other coagulation abnormalities may contribute to intestinal bleeding, but its relationship to intestinal bleeding during IBD is controversial Other investigations have shown enhanced local fibrinolytic activity in IBD patients which led to use tranaxemic acid, an antifibrinolytic agent, in the context of an increased intestinal bleeding tendency (Kondo et al., 1981)). This drug acts mainly preventing the interaction of tissue t - PA with fibrin which is required for its catalytic activity. However local fibrinolysis in IBD is related to u-PA, which is fibrin independent.

7. Serine proteases act via PARs

Four protease – activated receptors (PARs) 1-4 have been identified as mediators of cellular responses. It has been shown that coagulation activation may mediate inflammatory response, which support the concept of mutual activation of inflammatory and coagulation cascades in IBD. Thrombin is a key player of PARs activation as this enzyme can activate PAR1, 3 and 4, and in turn activates platelet and endothelial cells, whereas tissue factor can act due to PAR1 or 2 (Steinhoff et al., 2005). Recent study demonstrated that active factor X (FXa) may induce PAR -2 activation, and in turn may mediate inflammation and fibrosis, a features of IBD (Borensztajn et al., 2009). Interestingly, investigation revealed that PAR1 and PAR2 are present on intestinal epithelium, and PAR1 has been shown to mediate intestinal secretion (Oikonomopoulou et al., 2006). In addition tissue kallikrein may activate directly B2R independently of bradykinin release. Thus in addition to thrombin and trypsin which can affect tissues by activating a novel family of protease activated receptors (PARs 1-4), tissue kallikreins represent PAR regulator, and consequently B2R may belong to a new group of PARs. In animal studies a decreased plasma protein C activation was shown in DDS – induced colitis in mice (Yoshida et al., 2008), and APC administered to mouse colitis model also provided protection against thrombosis and accompanied colonic inflammation. In addition via thrombin generation platelets may by activated by PARs (Biloduane & Hamm, 2007). PARs activated coagulation cascade might participate in the progression of IBD suggesting that PARs blockade might provide a novel therapeutic target for the management of IBD.

8. Platelet as inflammatory cell in IBD

IBD patients have an increase of platelet numbers which correlate with both UC and Crohn's activity (Morowitz et al., 1968). In early 1990s it has been documented abnormal platelet aggregation in vitro, and activation in vivo expressed by elevation of tromboxane B2, tromboxane A2, and specific chemokines as platelet factor – 4 and β – tromboglobulin as well as higher expression of P– selectin and GP53 on platelets surface in both active and inactive IBD phases (Collins et al., 1994, Webberley et al., 1993). Thus platelet activation is a feature of IBD. During inflammation an increased endothelial exposure of adhesion glycoproteines may enhance binding of platelets and leukocyte. Later it has been (Danese et al., 2003 b) observed increased platelet expression of activation - dependent of CD40 – ligand (CD40L) as well as increased plasma level of soluble CD40 in both UC and Cronh's disease compared to normal controls. The increased of platelet-leukocyte aggregated (PLA) in systemic circulation account for platelet activation and platelet- leukocyte interaction in IBD patients (Irving et al., 2004). Taken together it seems that in IBD platelets show not only prothrombotic but also proinflammatory properties. Suppression of the adverse effect of thromboxane A2 can be achieved either by inhibiting its synthesis and/or antagonizing the receptor through which it acts. Selective antithromboxane agents have been shown to ameliorate experimental colitis (Vilaseca et al., 1990) however ridogrel not shown enough therapeutic effect (Tytgat et al., 2002). Unfortunately, ridogrel is a weaker thromboxane receptor antagonist than synthetase inhibitor, so that activation of the former by endoperoxides such as PGH-2 (accumulating after inhibition of thromboxane synthetase) activate thromboxane recepotors. New generation of antiplatelet compounds which selectively inhibit platelet activation rather than platelet aggregation merit future studies in IBD.

9. Thromboembolic complications in IBD

9.1 Risk factors for thromboembolism

Coagulation activation in IBD is one of significant feature to enhance prothrombotic potential, increased risk of thromboembolism is related to extension of intestinal inflammation, but coagulation system abnormalities found in IBD may also be caused by other acquired factors. Nutritional deficiencies of vitamins B6 and B12, and folic acid in Cronh's disease patients may be caused by ileitis, while sulfasalazine or methotrexate – induced folate deficiency may have similar effect in both Crohn' s disease and UC. Those deficiencies may lead to hyperhomocysteinemia which has been found in IBD patients (Bjerregaard et al., 2002). Increased level of lipoprotein (a) an independent risk factor for TE has been shown to account for tendency to thromboembolism in some Crohn'n disease patients (van Bodegraven & Meuwissen, 2001). Other ways that may predispose to thromboembolism in IBD include immobility, the need to undergo surgery, fluid depletion diarrhea – induced, and use central venous catheter for parenteral nutrition. At present no interaction between IBD and inherited factors of thrombophilia e.g. factor V gene (FV Leiden) mutation, prothrombin G20210A mutation, and methylenetetrahydrofolate reductase (MTHRF) gene mutation (related to hyperhomocysteinemia) were found (Guedon et al., 2001; Papa et al., 2001) .

9.2 Thrombotic manifestations

The thromboembolic complications are common extraintestinal manifestations in both Crohn's disease and UC, appear to have a 3-4 fold increased risk of developing compared to control patients), and also exist in quiescent disease (Bernstein et al., 2001). Importantly thromboembolic complications increased risk was found to be specific for IBD because neither in patient with rheumatoid arthritis, nor in patients with celiac disease had an increased thromboembolic risk compared with their controls (Miehsler et al., 2004). Deep venous thrombosis and pulmonary embolism are most common thrombotic complications in IBD, but there were also described in unusual sites *e.g.* portal vein, mesenteric vein, retinal vein, and cerebral sinus veins. In addition arterial thromboembolic events and ischemic heart disease risk is increased in IBD patients, (Bernstein et al., 2008). Systemic thrombotic events are life – threatening since mortality related to thromboembolism in IBD is described in high ranges between 8% - 25 % during acute thromboembolic episodes

(Quera & Shanahan, 2004). As unconventional IBD treatment heparin have paid attention because its anti- inflammatory effect, hence heparin interferes with anti-inflammatory cascade by influencing cell migration into tissue and modulates a release of proinflammatory cytokine. Early study indicated a beneficial effect of heparin in refractory ulcerative colitis (Gaffyney et al., 1995). In general better therapeutic efficacy of unfractionated heparin (UH) than low molecular weigh heparin (LMWH) in UC is probably related to more beneficial immunomodulatory effect of UH (Panes et al., 2000). In fact an efficacy of heparin treatment in UC is still controversial and not established. However a recent small open study demonstrated a reduction of inflammation using oral, slow- release LMWH (parnaparin) capsules in left- sided UC patients (Pastorelli et al., 2008). It appears that IBD is a thrombophilic syndrome, a risk of thromboembolic events in IBD is multifactoral including active intestinal inflammation and malnutrition, (Quera & Shanahan, 2004). Prophylactic anticoagulation against thromboembolism is currently not fully defined, and intestinal bleeding worsening may occur. In high – risk patients e.g. active IBD patients confined to bad, subjects with familial thrombosis, and patients with myocardial infraction, or stroke before age 50 in first degree relatives should be considered for using moderate dose of heparin (Zitomersky et al., 2011).

10. Coagulation, intestinal barrier and healing

The epithelium of the intestine creates a barrier to potentially immunogenic and noxious factors, including microorganisms and dietary components within the intestinal lumen. Healing of the intestinal surface is regulated by a complex mechanism that involves growth factors, cytokines, as well as intracellular matrix proteins and blood clotting factors to preserve homeostasis and integrity of the intestinal mucosa (Dignass & Podolsky, 2004). Once the intestinal epithelial barrier is damaged, luminal highly immunogenic bacterial antigens can enter the normally sterile submucosal layers and thus may play a role in the pathogenesis of IBD. The antibiotics, mainly tobramycin and metronidazole, have been found to be effective as adjunctive therapy not only in Crohn's disease but also in UC patients (Rahimi et al. 2007). Among the regulatory peptides that are expressed within the intestinal mucosa, transforming growth factor-β (TGF-β) and epidermal growth factor family peptides (EGFs) play especially important role. EGFs, potent stimulators of intestinal epithelial cells proliferation, and may increase the concentration of bioactive TGF-β, whereas TGF-β is capable of regulating growth, differentiation, and function of immune cells (Stadnicki et al., 2009). Interestingly, EGF enemas have been proved to be beneficial in UC patients (Dieckgraefe et al. 2007). Importantly, TGF-β1 that counteracts TNF-α and acts as negative regulator of mucosal inflammation is essential for wound healing (Blobe et al., 2000). The role of TNF-α, that occupies central position to generate the inflammatory cascade, has been well defined in Crohn's disease and recently in UC (Blonski et al., 2011). Infliximab administered with steroids, has been found to be effective in inducing responses and maintaining remissions in patients with moderate and severe stage of IBD. Interestingly treatment with infliximab, a chimeric antibody against TNF-α, has been reported not only induced clinical remission but also decreased thrombin generation in IBD patients (Hommes et al. 1997). Intestinal epithelial wound healing and tissue repair may also act trough growth factors independent pathway involved in cells interactions and blood coagulation factors. Besides fibrin, FXIIIa also cross-links actin, collagen, and fibronectin., thus it is as much connective tissue factor as a clotting factor. FXIII and other transglutaminases may be important in the maintenance of normal intestinal integrity and intestinal repair mechanism (D'Argenio et al. 1995). Our and others data suggested that interaction of factor XIII subunit A a with its natural plasmatic substrates e. g. fibronectin and α–2 plasmin inhibitor, plays a role in healing of UC lesions (Stadnicki et al., 1992). Consequently, factor XIIIa infusion has been shown to promote intestinal wound healing in both UC and Crohn's disease patients (Lorenz et al., 1991; Oshitani et al., 1996). In contrast vascular endothelial growth factor (VEGF) increases vascular permeability to activate metaloproteinases which participate in degradation of extracellular matrix, hence may have detrimental effect on intestinal barrier (Ferrara, 2004).

11. Kinins and angiogenesis in IBD

Recently it has been provided the direct evidences that angiogenesis has a role in the pathogenesis of both UC and Crohn's disease showing a higher density of microvessels within intestinal mucosa and sub-mucosa and increased expression of αvβ3 - integrin in endothelium with simultaneous increase of intestinal VEGF expression (Danese et al., 2006) . Most recent data demonstrated the increase of genes expression as well as protein levels for VEGF and its Flt-1 receptor in active inflammatory colonic tissue and increased VEGF levels in serum and plasma in active UC patients (Frysz – Naglak et al., 2011). TGF-β1 may directly stimulate angiogenesis in vivo; the stimulation can be blocked by TGF-β1 antibodies (Pepper, 1997). The influence of kinins in angiogenesis has recently been appreciated. Kinin promotes angiogenesis by upregulation of basic fibroblast growth factor through bradykinin - B1 receptor and by stimulation of VEGF formation by bradykinin both B1 and B2 receptors (Colman, 2006 b), and kinins may act synergistically with TGF-β1. Monoclonal antibody C11C1 which prevents binding HK to endothelial cells also limits its conversion to bradykinin thus downregulating angiogenesis (Colman et al. 2000). Thus, it is possible that kinins as proangiogenic may promote angiogenesis in IBD although the interaction between kinins and growth factors is highly complex, and requires future investigation. In contrast HKa or its domain 5 inhibit endothelial cells migration and proliferation needed for angiogenesis (Colman et al, 2003).

12. Conclusions

IBD appear to be immunologically mediated by activation of immune system cells and plasma proteolytic cascades. Products of activated cells such as cytokines, eicosanoids, lysosomal enzymes as well as kallikrein – kinin and coagulation system are reported to be increased in intestinal lesions and in the systemic circulation of IBD. The activation of coagulation has been recognized as important component of the inflammatory response in both Crohn's disease and UC, and also is significant in progression and possibly pathogenesis of these entities. A significance of coagulation in IBD was underestimated, now it appears that IBD is a thrombophilic syndrome in both active and quiescent phases. A risk of thromboembolic events in IBD is multifactoral including coagulation activation. Prophylactic anticoagulation against thromboembolic complications is currently not fully defined, however high – risk patients should be considered for using moderate dose of heparin. Kinins exert their biological effect by activating constitutive bradykinin receptor -2 (BR2), which are rapidly desensitized, and inducible by inflammatory cytokines bradykinin receptor -1 (BR1), resistant to densensitization. Intestinal tissue kallikrein (ITK) may hydrolyze growth factors and peptides whereas kinins increase capillary permeability, evoke pain, stimulate synthesis of nitric oxide and cytokines, and promote adhesion molecule – neutrophil cascade. Thus activation of intestinal kallikrein – kinin system may have relevance to idiopathic inflammatory bowel disease (IBD). These results promise to yield new insight in the pathogenesis of IBD. Currently it seems that upregulation of bradykinin B1 recepror (B1R) in human and animal intestinal inflammation provides a structural basis for the kinins function, and selective B1R antagonist may have potential in therapeutic trial of IBD patients.

13. References

Aadland E, Odegaard OR, Roseth A, Try K. (1994). Free protein S deficiency in patients with Cronh's disease. Scand J Gastroenterol, 29, 333- 5.

Andoh A, Tsujikawa T, Hata K, et al.(2005). Elevated circulating platelet – derived microplates in patients with active inflammatory bowel disease. Am J Gastroenterl, 100, 2042 – 8.

Arai Y, Takanashi H, Kitagawa H, et al. (1999). Effect of Icatibant, a bradykinin receptor -2 antagonist, on the development of experimental ulcerative colitis in mice. Dig Dis Sci, 44, 845 – 851.

Bachvarov DR, Houle S, Bachvarova M, et al.(2001). Bradykinin B(2) receptor endocytosis, recycling, and down-regulation assessed using green fluorescent protein conjugates. J Pharmacol Exp Ther, 297, 19-26.

Bachvarov DR, Landry M, Houle S, et al. (1998). Altered frequency of a promoter polymorphic allele of the kinin B1 receptor gene in inflammatory bowel disease. Gastroenterology 115, 1045 - 1058.

Baumgart DC, Carding SR. (2007). Gastroenterology 1. Inflammatory bowel disease: cause and immunobiology. Lancet, 369, 1627- 40.

Bernstein CN, Blanchard JF, Houston DS, Wajda A.(2001). The incidence of deep venous thrombosis and pulmonary embolism among patients with inflammatory bowel disease: a population-based cohort study. Thromb Haemost, 85, 430– 4.

Bernstein CN, Wajda A, Blanchard JF. (2008). The incidence of arterial thromboembolic disease in inflammatory bowel disease: a population based study. Clin Gastroenterol Hepatol, 6, 41-5.

Bhoola KD, Figueroa CD, Worthy K. (1992). Bioregulation of kinins: Kallikreins, kininogens, and Kininases. Pharmacol Rev, 44, 1- 80.

Biloduane LM, Hamm HE.(2007). Regulation of protease- activated receptor PAR1 and PAR4 signaling in human platelets by compartmentalized cyclic nucleotide action. J Pharm Exp Ther, 322, 778 – 88.

Binion DG, West GA, Volk EE, et al. (1998). Acquired increase in leucocyte binding by intestinal microvascular endothelium in inflammatory bowel disease. Lancet, 352, 1742 – 6.

Bjerregaard LT, Nederby NJ, Fredholm L, Brandslund I, Munkholm P, Hey H.(2002). Hyperhomocysteinaemia, coagulation pathway activation and thrombophilia in patients with inflammatory bowel disease. Scand J Gastroenterol, 37, 62-7.

Blobe GC, Schiemann WP, Lodish HF. (2000). Role of transforming growth factor beta in human disease.N Engl J Med, 342, 1350-1358.

Blonski W, Stadnicki A, Lichtenstein G, Burke A. Infliximab use in ulcerative colitis. In: Ulcerative Colitis. The complete quid to medical management. Editors: GR Lichtenstein and EJ Scherl. Slack Inc. 2011.

Boehme MW, Autschbach F, Zuna I, et al. (1997). Elevated serum levels and reduced immunohistochemical expression of thrombomodulin in active ulcerative colitis. *Gastroenterology*, 113, 107 – 17.

Borensztajn K, Peppelenbosch MP, Spek CA. (2009). Coagulation and factor Xa signaling: the link between coagulation and inflammatory bowel disease? *Trends Pharmacol Sci*, 30, 8-16.

Bouma BN, Mosnier LO. (2004). Thrombin activatable fibrinolysis inhibitor (TAFI) at the interface between coagulation and fibrinolysis. *Pathophysiol Haemost Thromb*, 33, 375- 81.

Calixto JB, Medeiros L, Fernandes ES, et al. (2004). Kinin B1 receptors: key G – protein coupled receptors and their role in inflammatory and painful processes. *Br J Pharmacol*, 143, 803 – 818.

Campbell D.(2001). The kallikrein – kinin system in humans. *Clin Exp Pharmacol Physiol*, 28, 1060-1065.

Chao J, Chao L.(2004). Kallikrein – kiinin in stroke, cardiovascular and renal disease. *Exp Physiol*, 90, 291 – 298.

Chao J, Schmaier AH, Chen LM, et al.(1996). Kallistatin, a novel human tissue kallikrein inhibitor: Levels in body fluids, blood cells, and tissues in health and disease. *J Lab Clin Med*, 127, 612-620.

Chen LM, Richards GP, Chao L, et al.(1995). Molecular cloning, purification and in situ localization of human colon kallikrein. *Biochem J*, 307, 481-486.

Chiarantini F, Valanzano R, Liotta AA, et al.(1996). Hemostatc abnormalities in inflammatory bowel disease. *Thromb Res*, 82, 137- 46.

Clements J, Mukhtar A, Ehrlich A, et al.(1992). A re-evaluation of the tissue-specific pattern of expression of the rat kallikrein gene family. *Agents Actions*, 38, 34-41.

Collins CE, Cahill MR, Newland AC, Rampton DS.(1994). Platelets circulate in an activated state in inflammatory bowel disease. *Gastroenterology*, 106, 840 – 45.

Collins CE, Rampton DS, Rogers J, et al. (1997). Platelet aggregation and neutrophil sequestration in the mesenteric circulation in inflammatory bowel disease. Eur J Gastroenterol Hepatol, 9, 1213-17.

Colman RW. (2006 a). Are hemostasis and thrombosis two sides of the same coin? *JEM*, 203, 493- 5.

Colman RW. (2006 b). Regulation of angiogenesis by the kallikrein-kinin system. *Cur Pharmaceut Des*, 12, 599-607.

Colman RW, Jameson BA, Lin Y, et al.(2000). Domain 5 of high molecular weight kininogen (kininostatin) down-regulates endothelial cell proliferation and migration and inhibits angiogenesis. *Blood*, 95, 543-550.

Colman RW, Pixley RA, Sainz IM, et al.(2003). Inhibition of angiogenesis by antibody blocking the action of proangiogenic high-molecular-weight kininogen. *Thromb Haemostas*, 1, 164- 170.

Colman RW. (2006 c). Contact activation (kallikrein – kinin) pathway: multiple physiologic and pathophysiologic activities. In: Colman RW, Marder VJ, Cloves AW, et al. ed.

Hemostasis and Thrombosis. Basic Principles and Clinical Practice.5th ed. Philadelphia: Lippincott Wiliams&Wilkins, pp.103 – 121.

Cuthbert AW. (2001). Kinins and epithelial ion transport in the alimentary tract. *Biol Chem*, 382, 57-60.

D'Argenio G, Biancone L, Cosenza V, *et al*.(1995). Transglutaminases in Cronh's disease. Gut, 37, 690 – 5.

Danese S, de La Motte C, Sturm A, *et al*. (2003 a). Platelets trigger a CD40 – dependent inflammatory response in the microvasculature of inflammatory bowel disease patients. Gastroenterology, 124, 1249 – 64.

Danese S, Katz JA, Saibeni S, *et al*. (2003 b). Activated platelets are the source of elevated levels of soluble CD40 ligand in the circulation of inflammatory bowel disease patients. Gut, 52, 1435 – 41.

Danese S, Papa A, Saibeni S, Repici A, Malesci A, Vecchi M. (2007). Inflammation and coagulation in inflammatory bowel disease: the clot thickens. *Am J Gastroenterol*, 102, 174- 86.

Danese S, Sans M, de LaMotte C, et al. (2006). Angiogenesis as a novel component of inflammatory bowel disease pathogenesis. *Gastroenterology*, 130: 2060-2073.

de Bruin PA, Crama-Bohbout G, Verspaget HW, *et al*. (1988). Plasminogen activators in the intestine of patients with inflammatory bowel disease. *Thromb Haemost*, 60, 262 6.

de Jong E, Porte RJ, Knot EA, Verheijen JH, Dees J.(1989). Disturbed fibrinolysis in patients with inflammatory bowel disease. A study of blood plasma, colon mucosa, and faeces. Gut, 30, 188 – 94.

DeLa Cadena R, Majluf - Cruz A, Stadnicki A, et al.(1998). Recombinant tumor necrosis factor receptor (TNFR: Fc) alters endotoxin – induced activation of the kinin, fibrinolytic, and coagulation system in normal human subjects. *Thromb Haemostas*, 80, 114 – 118.

Devani M, Cugno M, Vecchi M, et al.(2002). Kallikrein - kinin system activation in Crohn's disease: Differences in intestinal and systemic markers. *Amer J Gastroenterol*, 97: 2026 - 2032.

Devani M, Vecchi M, Ferrero S, et al. (2005). Kallikrein – kinin system in inflammatory bowel disease : intestinal involvement and correlation with the degree of tissue inflammation. *Dig Liver Dis*, 37, 665 – 673.

Dhillon AP, Anthony A, Sim R, *et al*. (1992). Mucosal capillary thrombi in rectal biopsies. *Histopathology*, 21: 127 – 33.

Dieckgraefe BK, Korzenik JR, Anant S.(2006). Growth factors as treatment options for intestinal inflammation. *Ann N Y Acad Sci*, 1072, 300-306.

Dignass AU, Podolsky DK.(2004). Epithelial restitution and intestinal repair. In: Sartor RB, Sandborn WJ, editors. Kirsner's inflammatory bowel diseases. Philadelphia: Saunders, pp. 18-29.

Drey A. (1997). Kinins and their receptors in hyperalgesia. *Br J Pharmacol*, 75, 704-712.

Edwards RL, Levine JB, Green R, *et al*.(1987). Activation of blood coagulation in Crohn's disease. Increased plasma fibrinopeptide A levels and enhanced generation of monocyte tissue factor activity. *Gastroenterology*, 92: 329 – 37.

Fagerstam JP, Whiss PA, Strom M, Andersson RG.(2000). Expression of platelet P – selectin and detection of soluble P-selectin, NPY and RANTES in patients with inflammatory bowel disease. Inflamm Res, 49, 466 – 72.

Faioni FM, Ferrero S, Fontana G, et al.(2004). Expression of endothelial protein C receptor and thromomodulin in the intestinal tissue of patients with inflammatory bowel disease. Crit Care Med, 32 (suppl 5): S266 – 70.

Fasth S, Hulten L.(1973). The effect of bradykinin on intestinal motility and blood flow. Acta Chir Scand, 139, 699 – 705.

Ferrara N.(2004). Vascular endothelial growth factor: basic science and clinical progress. Endocr Rev, 25, 581-611.

Figueroa CD, MacIver AG, Bhoola KD.(1998). Identification of tissue kallikrein in human polymorphonuclear leucocytes. Br J Haematol, 72, 321-328.

Frysz-Naglak D, Fryc B, Klimacka-Nawrot E, Mazurek U, Suchecka W, Kajor M, Kurek J Stadnicki A.(2011). Expression, localization and systemic concentration of vascular endothelial growth factor (VEGF) and its receptors in patients with ulcerative colitis. International Immunopharmacol, 11, 220-225.

Gaffyney PR, Doyle CT, Gaffyney A, et al.(1995). Paradoxical response to heparin in 10 patients with ulcerative colitis. Am J Gastroenterol, 90, 220 – 3.

Gaginella TS, Kachur J F. (1989). Kinins as mediators of intestinal secretion. Am J Physiol, 256:G1-15

Gardiner KR, Halliday MI, Barclay GR, et al. (1995). Significance of systemic endotoxemia in inflammatory bowel disease. Gut, 36, 897-901.

Gregory SA, Edgington TS.(1985). Tissue factor induction in human monocytes: Two distinct mechanisms displayed by different alloantigen responsive T cell clones. J Clin Invest, 76, 2440-2445.

Gris JC, Schved JF, Raffanel C, Dubois A, Ribard D, Balmes JL.(1991). Impaired fibrinolytic response to the venous occlusion test in patients with cryptogenic colitis.Gastroenterol Clin Biol, 15, 933-8.

Guedon C, Le Camp Duhes V, Lalaude O, Menard JF, Lerebous E, Borg JY.(2001). Prothrombotic inherited abnormalities other than factor V Leiden mutation do not play a role in venous thrombosis in inflammatory bowel disease. Am J Gastroenterol, 96, 1448- 54.

Hara DB, Fernandes ES, Campos MM, at al.(2007). Pharmacological and biochemical characterization of B2 receptors in the mouse colon :Influence of the TNBS-induced colitis. Regul Pept, 141, 25-34.

Hara DB, Leite DFP, Fernandes ES, et al.(2008). The relevance of kinin B1 receptor upregulation in a mouse model of colitis. Br J Pharmacol, 154, 1276 -1286.

Hayat M, Ariëns RA, Moayyedi P, Grant PJ, O' Mahony S.(2002). Coagulation factor XIII and markers of thrombin generation and fibrinolysis in patients with inflammatory bowel disease. Eur J Gastroenterol Hepatol, 14: 249-56.

He SH.(2004). Key role of mast cells and their major secretory products in inflammatory bowel disease. World J Gastroenterol, 10, 309-18.

Hoffman M, Monroe DM.(2007). Coagulation: A modern view of hemostasis. Hematol Oncol Clin North Am, 21: 1-11.

Hommes DW, van Dullemen HM, Levi M, et al. (1997). Beneficial effect of treatment with a monoclonal anti – tumor necrosis factor- α antibody on markers of coagulation and fibrinolysis in patients with Cronh's disease. Haemostasis, 27: 269 – 77.

Hudson M, Hutton RA, Wakefield AJ, Sawyerr AM, Pounder RE.(1992). Evidence for activation of coagulation in Crohn's disease. Blood Coagul Fibrinolysis, 3, 773 –8.

Hudson M, Wakefield AJ, Hutton RA, *et al*. (1993). Factor XIIIA subunit and Crohn's disease. *Gut*, 34, 75- 9.

Ichinose A, Fujikawa K, Suyama T.(1986). The activation of prourokinase by plasma kallikrein and its inactivation by thrombin. *J Biol Chem*, 261, 3486-3489.

Ichinose A.(2001). Physiopathology and regulation of factor XIII. *Thromb Haemost*, 86, 57 – 65.

Irving PM, Macey MG, Shah U, *et al*.(2004). Formation of platelet – leukocyte aggregates in inflammatory bowel disease. *Inflamm Bowel Dis*, 10, 361 – 72.

Isordia Salas I, Pixley RA, Parekh H, Li F, Kanapuli SP, Stadnicki A, Lin Y, Sartor RB, Colman RW. (2003). A single point mutation of serine S11 is responsible for the increased rate of cleavage of high molecular weight kininogen in Lewis rat which is genetically susceptible to inflammatory stimuli. *Blood*, 102, 2835 – 2842.

Khan MM, Bratford HN, Isordia – Salas I, et al .(2006). High molecular kininogen fragments stimulate the secretion of cytokines and chemokines through uPAR, Mac-1, and gC1qR in monocytes. *Arterioscler Thromb Vasc Biol*, 26, 2260-2266.

Knot EA, ten Cate JW, Bruin T, Iburg AH, Tytgat GN.(1985). Antithrombin III metabolism in two colitis patients wit acquired antithrombin III deficiency. *Gastroenterology*, 89: 421- 5.

Kondo M, Hotta T, Takemura S, Yoshikawa T, Fukumoto K.(1981). Treatment of ulcerative colitis by the direct administration o fan antifibrinolytic agent as an enema. *Hepatogastroenterology*, 28, 270 – 3.

Koutroubakis IE, Sfiridaki A, Tsiolakidou G, Coucoutsi C, Theodoropoulou A, Kouroumalis EA.(2008). Plasma thrombin-activatable fibrinolysis inhibitor and plasminogen activator inhibitor-1 levels in inflammatory bowel disease. *Eur J Gastroenterol Hepatol*, 20, 912- 6.

Kume K, Yamasaki M, Tashiro M, Yoshikawa I, Otsuki M.(2007). Activation of coagulation and fibrinolysis secondary to bowel inflammation in patients with ulcerative colitis. Internal Medicine, 46, 1323- 9.

Kyriakou DS, Aleksandrakis MG, Passam FH *et al*. (2002).Acquired inhibitors of coagulation factors in patients with gastrointestinal diseases. *Eur J Gastroenterol Hepatol*, 14, 1383- 7.

Lam A, Borda IT, Inwood MJ, Thomson S. (1975). Coagulation studies in ulcerative colitis and Chron's disease. *Gastroenterology* 68: 245 – 51.

Larsen TB, Nielsen JN, Fredholm L, *et al*. (2002). Platelets and anticoagulant capacity in patients with inflammatory bowel disease. *Pathophysiol Haemost Thromb*, 32, 92-6.

Lewis GP. (1964). Plasma kinins and inflammation. *Metabolism*, 13, 1256 – 1263.

Lichtenstein GR.(2000). Goblet cells make more than just mucus. *Gastroenterology*, 118, 1272 – 1274.

Lorenz R, Heinmullr M, Classen M, Tornieporth N, Gain T. (1991). Substitution of factor XIII: a therapeutic approach to ulcerative colitis. *Haemostasis*, 21, 5- 9.

Manning DC, Snyder SH, Kachur JF, et al. (1982). Bradykinin receptor-mediated chloride secretion in intestinal function. *Nature*, 299, 256-259.

Marceau F, Regoli D.(2008). Therapeutic options in inflammatory bowel disease: experimental evidence of a beneficial effect of kinin B1 receptor blockade. *Br J Pharmacol*, 154, 1163-1165.

Marceau F, Tremblay B (1986). Mitogenic effect of bradykinin and of des- Arg9- bradykinin on cultured fibroblast. *Life Sci,* 39, 2351 – 2358.

Mazlam MZ, Hodgson HJ.(1994). Interaction between interleukin – 6, interleukin-1 beta, plasma C-reactive protein values, and in virtro C-reactive protein generation in patients with inflammatory bowel disease. *Gut,* 35, 77- 86.

McLean PG, Ahluwalia A, Perretti M. (2000). Association between kinin B1 receptor expression and leukocyte trafficking across mouse mesenteric postcapillary venules. *J Exp Med,* 192, 367 – 380.

Meucci G, Pareti F, Vecchi M, *et al.* (1999). Serum von Willebrant factor levels in patients with inflammatory bowel disease are related to systemic inflammation. *Scand J Gastroenterol,* 34, 287 – 90.

Miehsler W, Reinisch W, Valic E, *et al.*(2004). Is inflammatory bowel disease an independent and disease specific risk factor for thromboembolism? *Gut,* 53, 542– 8.

Min B, Paul WE. (2008). Basophils in the spotlight at last. *Nature Immunol,* 9, 223-225.

More L, Sim R, Hudson M, *et al.* (1993). Immunohistochemical study of tissue factor expression in normal intestine and idiopathic inflammatory bowel disease. *J Clin Pathol,* 46: 703-8.

Moreau ME, Garbacki N, MolinaroG, et al.(2050). The kallikrein – kinin system: current and future pharmacological targets. *J Pharmacol Sci,* 99, 6-38.

Morowitz DA, Allen LW, Kirsner JB.(1968). Thrombocytosis in chronic inflammatory bowel disease. *Ann Intern Med,* 68, 1013 – 21.

Ni A, Chao L, Chao J. (1998). Trancriptional factor nuclear factor-kB regulates the inducible expression of the human receptor gene in inflammation. *J Biol Chem,* 273, 2784-2791.

Novacek G, Kapiotis S, Moser G, Speiser W, Gangl A, Vogelsang H. (1997). No evidence of activated blood coagulation in Crohn's disease. *Eur J Gastroenterol Hepatol,* 9, 963 – 7.

Oikonomopoulou K, Hansen KK, Saifeddine M, et al. (2006). Proteinase – activated receptors, targets for kallikrein signalling. *J Biol Chem,* 281, 32095 – 32112.

Okamoto H, Greenbaum LM. (1993). Isolation and stricture of T-kinin. *Biochem Biophys Res,* 112, 701 – 708

Oliver JA, Monroe DM, Roberts HR, Hoffman M.(1999). Thrombin activates factor XI on activated platelets in the absence of factor XII. *Arterioscler Thromb Vasc Biol,* 19, 170 – 7.

Oshitani N, Nakamura S, Matsumoto T, Kobyashi K, Kitano A. (1996). Treatment of Crohn's disease fistulas with coagulation factor XIII. *Lancet,* 347, 119- 20.

Panes J, Esteve M, Cabre E *et al.* (2000). Comparison of heparin and steroid in the treatment of moderate and severe ulcerative colitis. *Gastroenterology,* 119, 903-8.

Papa A, De Stefano V, Gasbarrini A, *et al.* (2000). Prelevalence of factor V Leiden and the G20210A prothrombin –gene mutation in inflammatory bowel disease *Blood Coagul Fibrinolysis,* 11, 499-503.

Pastorelli L, Saibeni S, Spina L, *et al.* (2008).Oral- colonic release low – molecular weight heparin: an initial open study of Parnaparin- MMX for the treatment of mild – to moderate left – sided ulcerative colitis. *Aliment Pharmacol Ther,* 28: 581- 88.

Peppers MS. (1997). Transforming grow factor-beta: vasculogenesis, angiogenesis, and vessel wall integrity. *Cytokine Growth Factor Rev,* 8, 21-43.

Pixley RA, Zellis S, Bankes P, et al. (1995). Prognostic value of assessing contact system activation and factor V in systemic inflammatory response syndrome. *Crit Care Med*, 23, 41- 51.

Quera R, Shanahan F. (2004). Thromboembolism – an important manifestation of inflammatory bowel disease. *Am J Gastroenterol*, 99:1971-3.

Rahimi R, Nikfar S, Rezaie A, Abdollahi M. (2007). A meta-analysis of antibiotic therapy for active ulcerative colitis. *Dig Dis Sci*, 52:2920-2925.

Rao AK, Schapira M, Clements ML, et al. (1988). A prospective study of Rocky Mountains spotted fever. *N Engl J Med*. 318, 1021 – 1028.

Rupniak NM, Boyce S, Webb JK, et al. (1997). Effect of the bradykinin B1receptor antagonist des – Arg9 (Leu 8) bradykinin and genetic disruption of the B2 receptor on nociception in rats and mice. *Pain*, 71, 89-97

Sabourin T, Bastien L, Bachvarov DR, et al. (2002). Agonist-induced translocation of the kinin B1 receptor to caveolae-related rafts. *Mol Pharmacol*, 61: 473-476.

Saibeni S, Bottasso B, Spina L, *et al.* (2004). Assessment of thrombin-activatable fibrilolysis inhibitor (TAFI) plasma levels in inflammatory bowel diseases. *Am J Gastroenterol*, 99, 1966-70.

Saibeni S, Ciscato C, Vecchi M, *at al.* (2006). Antibodies to tissue – type plasminogen activator (t-PA) in patients with inflammatory bowel disease: high prevalence, interaction with functional domains of t-PA and possible implications in thrombosis. *J Thromb Haemost*, 4, 1510-6.

Saibeni S, Vecchi M, Valsecchi C, *et al.* (2001). Reduced free protein S levels in patients with inflammatory bowel disease. Prelevalece, clinical relevance, and role of anti – protein S antibodies. Dig Dis Sci, 46, 637 – 43.

Sartor RB, DeLa Cadena RA, Green KD, Stadnicki A, Davis S, Schwab JH, Adam A, Raymond P, Colman RW. (1996). Selective kallikrein-kinin system activation in inbred rats differentially susceptible to granulomatous enterocolitis. *Gastroenterology*, 110, 1467-1481.

Sartor RB.(2006). Mechanism of disease: pathogenesis of Crohn's disease and ulcerative colitis. *Nature Clin Pract Gastroenterol Hepatol*, 3, 390- 407.

Schachter M, Longridge DJ, Wheleer GD, et al. (1986). Immunohistochemical and enzyme histochemical localization of killikrein – like enzymes in colon, intestine, and stomach of rat and cat. *J Histochem Cytochem*, 34, 926-934.

Schapira M, Despland E, Scott CF, et al. (1982). Purified human plasma kallikrein aggregates human blood neutrophils. *J Clin Invest*, 69, 1199-1202.

Souto JC, Martinez E, Roca M, *et al.* (1995). Prothrombotic state and signs of endothelial lesion in plasma of patients with inflammatory bowel disease. *Dig Dis Sci*, 40, 1883-9.

Souza DG, Lomez ES, Pinho V, et al. (2004). Role of bradykinin B(2) and B(1) receptors in the local, remote, and systemic inflammatory responses that follow intestinal ischemia and reperfusion injury. *J Immunol*, 172, 2542-2548.

Stadnicki A, Chao J, Stadnicka I, et al.(1998 a). Localization and secretion of tissue kallikrein in peptidoglycan-induced enterocolitis in Lewis rats. *Am J Physiol*, 275, G854-G861.

Stadnicki A, DeLa Cadena R, Sartor RB, et al (1996). A selective plasma kallikrein inhibitor attenuates acute enterocolitis in the Lewis rats. *Dig Dis Sci*, 41, 912 – 920.

Stadnicki A, Gonciarz M, Niewiarowski TJ, et al.(1997). Activation of plasma contact and coagulation systems and neutrophils in the active phase of ulcerative colitis. *Dig Dis Sci*, 42, 2356-2366.

Stadnicki A, Kloczko J, Nowak A, Sierka E, Sliwinski Z.(1991). Factor XIII subunits in relation to some other hemostatic parameters in ulcerative colitis. *Am J Gastroenterol*, 86, 690 – 3.

Stadnicki A, Kłoczko J, Nowak A, Sierka E.(1992) Alterations of haemostatic parameters in special references to factor XIII and fibronectin in patients with ulcerative colitis. *Eur J Gastroenterol Hepatol*, 4, 743- 6.

Stadnicki A, Machnik G, Klimacka-Nawrot E, et al. (2009). Expression, immunolocalization and systemic concentration of transforming grow factor - β1 and its receptors in human ulcerative colitis. *Int Immunopharmacol*, 9, 761-766.

Stadnicki A, Mazurek U, Gonciarz M, et al.(2003) Immunolocalization and expression of kallistatin and tissue kallikrein in human inflammatory bowel disease. *Dig Dis Sci*, 48, 615-623.

Stadnicki A, Pastucha E, Nowaczyk G, et al.(2005). Immunolocalization and expression of kinin B1 and B2 receptors in human inflammatory bowel disease. *Am J Physiol*, 289, G361-G366.

Stadnicki A, Sartor RB, Fengling Li, et al (1999). Bradykinin B-2 recepror antagonist attenuates arthritis, but not gut inflammation in Lewis rats. *Gut*, Suppl. 5, Abs. 1094.

Stadnicki A, Sartor RB, Janardham R, at al. (1998 b). Specific inhibition of plasma kallikrein modulates chronic granulomatous intestinal and systemic inflammation in genetically susceptible rats. *FASEB J*, 12, 325-333.

Stadnicki A, Sartor RB, Janardham R, et al.(1998 c). Kallikrein-kininogen system activation and bradykinin (B2) receptors in indomethacin-induced enterocolitis in genetically susceptible Lewis rats. *Gut*, 43, 365-374.

Stanley CM, Philips TE.(1994). Bradykinin modulates mucin secretion but not synthesis from an intestinal goblet cell line. *Agents Actions*, 42, 141-145.

Steinhoff M, Buddenkotte J, Shpacovitch V, *et al*. (2005). Proteinase activated receptors: transducers of proteinase mediated signaling in inflammation and immune response. *Endoc Rev*, 26, 1- 43.

Techesche H, Kohnerty V, Fedowitz J, et al. (1983) Tissue kallikrein effectively activates latent matrix degrading matalloenzymes. *Adv Exp Med Biol*, 247A, 545-548.

Tiffany C, Burch RM.(1989). Bradykinin stimulates tumor necrosis factor and interleukin-1 release from macrophages. *FEBS Lett*, 247, 189-192.

Tytgat GN, Van Nueten L, Ven de Velde I, *et al*. (2002). Efficacy and safety of oral ridogrel in the treatment of ulcerative colitis: two multicenter randomized , double blind studies. *Aliment Pharmacol Ther*, 16, 87 – 99.

Ulbrich H, Eriksson EE, Lindbom L.(2003). Leucocyte and endothelial cell adhesion molecules as targets for therapeutic interventions in inflammatory disease. *Trends Pharmacol Sci*, 24, 640-647.

van Bodegraven AA, Meuwissen SG. (2001) Lipoprotein (a), thrombophilia and inflammatory bowel disease. *Eur J Gastroenterol Hepatol*, 13, 1407- 9.

van Bodegraven AA, Schoorl M, Linskens RK, Bartels PC, Tuynman HA. (2002). Persistent activation of coagulation and fibrinolysis after treatment of active ulcerative colitis. *Eur J Gastroenterol Hepatol,* 14, 413- 8.

van Bodegraven AA, Tuynman HA, Schoorl M, Kruishoop AM, Bartels PC.(1995). Fibrinolytic split product, fibrinolysis and factor XIII activity in inflammatory bowel disease. *Scand J Gastroenterol,* 30, 580-5.

Vilaseca J, Salas A, Guarner F,Rodriguez R, Malagelada JR. (1990). Participation of thromboxane and other eicosanoid synthesis in the course of experimental inflammatory colitis. *Gastroenterology,* 98, 269-277.

Wachtfogel YT, Kucich U, James HL, et al. (1983). Human plasma kallikrein releases neutrophil elastase during blood coagulation. *J Clin Invest, 72,* 1672-1677.

Wakefield A, Sabkey EA, Dhillon A, *et al.* (1991). Granulomatous vasculitis in Crohn's disease. *Gastroenterology,* 100, 1279- 87.

Wakefield A, Sawyerr A, Dhillon A, *et al.* (1989). Pathogenesis of Crohn's disease: multifocal gastrointestinal infarction. *Lancet, 2,* 1057 -62.

Wan der Wouwer D, Collen D, Conway EM.(2004). Thrombomodulin- protein C – EPCR system: integrated to regulate coagulation and inflammation. *Arterioscler Thromb Vasc Biol,* 24: 1374 – 83.

Webberley MJ, Hart MT, Melikian V, *et al.* (1993). Thromboembolism in inflammatory bowel disease: role of platelets. *Gut,* 34, 247 – 51.

Werle E. (1960). Kallikrein, kallidin and related substances. In: Schachter M ed. Polypeptides which affect smooth muscles and blood vessels. Pergamon Press, Oxford, England.

Wolf WC, Harley RA, Sluce D,et al. (1998). Cellular localization of kallistatin and tissue kallikrein in human pancreas and salivary glands. *Histochem Cell Biol,* 110, 477-84.

Xiong W, Tang CQ, ZhouGX et al. (1992). In vivo catabolism of human kallikrein – binding protein and its complex with tissue kallikrein. *J Lab Clin Med,* 119, 514-521.

Yoshida H, Russell J, Stokes KY, et al. (2008). Role of the protein C pathway in the extraintestinal thrombosis associated with murine colitis. Gastroenterology, 135: 882-8.

Zeitlin IJ, Smith AN.(1973). Mobilization of tissue kallikrein in inflammatory disease of the colon. *Gut,* 14, 133-138.

Zipser R, Patterson J, Kao H, et al. (1985). Hypersentive prostaglandin and thromboxane response to hormones in rabbit colitis. *Am J Physiol,* 249: G457-G463.

Zitomersky NL, Verhave M, Trenor CC. (2011). Thrombosis and inflammatory bowel disease: a call for improved awareness and prevention. *Inflamm Bowel Dis,* 17, 458- 70.

12

Inflammatory Bowel Disease and Primary Sclerosing Cholangitis

Gulbanu Erkan

*Ufuk University Faculty of Medicine, Department of İnternal Medicine,
Division of Gastroenterology
Turkey*

1. Introduction

Inflammatory bowel disease (IBD) is a chronic condition which is characterized by recurrent immune-mediated inflammation of the gastrointestinal system. IBD is frequently associated with extraintestinal manifestations (EIM) characterized by involvement of multiple organs. EIM occur in 21% to 47% of IBD patients (Navaneethan & Shen, 2010). While some extraintestinal manifestations are encountered more frequently in Crohn's disease (CD) than in ulcerative colitis (UC), some are encountered equally in CD and UC. While the degree of involvement of the skin, eyes, and joints is parallel to disease activity, hepatobiliary and pulmonary involvement is independent of disease activity and intestinal inflammation (Greenstein AJ, et al., 1996).

Hepatopancreatobiliary (HPB) manifestations are the most frequently encountered EIM in patients with IBD. They can be encountered in various ways:

1. HPB conditions sharing the same pathological mechanisms with IBD (Primary Sclerosing Cholangitis (PSC), small-duct PSC/pericholangitis, and PSC/autoimmune hepatitis overlap, IBD associated acute or chronic idiopathic pancreatitis)
2. HPB conditions that reflect the degree of pathophysiologic damage seen in IBD (Cholelithiasis and portal vein thrombosis)
3. HPB conditions related to side effects of drugs used in treatment of IBD (Drug induced or associated hepatitis, pancreatitis, cirrhosis, Hepatitis B reactivation, hepatosplenic T cell lymphoma)
4. HPB conditions possibly related to IBD (Autoimmune pancreatitis, IgG4-associated cholangitis, fatty liver, hepatic amiloidosis, granulomatous hepatitis, primary biliary cirrhosis) (Navaneethan & Shen, 2010)

The various HPB manifestations and their associations are summarized in Tables 1 and 2.

The aim of this chapter is to cover in detail primary sclerosing cholangitis, which is an important and frequently encountered HPB manifestation of ulcerative colitis.

2. The association of Inflammatory Bowel Disease and Primary Sclerosing Cholangitis

PSC is a chronic cholestatic hepatobiliary disease that often develops in the setting of IBD and which affects predominantly young to middle-aged patients (Olsson et al., 1991).

HBP manifestations with a possibly shared pathogenesis and mechanism as IBD	Primary sclerosing cholangitis(PSC) Small- duct PSC Cholangiocarcinoma Autoimmune hepatitis/PSC overlap IgG4 associated cholangitis Acute and chronic idiopathic pancreatitis
HPB manifestations parallel the pathophysiology associated with IBD	Gallstones Portal vein thrombosis and hepatic abscess
HPB manifestations associated with treatment of IBD	Drug induced hepatitis(azathioprine, 6-mercaptopurine, methotrexate, cyclosporine, infliximab) Reactivation of hepatitis B(infliximab) Drug induced pancreatitis(azathioprine, 6-mercaptopurine), Hepatosplenic T-cell lymphoma
HPB manifestations possibly associated with IBD	Fatty liver Hepatic amyloidosis Granulomatous hepatitis Primary biliary cirrhosis Autoimmune pancreatitis

Table 1. Association Between Inflammatory Bowel Disease (IBD) and Hepatopancreatobiliary (HPB) Manifestations. Adapted from Navaneethan & Shen, 2010

HPB manifestation	Ulcerative Colitis	Crohn's Disease
Primary sclerosing cholangitis(PSC)	++	+(colonic or ileocolonic)
Small duct PSC	++	+
Cholangiocarcinoma	++	+
Autoimmunehepatitis/PSC overlap	++	+
IgG4- associated cholangitis	++	+
Acute and chronic pancreatitis	+	++
Gall stones	-	++
Portal vein thrombosis and hepatic abscess	+	++
Drug induced hepatitis	++	++
Reactivation of hepatitis B(infliximab)	++	++
Drug induced pancreatitis	+	++
Hepatosplenic T-cell lymphoma	+/-	+
Autoimmune pancreatitis	++	+
Fatty liver	++	++
Hepatic amyloidosis	-	++
Granulomatous hepatitis	-	++
Primary biliary cirrhosis	++	+

Table 2. HPB Manifestations Associated with IBD. Adapted from Navaneethan & Shen, 2010

The association of primary sclerosing cholangitis (PSC) and ulcerative colitis (UC) was first reported by Smith and Loe in 1965 (Smith&Loe, 1965). The incidence of IBD in patients with PSC is 25-30%. Increasing awareness of association of PSC and UC led to more widespread use of endoscopic retrograde cholangiopancreatography (ERCP) and hence more cases were diagnosed with PSC (Broome & Bergquist, 2006).

The association of PSC and Crohn's disease, which was first described by Atkinson and Carroll in 1964 (Atkinson & Carroll, 1964) , is relatively rare. The incidence of CD in PSC varies between 1.3-14% (Wiesner & LaRusso, 1980; Chapman et al., 1980; Rasmussen et al., 1997; McGarity et al., 1991; Faubion et al., 2001; Loftus et al., 2005; Tobias et al., 1983). The most eminent finding is rectal sparing. Colonic stricture and perianastomotic ulcers are relatively rare in this patient group. Patients with PSC and CD almost always have extensive colitis or ileocolitis, but never have isolated ileitis (Broome & Bergquist, 2006).

About 85-90% of patients with PSC and IBD are comprised of UC patients and the remainder are comprised of patients with Crohn's colitis or Crohn's ileocolitis (Olsson et al., 1991).

IBD can be diagnosed at any time throughout the course of PSC, and PSC can develop at any time throughout the course of IBD (Fausa et al., 1991; Broome et al., 1990). However, IBD is often diagnosed many years before the diagnosis of PSC. PSC can occur many years after proctocolectomy for colitis; IBD can be diagnosed many years after liver transplantation for advanced PSC (Fausa et al., 1991; Wiesner & LaRusso, 1980; Aadland et al., 1987; Chapman et al., 1980; Riley et al., 1997) . As IBD and PSC can be asymptomatic, the time of diagnosis depends on the diagnostic alertness of the physician (Broome & Bergquist, 2006).

PSC has a variable natural course. Nevertheless, PSC is typically characterized by progressive inflammation, obliterative fibrosis, damage to the intrahepatic and extrahepatic biliary tree and eventually biliary fibrosis, cirrhosis and finally liver failure. PSC is often diagnosed between the 3rd and 5th decades and male to female gender ratio is 2:1 (Chapman et al., 1980; Lee & Kaplan, 1995; Navaneethan & Shen, 2010) . Freeman et al. observed that patients with PSC had more extensive endoscopic and histological inflammation of the afferent limb who had restorative proctocolectomy with ileal pouch-anal anastomosis (IPAA) for UC than those with no concurrent PSC (Freeman et al., 2008).

A report from Mayo Clinic has identified characteristic clinical, endoscopic, and histological findings in IBD accompanied by PSC as quiescent colitis, substantial preclinical phase, pancolitis, rectal sparing, backwash ileitis, pouchitis, and colorectal dysplasia/carcinoma (Loftus et al., 2005) (Table 3).

Clinical, Endoscopic, and Histological Findings that Characterize IBD-PSC
Quiescent colitis
Substantial preclinical phase
Pancolitis
Rectal sparing
Backwash ileitis
Pouchitis
Colorectal dysplasia/carcinoma

Table 3. Clinical, Endoscopic, and Histological Findings that Characterize IBD-PSC.
Adapted from Broome & Bergquist, 2006

2.1 Prevalence of IBD in patients with PSC

The prevalence of UC in patients with PSC varies from country to country in the range of 21-80% (Takikawa & Manabe, 1997; Bergquist A et al., 2002). The prevalence of PSC in patients with Crohn's disease varies between 1.4-3.4% (Rasmussen et al., 1997; Schrumpf et al., 1980; Shepherd et al., 1983). Colitis in PSC is often quiescent or mild. Therefore, all patients with PSC should undergo colonoscopy and multiple biopsies should be taken to estimate the true prevalence (Broome & Bergquist, 2006). An algorithm for screening for IBD in patients with PSC is given in Figure 1.

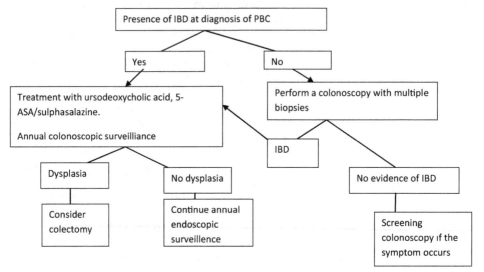

Fig. 1. Screening for IBD in patients with PSC.
Adapted from Navaneethan U, Shen B, 2010, and Broome U, Bergquist A, 2006

2.2 Prevalence of PSC in patients with IBD

The prevalence of PSC in patients with IBD and persistently abnormal liver function tests is 2.4-7.5% (Olson R, et al., 1991; Aadland E et al., 1987). PSC prevalence is 5.5 % in patients with substantial colitis, and 0.5% in patients with distal colitis (Olsson et al., 1991). 1.3 to 14% of patients with Crohn's disease have PSC (Wiesner &LaRusso 1980; Chapman et al., 1980; Rasmussen et al 1997; McGarity et al., 1991; Faubion et al., 2001; Loftus et al., 2005).
PSC can present as an asymptomatic disease characterized by mild increases in aminotransferases, episodes of normal liver function tests can also occur. The frequency of liver function test screening is decisive in determining the prevalence of this disease. However, there may also be liver enzyme elevations due to autoimmune hepatitis, fatty liver, colonic disease activation, total parenteral nutrition and steroid use (Loftus et al., 1997; Broome et al., 1994). Therefore, liver function tests at presentation may be misguiding. Ideally, liver function tests must be assessed when the colonic disease is in the inactive phase (Broome & Bergquist, 2006). An algorithm for PSC screening in a patient with IBD is presented below in Figure 2.
Enlargement of perihepatic lymph nodes is a common finding in PSC (Outwater et al., 1992). The presence of enlarged perihepatic lymph nodes in a patient with UC should alert the

clinician for PSC. A prospective study by Hirche et al that involved 310 IBD patients showed that the detection of enlarged perihepatic lymph nodes by ultrasonography (US) was a better predictor of PSC when compared to serum parameters alone (Hirche et al., 2004).

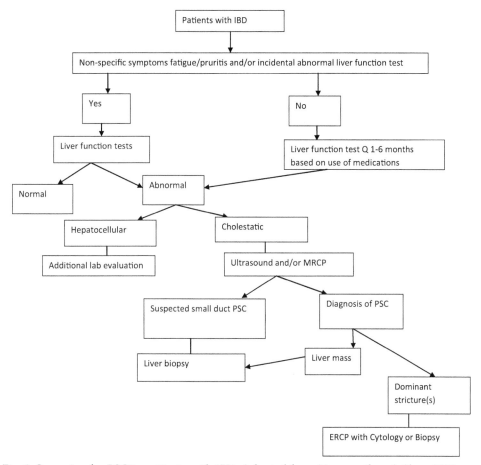

Fig. 2. Screening for PSC in patients with IBD. Adapted from Navaneethan & Shen, 2010

Rabinowitz et al., who investigated patients with advanced PSC , found that patients with PSC and UC are predominantly male and the first presentation is often mild liver enzyme elevation. Bile duct involvement is different among patients with PSC plus UC and those with PSC only. While the prevalence of combined intrahepatic and extrahepatic bile duct strictures is 82% in patients with PSC and UC, it is 46% in those with only PSC. Isolated extrahepatic duct involvement is 38% in PSC, and 7% in those with PSC and UC (Rabinovitz et al., 1990). Among 305 Swedish PSC patients, no difference between patients with and without IBD could be found (Broome et al., 1996). Currently, we do not have enough data to arrive at a conclusion that PSC in patients without IBD is an entity different from PSC that accompanies IBD.

Rectal sparing and backwash ileitis are more common in patients with UC and PSC (Loftus et al., 2005). As rectal sparing is common in these patients, rectosigmoidoscopy is not adequate in demonstrating the association of UC and PSC, a colonoscopy is often recommended (Faubion et al., 2001; Perdigoto et al., 1991).

The clinical course of colitis is variable in patients who undergo OLT for PSC. MacLean et al have reported clinical healing in one third of patients, unchanged clinical course in one third, and worsening in the last one third (MacLean et al., 2003).

In UC patients operated on with an ileal pouch-anal anastomosis, nonspecific inflammation of the pouch (pouchitis) is the most frequent long-term complication. Chronic pouchitis is more common in patients with PSC and UC when compared to those with UC only (60% vs 15%)(Penna et al., 1996). Pouchitis continues to occur after OLT in patients with PSC (Zins BJ et al., 1995).

3. Impact of coexisting PSC on the disease behavior and course of IBD

Patients with PSC and IBD have a different clinical course when compared to IBD patients not complicated with PSC, and this patient group has been defined by the Mayo clinic as a different clinical entity (Loftus et al., 2005). While UC can be diagnosed many years after PSC diagnosis and even after orthotopic liver transplantation(OLT), a patient with UC, who had a proctocolectomy or not, can be diagnosed with PSC many years later (Joo et al.,2009).

Patients with UC and PSC more frequently experience rectal sparing, backwash ileitis, pancolitis, colorectal neoplasia when compared to patients with UC alone, and their prognosis is worse (Faubion et al., 2001; Loftus et al., 2005; Loftus et al., 1997; Penna et al.; 1996; Heuschen et al., 2001; Lundkvist & Broome, 1997; Broome et al., 1995; Soetikno et al., 2002). However, there are studies reporting different results. A recent case -control study found no difference between patients with PSC plus IBD and IBD alone in terms of rectal sparing. The same investigators found similar backwash ileitis prevalences in the PSC plus UC group and the UC alone group (Joo et al., 2009).

It was suggested that patients with PSC and UC may more likely run a quiescent course of colitis than UC patients without coexistent PSC. PSC-UC patients have colitis with a lower histopathological grade of inflammation (Joo et al.,2009). In a study from Sweden that included 76 patients with PSC, 7 of 11 asymptomatic patients had a histopathological diagnosis of IBD, and 2 of these 7 patients had colonic dysplasia. In the follow-up, these 2 patients died before developing any IBD symptoms while 3 patients developed IBD symptoms (Broome et al.,1995).

A colonoscopy must be performed at the time of PSC diagnosis for IBD screening (Faubion et al., 2001). Currently, there is no guideline about the necessity and frequency of colonoscopic screening in asymptomatic patients with a normal baseline screening colonoscopy. However, patients with PSC and UC/Crohn's colitis should undergo annual colonoscopy (Kornbluth & Sachar,1997).

The risk of pouchitis after restorative proctocolectomy is higher in patients with PSC and UC when compared to patients with UC alone (Faubion et al.,2001; Loftus et al., 2005; Penna et al., 1996) . On the other hand, there is no correlation between the severity of liver disease and the risk of pouchitis (Penna et al., 1996).

While there are conflicting reports in the literature, it is generally agreed upon that the risk of IBD-associated colonic dysplasia is increased in the presence of PSC. In a meta-analysis, the presence of PSC was an independent risk factor for colorectal dysplasia/cancer in UC patients with an odds ratio of 4.79 (Soetikno et al.,2002). Screening colonoscopy is associated with a survival benefit in patients with PSC and UC or Crohn's colitis (Rutter et al., 2004), and a yearly colonoscopy is recommended beginning from the time of PSC diagnosis (Kornbluth & Sachar,1997). The risk for dyplasia seems to remain high after colectomy in patients with PSC and UC (Ståhlberg et al.,2003). According to histological and flow cytometry studies, atrophy in the pouch mucosa, dysplasia, and DNA aneuploidia are more common in PSC plus UC patients with IPAA when compared to patients with UC only with IPAA (Ståhlberg et al.,2003).

4. The impact of coexisting IBD on the disease behavior and course of PSC

In a liver biopsy study that compared PSC patients with and without accompanying IBD no difference was found in terms of liver histopathology (Ludwig et al.,1981). Two other studies were unable to define any specific clinical or radiological criteria to distinguish patients with UC plus PSC from those with PSC alone (Broome et al., 1996; MacCarty et al., 1985). On the other hand, Rabinovitz et al showed that the first sign of liver disease was often liver enzyme abnormality in PSC accompanied by IBD. In contrast, liver disease more often presented with jaundice, pruritus, and fatigue in patients with PSC alone (Rabinowitz et al., 1990).

5. Pathogenesis

As IBD tends to coexist with other autoimmune diseases such as Type I diabetes mellitus and Graves' disease (Saarinen S et al., 2000), genetic and immunological mechanisms have been extensively studied (Navaneethan & Shen, 2010). HLA-B8, HLA-DRB1*0301(DR3), HLA-DR3*0101(DRw52a), and HLA-DRB1*0401(DR4) are among genetic variants that are associated with susceptibility to IBD (Farrant et al., 1992; Olerup et al., 1995). Many antibodies have been detected in PSC patients with varying prevalences, including antinuclear antibodies (24-53%), smooth muscle antibodies (13-20%), anti-perinuclear cytoplasmic antibody (65-88%) (Mulder et al., 1993; Bansi et al., 1996; Terjung & Spengler, 2005; Terjung et al., 2000). However, in contrast to other autoimmune diseases, PSC is more frequently encountered in male subjects, and it does not respond to immunosuppressive therapy (O'Mahony & Vierling, 2006). One hypothesis that aims to explain the increased incidence of PSC in IBD patients postulates that the transportation of bacterial endotoxins from the inflamed colonic mucosa to the liver via the portal circulation stimulates the Kupffer cells (Fausa et al., 1991; Aoki et al., 2005). However, another study showed that there is no evidence of altered intestinal permeability or bacterial overgrowth in PSC patients (Björnsson et al.,2000). Other factors that are suspected to play a role in pathogenesis are ANCA autoantigen Beta-tubulin isotype 5 (TBB5) that shares epitopes with microbial antigens and human autoantigens (Erickson,1995) and leaky gut (Terjung & Spengler,2009).

6. Diagnosis

Most PSC patients are asymptomatic at the time of diagnosis. Fatigue, pruritus, jaundice, abdominal pain, and weight loss are the presenting symptoms in 10-15% of the patients (Tischendorff et al., 2007; Wiesner et al., 1989). A cholestatic pattern of abnormal liver function tests in the form of elevation in alkaline phosphatase is a biochemical feature for PSC (Rasmussen HH et al., 1997; Talwalkar & Lindor, 2005).The most frequent cause of persistent liver enzyme elevation in a patient with IBD is PSC (Heikius et al., 1997). PSC is also the most frequent cause of persistent liver enzyme elevation in an IBD patient with proctocolectomy (Navaneethan et al.,2009). Various antibodies may be detected with varying prevalences (antinuclear antibodies 24-53%, antismooth muscle antibodies 13-20%, p-ANCA 65-88%). Nevertheless, the role of these antibodies in diagnosis and discrimination between isolated PSC and PSC accompanied by IBD remains unclear (Mulder et al., 1993; Bansi et al., 1996; Terjung & Spengler, 2005; Terjung et al., 2000).

Diffuse, multifocal strictures involving the medium- sized intrahepatic and/or medium or large- sized extrahepatic ducts demonstrated by cholangiography constitutes the gold standard in the diagnosis of PSC (MacCarty et al.,1983) (Pictures 1 and 2). ERCP may be used both for diagnostic and therapeutic purposes, but is associated with procedure-related complications such as cholangitis and pancreatitis (Moreno & Gores, 2006). Magnetic Resonance Cholangiopancreatography (MRCP) is a non-invasive alternative tool for PSC diagnosis. MRCP has a sensitivity of 80-91%, specifity of 85-99%, and diagnostic accuracy of 83-93% for diagnosis of PSC, all of which are slightly lower than those of ERCP (Fulcher et al., 2000; Angulo et al., 2000; Moff et al., 2006; Berstad et al., 2006; Textor et al., 2002).

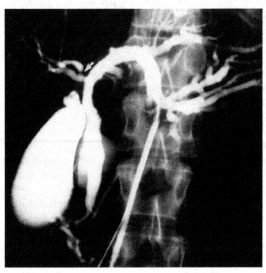

Picture 1. Percutaneus cholangiogram displaying early PSC in a 45-year-old man with ulcerative colitis and elevated results of liver function tests. (Vitellas et al., 2000)

Liver biopsy is useful for the diagnosis of small-duct PSC or pericholangitis in IBD patients with cholestatic enzyme elevation and a normal cholangiogram (Burak et al., 2003). US examination of the liver may be used for screening in patients with liver enzyme elevation. The demonstration of dilated bile ducts by US may guide the clinician for further evaluations such as ERCP or liver biopsy. Nevertheless, there is no published data about the value of abdominal US for screening purposes in PSC (Navaneethan U, Shen B, 2010).

Another clinical scenario that may be encountered throughout the clinical course of PSC is cholangiocarcinoma (Picture 3) .Current imaging methods have limited capability in the early diagnosis of cholangiocarcinoma and most patients are diagnosed at advanced stages of the disease. Computerized tomography (CT) and magnetic resonance imaging (MRI) have higher sensitivity than US, but US examination may provide better accuracy than CT and MRI in distinguishing cholangiocarcinoma from underlying PSC (Charatcharoenwitthaya et al., 2008). When a mass lesion is detected by US ,CT or MRI may be performed to assess the extent of the mass.

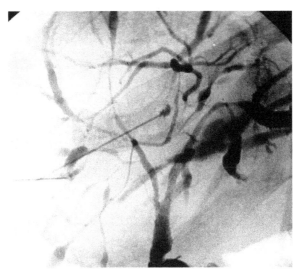

Picture 2. Percutaneus cholangiogram displaying PSC in a 67-year-old man with ulcerative colitis and jaundice. (Vitellas et al., 2000)

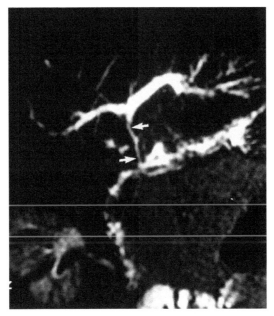

Picture 3. MRCP image of cholangiocarcinoma in a 29-year-old man with ulcerative colitis and primary sclerosing cholangitis who presented with jaundice and abdominal pain. (Vitellas et al., 2000)

ERCP with brush cytology or CT/ US guided biopsy of the mass may be required to accurately establish the diagnosis. ERCP is especially useful for the final diagnosis of cholangiocarcinoma, as it provides opportunities such as brush cytology and obtaining a biopsy sample (Charatcharoenwitthaya et al.,2008). The application of advanced cytological techniques such as digital imaging analysis (DIA) and fluorescent in situ hybridization (FISH) in brush cytology and biopsy samples obtained by ERCP may further facilitate the early diagnosis of cholangiocarcinoma (Moreno & Gores, 2006; Rea et al., 2005; Parsi et al., 2008). The sensitivity of combined use of cytology, FISH and DIA is 50-64%, spesicifity and positive predictive value is 100% (Charatcharoenwitthaya et al.,2008). The National Institutes of Health consensus statement on the role of diagnostic and therapeutic ERCP described the role of ERCP in the diagnosis of biliary cancers in patients with PSC (Cohen et al.,2002). It is not clear whether a different surveilliance program is needed in case PSC is accompanied by IBD. An algorithm for cholangiocarcinoma screening in patients with IBD and PSC is given below (Figure 3). The advantages and disadvantages of diagnostic modalities are summarized in Table 4.

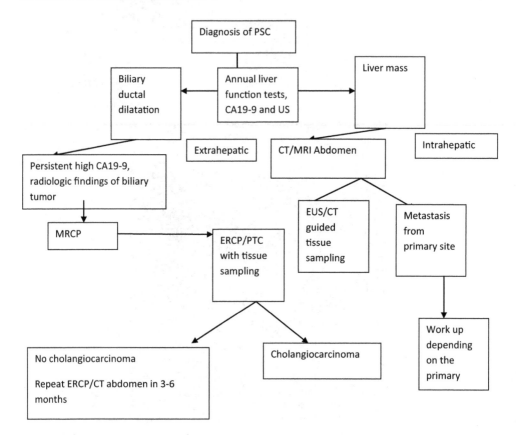

Fig. 3. Surveilliance of cholangiocarcinoma in patients with IBD-PSC
(Adapted from Charatcharoenwitthaya P and Lindor KD, 2007)

Diagnostic modality	Advantages	Disadvantages
Endoscopic retrograde cholangiopancreatography(ERCP)	-Can be both diagnostic and therapeutic Gold standart for diagnosis of PSC	-Complications, including post-ERCP pancreatitis. -Procedure associated cholangitis
Magnetic resonance retrograde cholangiopancreatography (MRCP)	-Visualizing bile ducts proximal to a complete bile duct obstruction -Useful in patients with gastric bypass or biliary-enteric anastomosis without radiation exposure	-Purely diagnostic -PSC limited to the peripheral ducts -Sensitivity and specificity slightly inferior to ERCP
Liver biopsy	-Diagnosis of small duct PSC in suspected patients with a normal cholangiography	-Patchy nature of PSC which leads to sampling error
Abdominal ultrasound	Screening for biliary ductal dilatation	Insensitive for diagnosis of PSC

Table 4. Diagnostic modalities in primary sclerosing cholangitis
(Adapted from Navaneethan & Shen 2010)

7. Natural history

Both symptomatic and asymptomatic PSC patients have decreased survival rates when compared to healthy population (Porayko et al., 1990). Median survival from time of diagnosis to death or liver transplantation was reported as 10 years (Farrant et al., 1991). In a Dutch cohort, transplantation free survival was 18 years on average (Ponsioen et al.,2002). PSC patients are prone to end stage liver disease complications such as esophageal varices, ascites, and hepatic encephalopathy. There are no guidelines on timing of screening for esophageal varices in PSC with or without IBD except for patients with cirrhosis. Because of the patchy nature of PSC, liver biopsy is limited by sampling error. Thus, non-invasive diagnostic methods were explored. A platelet count less than 150000/mm^3 may be a marker for the presence of esophageal varices (Zein et al.,2004). The composite Mayo Risk Score based on age, serum bilirubin, albumin, aspartate aminotransferase and variceal bleeding has been used to assess disease progression and prognosis (Kim et al., 2000). Cholangiocarcinoma is another complication of PSC and annual incidence is 0.6%-1%(Bergquist el al., 2007). It can develop at any stage of PSC, it can present as an intraductal tumor in the biliary system or rarely as a hepatic mass (Fevery et al.,2007). The risks of colorectal cancer and pancreatic cancer are also increased in patients with PSC when compared to the general population (Kim et al., 2000).

8. Management

The presence of accompanying IBD does not change the therapeutic approach in patients with PSC. Currently, there is no treatment option capable of halting progression to PSC or modifying the natural course of the disease. Ursodeoxycholic acid (UDCA) is widely used for the treatment of PSC. A randomized trial which tested a UDCA dose of 13-15 mg/kg/day showed normalization in liver enzyme levels, however, there was no improvement of liver histology or liver transplant free survival (Lindor,1997). In another randomized trial that included 219 patients, a higher dosage of UDCA treatment (17-23 mg/kg/day) did not result in any benefit in terms of mortality, need for OLT, or cholangiocarcinoma risk (Olsson, 2005). A pilot study reported that a very high dosage of UDCA (28-30 mg/kg/day) might improve survival (Cullen et al., 2008) ,however, a large multicenter randomized controlled trial was terminated prematurely due to side effects in the treatment arm (Lindor et al., 2009).

UDCA treatment can prevent colonic neoplasia in PSC-IBD patients (Tung et al., 2001). On the other hand, high dose UDCA treatment was reported to increase the risk of colon cancer in PSC-UC patients (Eaton et al., 2011).

The treatment of choice in end stage PSC or cholangiocarcinoma-PSC is OLT. The 5 and 10 year survival rates in PSC patients are 85% and 70%, repectively (Rea et al., 2005 and Graziadei et al., 1999a). On the other hand, the rate of PSC recurrence in the transplanted liver is 20%-25% (Graziadei et al., 1999b).

Small-duct PSC: This entity was previously termed pericholangitis. These patients have biochemical and histopathological features compatible with PSC despite normal cholangiograms (Wee et al., 1985). The Mayo Clinic's criteria for the diagnosis of small-duct PSC mandates the presence of coexisting IBD (Angulo et al., 2002). On the other hand, European criteria for small duct PSC does not include the presence of IBD (Björnsson et al., 2002 and, Broome et al., 2002). Initial studies with limited follow-up suggested that patients with small-duct PSC have a better prognosis than those with its large-duct counterpart (Angulo P et al., 2002; Björnsson et al., 2002 and, Broome et al., 2002). A large multicenter study with a longer follow-up period showed that the incidence of IBD is 80% in patients with small-duct PSC. Accompanying IBD was UC in 78%, Crohn's colitis in 21%, and collagenous colitis in one patient (Björnsson et al., 2008).

The presence of IBD does not seem to have an effect on the course of liver disease in patients with small-duct PSC. 12-23% of patients with small-duct PSC progress to large-duct PSC. Cholangiocarcinoma developing in the setting of isolated small-duct PSC has never been reported in the literature, unless it progresses to large-duct PSC (Björnsson et al., 2008). In some patients, OLT may be necessary because of progressive disease and disease recurrence may be encountered in the transplanted liver. If the alkalene phosphatase level is elevated, cholangiogram is normal, and other hepatobiliary diseases are ruled out in an IBD patient, liver biopsy may be required to rule out small-duct PSC (Navaneethan & Shen, 2010).

9. Disease course of IBD following liver transplantation for PSC

OLT for PSC or PSC-associated cholangiocarcinoma may affect the clinical course of UC, as corticosteriods and other immunosuppressive agents used following OLT may theoretically improve coexisting UC. However, while some studies report alleviation of UC-associated symptoms after OLT (Saldeen et al., 1999 and Befeler et al., 1998) , some studies report exacerbation of symptoms after OLT (Riley et al., 1997; Papatheodoridis et al., 1998 and Verdonk et al., 2006).

The effect of OLT on the natural course of ileal pouch in UC patients undergoing restorative proctocolectomy seems to be minor. In some case series, OLT and subsequent immunosuppressive therapy did not have a significant effect on the severity of pouchitis (Zins BJ et al.,1995). In a recent study investigating the modification of chronic pouchitis course by PSC and/or OLT performed for PSC, 14 of 32 patients who underwent both IPAA and OLT for PSC experienced chronic pouchitis and in 8 patients PSC recurred, with 4 of them requiring retransplantation (Mathis et al., 2008). Large scale studies are needed to clarify the disease nature of pouchitis and the interaction of it with OLT and OLT related procedures.

10. Course of liver disease following IPAA

IPAA does not appear to affect the disease course of PSC and PSC appears to follow an independent disease course in spite of proctocolectomy (Poritz & Koltun, 2003). In a study of 214 patients with UC undergoing IPAA including 13 (6.1%) with PSC, 4 patients with PSC showed clinical progression, while none of these patients with minor histological changes progressed with a follow-up over 9 years (Mikkola et al., 1995). In a study of PSC in 68 patients with UC with 30 having follow-up examinations, the staging of PSC on liver biopsy after IPAA showed disease progression in 4 (13%), regression in 15 (50%), and stable in 11 (37%) from baseline liver histology at the time of proctocolectomy. Six of the 68 patients (8.8%) developed cholangiocarcinoma. The progression of PSC in patients with minor ductal changes appeared to be uncommon after IPAA surgery (Lepistö et al., 2009).

11. Colorectal Dysplasia and carcinoma in patients with Ulcerative Colitis and Primary Sclerosing Cholangitis

It is well-known that the risk of developing colorectal carcinoma is increased in patients with UC. Disease duration and extensive colitis are two major risk factors for this serious complication. The mechanism of developing malignancy in UC is not fully understood. Recent studies have shown that family history of sporadic colorectal carcinoma (Askling et al., 2001), presence of active inflammation in the mucosa (Rutter et al., 2004), and presence of PSC increase the risk of dysplasia and colorectal carcinoma in patients with UC (Kornfeld et al., 1997; Brentnall et al., 1996). A study from Sweden has shown that the incidence of colorectal dysplasia and carcinoma in patients with UC and PSC at 10, 20, and 25 years is 9%, 31% and 50% respectively (Broome et al., 1995). A meta-analysis of 11 studies has shown that the presence of PSC is an independent risk factor for colorectal dysplasia/carcinoma in patients with UC (Soetikno et al.,2002).

The incidence of colorectal dysplasia/cancer is high after orthotopic liver transplantation (OLT) in patients with UC and PSC (Bleday et al., 1993; Higashi et al., 1990). The risk of developing colorectal carcinoma increases over time after OLT. Vera et al. have identified three risk factors for developing colorectal carcinoma after OLT; colitis duration of more than 10 years, pancolitis, and dysplasia after OLT (Vera et al., 2003). A yearly colonoscopy is adequate in patients with PSC and UC, beginning from the time of PSC diagnosis (Broome & Bergquist, 2006).

12. References

Aadland E, Schrumpf E, Fausa O, Elgjo K, Heilo A, Aakhus T, Gjone E. Primary sclerosing cholangitis: a long-term follow-up study. *Scand J Gastroenterol*. 1987 Aug;22(6):655-64.

Angulo P, Maor-Kendler Y, Lindor KD.Small-duct primary sclerosing cholangitis: a long-term follow-up study. *Hepatology*. 2002 Jun;35(6):1494-500.

Angulo P, Pearce DH, Johnson CD, Henry JJ, LaRusso NF, Petersen BT, Lindor KD. Magnetic resonance cholangiography in patients with biliary disease: its role in primary sclerosing cholangitis.*J Hepatol*. 2000;33(4):520-7.

Aoki CA, Bowlus CL, Gershwin ME.The immunobiology of primary sclerosing cholangitis. *Autoimmun Rev*. 2005;4(3):137-43.

Askling J, Dickman PW, Karlén P, Broström O, Lapidus A, Löfberg R, Ekbom A. Family history as a risk factor for colorectal cancer in inflammatory bowel disease. Gastroenterology. 2001 May;120(6):1356-62.

Atkinson AJ, Carroll WW. Sclerosing cholangitis, association with regional enteritis. JAMA 1964;188:183-4.

Bansi DS, Fleming KA, Chapman RW. Importance of antineutrophil cytoplasmic antibodies in primary sclerosing cholangitis and ulcerative colitis: prevalence, titre, and IgG subclass. Gut. 1996 Mar;38(3):384-9.

Befeler AS, Lissoos TW, Schiano TD, Conjeevaram H, Dasgupta KA, Millis JM, Newell KA, Thistlethwaite JR, Baker AL. Clinical course and management of inflammatory bowel disease after liver transplantation.*Transplantation*. 1998 Feb 15;65(3):393-6.

Bergquist A, Ekbom A, Olsson R, Kornfeldt D, Lööf L, Danielsson A, Hultcrantz R, Lindgren S, Prytz H, Sandberg-Gertzén H, Almer S, Granath F, Broomé U. Hepatic and extrahepatic malignancies in primary sclerosing cholangitis. *J Hepatol*. 2002 Mar;36(3):321-7.

Berstad AE, Aabakken L, Smith HJ, Aasen S, Boberg KM, Schrumpf E. Diagnostic accuracy of magnetic resonance and endoscopic retrograde cholangiography in primary sclerosing cholangitis. *Clin Gastroenterol Hepatol*. 2006;4(4):514-20.

Björnsson E, Boberg KM, Cullen S, Fleming K, Clausen OP, Fausa O, Schrumpf E, Chapman RW.Patients with small duct primary sclerosing cholangitis have a favourable long term prognosis.*Gut*. 2002 Nov;51(5):731-5.

Björnsson E, Olsson R, Bergquist A, Lindgren S, Braden B, Chapman RW, Boberg KM, Angulo P. The natural history of small-duct primary sclerosing cholangitis. *Gastroenterology*. 2008 Apr;134(4):975-80.

Björnsson ES, Kilander AF, Olsson RG. Bile duct bacterial isolates in primary sclerosing cholangitis and certain other forms of cholestasis--a study of bile cultures from ERCP. *Hepatogastroenterology*. 2000;47(36):1504-8.

Bleday R, Lee E, Jessurun J, Heine J, Wong WD. Increased risk of early colorectal neoplasms after hepatic transplant in patients with inflammatory bowel disease. *Dis Colon Rectum*. 1993 Oct;36(10):908-12.

Brentnall TA, Haggitt RC, Rabinovitch PS, Kimmey MB, Bronner MP, Levine DS, Kowdley KV, Stevens AC, Crispin DA, Emond M, Rubin CE.Risk and natural history of colonic neoplasia in patients with primary sclerosing cholangitis and ulcerative colitis. *Gastroenterology*. 1996 Feb;110(2):331-8.

Broome U, Bergquist A. Primary sclerosing cholangitis, inflammatory bowel disease, and colon cancer. *Semin Liver Dis* 2006;26(1):31-41.

Broome U, Glaumann H, Hellers G, Nilsson B, Sörstad J, Hultcrantz R. Liver disease in ulcerative colitis: an epidemiological and follow up study in the county of Stockholm. *Gut*. 1994 Jan;35(1):84-9.

Broomé U, Glaumann H, Lindstöm E, Lööf L, Almer S, Prytz H, Sandberg-Gertzén H, Lindgren S, Fork FT, Järnerot G, Olsson R. Natural history and outcome in 32 Swedish patients with small duct primary sclerosing cholangitis (PSC). *J Hepatol.* 2002 May;36(5):586-9.

Broomé U, Löfberg R, Lundqvist K, Veress B. Subclinical time span of inflammatory bowel disease in patients with primary sclerosing cholangitis. *Dis Colon Rectum.* 1995 ;38(12):1301-

Broomé U, Löfberg R, Veress B, Eriksson LS. Primary sclerosing cholangitis and ulcerative colitis: evidence for increased neoplastic potential.*Hepatology.* 1995 Nov;22(5):1404-8.

Broomé U, Olsson R, Lööf L, Bodemar G, Hultcrantz R, Danielsson A, Prytz H, Sandberg-Gertzén H, Wallerstedt S, Lindberg G. Natural history and prognostic factors in 305 Swedish patients with primary sclerosing cholangitis. *Gut.* 1996 ;38(4):610-5.

Broomé U, Glaumann H, Hultcrantz R. Liver histology and follow up of 68 patients with ulcerative colitis and normal liver function tests. *Gut* 1990;31:468-71.

Burak KW, Angulo P, Lindor KD. Is there a role for liver biopsy in primary sclerosing cholangitis? *Am J Gastroenterol.* 2003;98(5):1155-8.

Chapman RW, Arborgh BA, Rhodes JM, Summerfield JA, Dick R, Scheuer PJ, Sherlock S. Primary sclerosing cholangitis: a review of its clinical features, cholangiography, and hepatic histology. *Gut.* 1980;21(10):870-7.

Charatcharoenwitthaya P, Enders FB, Halling KC, Lindor KD. Utility of serum tumor markers, imaging, and biliary cytology for detecting cholangiocarcinoma in primary sclerosing cholangitis.*Hepatology.* 2008;48(4):1106-17.

Cohen S, Bacon BR, Berlin JA, Fleischer D, Hecht GA, Loehrer PJ Sr, McNair AE Jr, Mulholland M, Norton NJ, Rabeneck L, Ransohoff DF, Sonnenberg A, Vannier MW.National Institutes of Health State-of-the-Science Conference Statement: ERCP for diagnosis and therapy, January 14-16, 2002. Gastrointest Endosc. 2002 ;56(6):803-9.

Cullen SN, Rust C, Fleming K, Edwards C, Beuers U, Chapman RW. High dose ursodeoxycholic acid for the treatment of primary sclerosing cholangitis is safe and effective.*J Hepatol.* 2008 May;48(5):792-800.

Eaton JE, Silveira MG, Pardi DS, Sinakos E, Kowdley KV, Luketic VA, Harrison ME, McCashland T, Befeler AS, Harnois D, Jorgensen R, Petz J, Lindor KD. High-Dose Ursodeoxycholic Acid Is Associated With the Development of Colorectal Neoplasia in Patients With Ulcerative Colitis and Primary Sclerosing Cholangitis. *Am J Gastroenterol.* 2011 May 10 [Epub ahead of print].

Erickson HP. FtsZ, a prokaryotic homolog of tubulin? *Cell.* 1995 Feb 10;80(3):367-70.

Farrant JM, Doherty DG, Donaldson PT, Vaughan RW, Hayllar KM, Welsh KI, Eddleston AL, Williams R. Amino acid substitutions at position 38 of the DR beta polypeptide confer susceptibility to and protection from primary sclerosing cholangitis. *Hepatology.* 1992 ;16(2):390-5.

Farrant JM, Hayllar KM, Wilkinson ML, Karani J, Portmann BC, Westaby D, Williams R. Natural history and prognostic variables in primary sclerosing cholangitis. *Gastroenterology.* 1991 ;100(6):1710-7.

Faubion WA Jr, Loftus EV, Sandborn WJ, Freese DK, Perrault J.Pediatric "PSC-IBD": a descriptive report of associated inflammatory bowel disease among pediatric patients with PSC. *J Pediatr Gastroenterol Nutr.* 2001;33(3):296-300.

Fausa O, Schrumpf E, Elgjo K. Relationship of inflammatory bowel disease and primary sclerosing cholangitis. *Semin Liver Dis.* 1991 ;11(1):31-9.

Fevery J, Verslype C, Lai G, Aerts R, Van Steenbergen W. Incidence, diagnosis, and therapy of cholangiocarcinoma in patients with primary sclerosing cholangitis.*Dig Dis Sci.* 2007 Nov;52(11):3123-35.

Freeman K, Bennett AE, Lopez R, Shen B. Primary sclerosing cholangitis is associated with endoscopic and histologic backwash ileitis in patients with ileal pouch-anal anastomosis. *Gastroenterology.* 2008;134(suppl 1):A344.

Fulcher AS, Turner MA, Franklin KJ, Shiffman ML, Sterling RK, Luketic VA, Sanyal AJ. Primary sclerosing cholangitis: evaluation with MR cholangiography-a case-control study. *Radiology.* 2000;215(1):71-80.

Graziadei IW, Wiesner RH, Batts KP, Marotta PJ, LaRusso NF, Porayko MK, Hay JE, Gores GJ, Charlton MR, Ludwig J, Poterucha JJ, Steers JL, Krom RA. Recurrence of primary sclerosing cholangitis following liver transplantation. *Hepatology.* 1999 Apr;29(4):1050-6.

Graziadei IW, Wiesner RH, Marotta PJ, Porayko MK, Hay JE, Charlton MR, Poterucha JJ, Rosen CB, Gores GJ, LaRusso NF, Krom RA. Long-term results of patients undergoing liver transplantation for primary sclerosing cholangitis. *Hepatology.* 1999 Nov;30(5):1121-7.

Greenstein AJ, Janowitz HD, Sachar DB. The extra-intestinal complications of Crohn's disease and ulcerative colitis: a study of 700 patients. *Medicine(Baltimore)* 1996;55:401-12.

Heikius B, Niemelä S, Lehtola J, Karttunen T, Lähde S. Hepatobiliary and coexisting pancreatic duct abnormalities in patients with inflammatory bowel disease. *Scand J Gastroenterol.* 1997 Feb;32(2):153-61.

Heuschen UA, Hinz U, Allemeyer EH, Stern J, Lucas M, Autschbach F, Herfarth C, Heuschen G. Backwash ileitis is strongly associated with colorectal carcinoma in ulcerative colitis. Gastroenterology. 2001;120(4):841-7.

Higashi H, Yanaga K, Marsh JW, Tzakis A, Kakizoe S, Starzl TE. Development of colon cancer after liver transplantation for primary sclerosing cholangitis associated with ulcerative colitis. *Hepatology.* 1990 Mar;11(3):477-80.

Hirche TO, Russler J, Braden B Schuessler G, Zeuzem S, Wehrmann T, Seifert H, Dietrich CF. Sonographic detection of perihepatic lymphadenopathy is an indicator for primary sclerosing cholangitis in patients with inflammatory bowel disease. *Int J Colorectal Dis.* 2004 Nov;19(6):586-94.

Joo M, Abreu-e Lima P, Farreye F, Smith T, Swaroop P, Gardner L, Lauwers GY, Odze RD. Pathologic features of ulcerative colitis in patients with primary sclerosing cholangitis: a case-control study. *Am J Surg Pathol.* 2009 Jun;33(6):854-62.

Kornbluth A, Sachar DB. Ulcerative practice guidelines in adults. American College of Gastroenterology, Practice Parameters Committee. *Am J Gastroenterol* 1997;92:204-211.

Kim WR, Therneau TM, Wiesner RH, Poterucha JJ, Benson JT, Malinchoc M, LaRusso NF, Lindor KD, Dickson ER. A revised natural history model for primary sclerosing cholangitis.*Mayo Clin Proc.* 2000 ;75(7):688-94.

Kornfeld D, Ekbom A, Ihre T. Is there an excess risk for colorectal cancer in patients with ulcerative colitis and concomitant primary sclerosing cholangitis? A population based study. *Gut.* 1997 Oct;41(4):522-5.

Lee YM, Kaplan MM. Primary sclerosing cholangitis. *N Engl J Med.* 1995;332:924-33.

Lepistö A, Kivistö S, Kivisaari L, Arola J, Järvinen HJ. Primary sclerosing cholangitis: outcome of patients undergoing restorative proctocolecetomy for ulcerative colitis. *Int J Colorectal Dis.* 2009 Oct;24(10):1169-74.

Lindor KD, Kowdley KV, Luketic VA, Harrison ME, McCashland T, Befeler AS, Harnois D, Jorgensen R, Petz J, Keach J, Mooney J, Sargeant C, Braaten J, Bernard T, King D, Miceli E, Schmoll J, Hoskin T, Thapa P, Enders F. High-dose ursodeoxycholic acid for the treatment of primary sclerosing cholangitis.*Hepatology.* 2009;50(3):808-14.

Lindor KD. Ursodiol for primary sclerosing cholangitis. Mayo Primary Sclerosing Cholangitis-Ursodeoxycholic Acid Study Group. *N Engl J Med.* 1997 Mar 6;336(10):691-5.

Loftus EV Jr, Harewood GC, Loftus CG, Tremaine WJ, Harmsen WS, Zinsmeister AR, Jewell DA, Sandborn WJ.PSC-IBD: a unique form of inflammatory bowel disease associated with primary sclerosing cholangitis. *Gut.* 2005;54(1):91-6.

Loftus EV, Sandborn WJ, Lindor KD, La Russo NF. Interactions between chronic liver disease and inflammatory bowel disease. Inflamm Bowel Dis 1997;3:288-302.

Ludwig J, Barham SS, LaRusso NF, Elveback LR, Wiesner RH, McCall JT. Morphologic features of chronic hepatitis associated with primary sclerosing cholangitis and chronic ulcerative colitis. *Hepatology.* 1981;1(6):632-40.

Lundqvist K, Broomé U. Differences in colonic disease activity in patients with ulcerative colitis with and without primary sclerosing cholangitis: a case control study. Dis Colon Rectum. 1997 Apr;40(4):451-6.

MacCarty RL, LaRusso NF, May GR, Bender CE, Wiesner RH, King JE, Coffey RJ. Cholangiocarcinoma complicating primary sclerosing cholangitis: cholangiographic appearances. *Radiology.* 1985;156(1):43-6.

MacCarty RL, LaRusso NF, Wiesner RH, Ludwig J.Primary sclerosing cholangitis: findings on cholangiography and pancreatography. Radiology. 1983 ;149(1):39-44.

MacLean AR, Lilly L, Cohen Z, O'Connor B, McLeod RS. Outcome of patients undergoing liver transplantation for primary sclerosing cholangitis. *Dis Colon Rectum* 2003;46:1124-1128.

Mathis KL, Dozois EJ, Larson DW, Cima RR, Sarmiento JM, Wolff BG, Heimbach JK, Pemberton JH.Ileal pouch-anal anastomosis and liver transplantation for ulcerative colitis complicated by primary sclerosing cholangitis.*Br J Surg.* 2008 Jul;95(7):882-6.

McGarity B, Bansi DS, Robertsson DAF, Millward-Sadler GH, Shepherd HA. Primary sclerosing cholangitis: an important and prevalent complication of Crohn's disease. *Eur J Gastroenterol Hepatol* 1991;3:361-364.

Mikkola K, Kiviluoto T, Riihelä M, Taavitsainen M, Järvinen HJ. Liver involvement and its course in patients operated on for ulcerative colitis. *Hepatogastroenterology.* 1995 Feb;42(1):68-72.

Moff SL, Kamel IR, Eustace J, Lawler LP, Kantsevoy S, Kalloo AN, Thuluvath PJ. Diagnosis of primary sclerosing cholangitis: a blinded comparative study using magnetic resonance cholangiography and endoscopic retrograde cholangiography. *Gastrointest Endosc.* 2006 ;64(2):219-23.

Moreno Luna LE, Gores GJ. Advances in the diagnosis of cholangiocarcinoma in patients with primary sclerosing cholangitis. *Liver Transpl.* 2006 ;12(11 Suppl 2):15-9.

Mulder AH, Horst G, Haagsma EB, Limburg PC, Kleibeuker JH, Kallenberg CG. Prevalence and characterization of neutrophil cytoplasmic antibodies in autoimmune liver diseases. *Hepatology.* 1993;17(3):411-7.

Navaneethan U, Remzi FH, Nutter B, Fazio VW, Shen B. Risk factors for abnormal liver function tests in patients with ileal pouch-anal anastomosis for underlying inflammatory bowel disease. *Am J Gastroenterol.* 2009 Oct;104(10):2467-75.

Navaneethan U, Shen B.Hepatopancreatobiliary manifestations and complications associated with inflammatory bowel disease. İnflamm Bowel Dis 2010;16:1598-1619.

Olerup O, Olsson R, Hultcrantz R, Broome U. HLA-DR and HLA-DQ are not markers for rapid disease progression in primary sclerosing cholangitis. *Gastroenterology.* 1995;108(3):870-8.

Olsson R, Boberg KM, de Muckadell OS, Lindgren S, Hultcrantz R, Folvik G, Bell H, Gangsøy-Kristiansen M, Matre J, Rydning A, Wikman O, Danielsson A, Sandberg-Gertzén H, Ung KA, Eriksson A, Lööf L, Prytz H, Marschall HU, Broomé U. High-dose ursodeoxycholic acid in primary sclerosing cholangitis: a 5-year multicenter, randomized, controlled study. *Gastroenterology.* 2005 ;129(5):1464-72.

Olsson R, Danielsson A, Jarnerot G, Lindström E, Lööf L, Rolny P, Rydén BO, Tysk C, Wallerstedt S. Prevalence of primary sclerosing cholangitis in patients with ulcerative colitis. *Gastroenterology.* 1991 May;100(5 Pt 1):1319-23.

O'Mahony CA, Vierling JM. Etiopathogenesis of primary sclerosing cholangitis. *Semin Liver Dis.* 2006 Feb;26(1):3-21.

Outwater E, Kaplan MM, Bankoff MS. Lymphadenopathy in sclerosing cholangitis: pitfall in the diagnosis of malignant biliary obstruction. *Gastrointest Radiol.* 1992 ;17(2):157-60.

Papatheodoridis GV, Hamilton M, Mistry PK, Davidson B, Rolles K, Burroughs AK.Ulcerative colitis has an aggressive course after orthotopic liver transplantation for primary sclerosing cholangitis. *Gut.* 1998 Nov;43(5):639-44.

Parsi MA, Li A, Li CP, Goggins M. DNA methylation alterations in endoscopic retrograde cholangiopancreatography brush samples of patients with suspected pancreaticobiliary disease. *Clin Gastroenterol Hepatol.* 2008; 6(11):1270-8.

Penna C, Dozois R, Tremaine W. Sandborn W, LaRusso N, Schleck C, Ilstrup D. Pouchitis after ileal pouch-anal anastomosis for ulcerative colitis occurs with increased frequency in patients with associated primary sclerosing cholangitis. *Gut.* 1996 Feb;38(2):234-9.

Perdigoto R, Wiesner RH, La Russo N, Dozois R. Inflammatory bowel disease associated with primary sclerosing cholangitis: incidence, severity and relationship to liver disease. *Gastroenterology* 1991;100:1319-1323.

Ponsioen CY, Vrouenraets SM, Prawirodirdjo W, Rajaram R, Rauws EA, Mulder CJ, Reitsma JB, Heisterkamp SH, Tytgat GN. Natural history of primary sclerosing cholangitis and prognostic value of cholangiography in a Dutch population. *Gut.* 2002;51(4):562-6.

Porayko MK, Wiesner RH, LaRusso NF, Ludwig J, MacCarty RL, Steiner BL, Twomey CK, Zinsmeister AR. Patients with asymptomatic primary sclerosing cholangitis frequently have progressive disease.*Gastroenterology.* 1990 ;98(6):1594-602.

Poritz LS, Koltun WA. Surgical management of ulcerative colitis in the presence of primary sclerosing cholangitis.*Dis Colon Rectum.* 2003 Feb;46(2):173-8.

Rabinovitz M, Gavaler JS, Schade RR, Dindzans VJ, Chien MC, Van Thiel DH. Does primary sclerosing cholangitis occurring in association with inflammatory bowel disease differ from that occurring in the absence of inflammatory bowel disease? A study of sixty-six subjects.*Hepatology.* 1990;11(1):7-11.

Rasmussen HH, Fallingborg JF, Mortensen PB, Vyberg M, Tage-Jensen U, Rasmussen SN. Hepatobiliary dysfunction and primary sclerosing cholangitis in patients with Crohn's disease. *Scand J Gastroenterol.* 1997 Jun;32(6):604-10.

Rea DJ, Heimbach JK, Rosen CB, Haddock MG, Alberts SR, Kremers WK, Gores GJ, Nagorney DM. Liver transplantation with neoadjuvant chemoradiation is more effective than resection for hilar cholangiocarcinoma.*Ann Surg.* 2005;242(3):451-8.

Riley TR, Schoen RE, Lee RG, Rakela J. A case series of transplant recipients who despite immunosuppression developed inflammatory bowel disease. *Am J Gastroenterol* 1997;92:279-82.

Rutter M, Saunders B, Wilkinson K, Rumbles S, Schofield G, Kamm M, Williams C, Price A, Talbot I, Forbes A.Severity of inflammation is a risk factor for colorectal neoplasia in ulcerative colitis.*Gastroenterology.* 2004 Feb;126(2):451-9.

Rutter MD, Saunders BP, Wilkinson KH, Rumbles S, Schofield G, Kamm MA, Williams CB, Price AB, Talbot IC, Forbes A. Cancer surveillance in longstanding ulcerative colitis: endoscopic appearances help predict cancer risk. *Gut.* 2004 Dec;53(12):1813-6.

Saarinen S, Olerup O, Broome U. Increased frequency of autoimmune disease in patients with primary sclerosing cholangitis. *Am J Gastroenterol.* 2000;95:3195-3199.

Saldeen K, Friman S, Olausson M, Olsson R.Follow-up after liver transplantation for primary sclerosing cholangitis: effects on survival, quality of life, and colitis.*Scand J Gastroenterol.* 1999 May;34(5):535-40.

Schrumpf E, Elgjo K, Fausa K, Gjone E, Kolmannskog F, Ritland S. Sclerosing cholangitis in ulcerative colitis. *Scand J Gastroenterol* 1980;15:689-97.

Shen B, Bennett AE, Navaneethan U, Lian L, Shao Z, Kiran RP, Fazio VW, Remzi FH. Primary sclerosing cholangitis is associated with endoscopic and histologic inflammation of the distal afferent limb in patients with ileal pouch-anal anastomosis. *Inflamm Bowel Dis.* 2010 Dec 27. [Epub ahead of print]

Shepherd HA, Selby WS, Chapman RW, Nolan D, Barbatis C, McGee JO, Jewell DP. Ulcerative colitis and persistent liver dysfunction. *Q J Med.* 1983 Autumn;52(208):503-13.

Smith M, Loe S. Sclerosing cholangitis:review of recent case reports and associated diseases and four new cases. Am J Surg 1965;110:239-246.

Soetikno RM, Lin OS, Heidenreich PA, Young HS, Blackstone MO. Increased risk of colorectal neoplasia in patients with primary sclerosing cholangitis and ulcerative colitis: a meta-analysis. *Gastrointest Endosc.* 2002 Jul;56(1):48-54.

Ståhlberg D, Veress B, Tribukait B, Broomé U. Atrophy and neoplastic transformation of the ileal pouch mucosa in patients with ulcerative colitis and primary sclerosing cholangitis: a case control study. *Dis Colon Rectum.* 2003 ;46(6):770-8.

Takikawa H, Manabe T. Primary sclerosing cholangitis in Japan--analysis of 192 cases. *J Gastroenterol.* 1997 Feb;32(1):134-7.

Talwalkar JA, Lindor KD. Primary sclerosing cholangitis. Inflamm Bowel Dis. 2005;11:62-72.

Terjung B, Spengler U, Sauerbruch T, Worman HJ. "Atypical p-ANCA" in IBD and hepatobiliary disorders react with a 50-kilodalton nuclear envelope protein of neutrophils and myeloid cell lines.*Gastroenterology.* 2000 Aug;119(2):310-22.

Terjung B, Spengler U. Atypical p-ANCA in PSC and AIH: a hint toward a "leaky gut"?. *Clin Rev Allergy Immunol* 2009;36(1):40-51.

Terjung B, Spengler U. Role of auto-antibodies for the diagnosis of chronic cholestatic liver diseases. *Clin Rev Allergy Immunol*. 2005 Apr;28(2):115-33.

Textor HJ, Flacke S, Pauleit D, Keller E, Neubrand M, Terjung B, Gieseke J, Scheurlen C, Sauerbruch T, Schild HH. Three-dimensional magnetic resonance cholangiopancreatography with respiratory triggering in the diagnosis of primary sclerosing cholangitis: comparison with endoscopic retrograde cholangiography. *Endoscopy*. 2002;34(12):984-90.

Tischendorf JJ, Hecker H, Krüger M, Manns MP, Meier PN. Characterization, outcome, and prognosis in 273 patients with primary sclerosing cholangitis: A single center study. *Am J Gastroenterol*. 2007 Jan;102(1):107-14. Epub 2006 Oct 13.

Tobias R, Wright JP, Kottler RE, Bornman PC, Price SK, Hatfield A, Marks IN. Primary sclerosing cholangitis associated with inflammatory bowel disease in Cape Town, 1975 - 1981.*S Afr Med J*. 1983 Feb 12;63(7):229-35.

Tung BY, Emond MJ, Haggitt RC, Bronner MP, Kimmey MB, Kowdley KV, Brentnall TA.Ursodiol use is associated with lower prevalence of colonic neoplasia in patients with ulcerative colitis and primary sclerosing cholangitis. *Ann Intern Med*. 2001 Jan 16;134(2):89-95.

Vera A, Gunson BK, Ussatoff V, Nightingale P, Candinas D, Radley S, Mayer AD, Buckels JA, McMaster P, Neuberger J, Mirza DF. Colorectal cancer in patients with inflammatory bowel disease after liver transplantation for primary sclerosing cholangitis.*Transplantation*. 2003 Jun 27;75(12):1983-8.

Verdonk RC, Dijkstra G, Haagsma EB, Shostrom VK, Van den Berg AP, Kleibeuker JH, Langnas AN, Sudan DL. Inflammatory bowel disease after liver transplantation: risk factors for recurrence and de novo disease.*Am J Transplant*. 2006 Jun;6(6):1422-9.

Wee A, Ludwig J, Coffey RJ Jr, LaRusso NF, Wiesner RH.Hepatobiliary carcinoma associated with primary sclerosing cholangitis and chronic ulcerative colitis.*Hum Pathol*. 1985 Jul;16(7):719-26.

Wiesner RH, Grambsch PM, Dickson ER, Ludwig J, MacCarty RL, Hunter EB, Fleming TR, Fisher LD, Beaver SJ, LaRusso NF. Primary sclerosing cholangitis: natural history, prognostic factors and survival analysis. *Hepatology*. 1989;10(4):430-6.

Wiesner RH, LaRusso NF.Clinicopathologic features of the syndrome of primary sclerosing cholangitis.*Gastroenterology*. 1980;79(2):200-6.

Wiesner RH, Grambsch PM, Dickson ER, Ludwig J, MacCarty RL, Hunter EB, Fleming TR, Fisher LD, Beaver SJ, LaRusso NF. Primary sclerosing cholangitis: natural history, prognostic factors and survival analysis. *Hepatology*. 1989 Oct;10(4):430-6.

Worthington J, Cullen S, Chapman R. Immunopathogenesis of primary sclerosing cholangitis. *Clin Rev Allergy Immunol*. 2005;28(2):93-103. Review.

Zein CO, Lindor KD, Angulo P. Prevalence and predictors of esophageal varices in patients with primary sclerosing cholangitis.*Hepatology*. 2004 ;39(1):204-10.

Zins BJ, Sandborn WJ, Penna CR, Landers CJ, Targan SR, Tremaine WJ, Wiesner RH, Dozois RR. Pouchitis disease course after orthotopic liver transplantation in patients with primary sclerosing cholangitis and an ileal pouch-anal anastomosis. *Am J Gastroenterol*. 1995;90(12):2177-81.

13

Neoplasia in IBD

Joel Pekow and Marc Bissonnette

Department of Medicine, Section of Gastroenterology, University of Chicago
USA

1. Introduction

Longstanding inflammation of the colonic mucosa places patients with ulcerative colitis (UC) at increased risk for the development of colon cancer. As such, there has been significant research over the last 20 years into efforts to understand the natural history of neoplastic lesions in UC in order to modify this risk. This chapter will focus on the epidemiology of neoplasia in UC, the biology of IBD-associated cancer, outcomes after a diagnosis of a dysplastic lesion, as well as strategies for surveillance and chemoprevention.

2. Epidemiology

The majority of studies examining the development of cancer in IBD have demonstrated an increased risk for neoplasia in patients with long-standing UC (1-6). A 2001 meta-analysis involving 116 studies and over 50,000 patients calculated the cumulative risk of CRC in UC as 8.3% at 20 years and 18.4% at 30 years (7). However, two recent population based studies, one from Denmark and the other from Olmstead County in Minnesota, did not find a significant increase in risk (3, 8). The discrepancy in results between these more recent studies and older analyses may be secondary to the effects of newer, more effective anti-inflammatory agents for IBD or the implementation of surveillance programs and removal of colons with dysplastic lesions prior to the development of cancer.

3. Risk factors

It is postulated that cancer develops in patients with IBD secondary to prolonged inflammation. The evidence to support inflammation driving neoplastic transformation stems from studies demonstrating that patients with longer disease duration, extensive colitis, and uncontrolled inflammation are at increased risk for neoplastic changes. Risk of colorectal cancer (CRC) development rises with increased interval from diagnosis of IBD-associated colitis (2, 9). In fact, CRC is uncommon in patients who have had colitis for less than 7 years, and more commonly develops in patients who are diagnosed with IBD at a younger age (5, 7). Several studies have also demonstrated that cancer develops more frequently in those with an increased extent of colitis (2, 4). A Swedish population-based study using barium enemas quantified this risk by standardized incidence ratio as 1.7 for individuals with proctitis, 2.8 for those with left-sided colitis, and 14.8 for those with pancolitis (2).

Two recent publications have established that severity of inflammation is associated with an increased risk for cancer in IBD. In a retrospective cohort from the St. Mark's hospital, severity of inflammation by histology was significantly associated with neoplasia in patients with extensive colitis (10). Interestingly, in this multivariate analysis only histologic inflammatory activity and not endoscopic inflammation was associated with neoplasia. A second retrospective study from Mt. Sinai hospital in New York confirmed severity of inflammation over time as a risk for neoplasia (11).

Two other well-described risk factors for neoplastic development in IBD include a family history of colorectal cancer and a history of primary sclerosing cholangitis (PSC). Several retrospective analyses have reported that patients with IBD who develop neoplasia have an odds ratio between 2.3 and 5.0 for having a family history of CRC (5, 12-14). A large population-based cohort also demonstrated a relative risk for the development of neoplasia of 2.5 for patients with a family history of colon cancer (15). As in the case of sporadic colon cancer with positive family history, this association was stronger for patients with a first-degree relative with CRC less than 50 years of age (15). Potentially, the most significant risk factor for neoplasia in patients with UC is a concomitant diagnosis of PSC. Although the reported frequency of neoplastic changes in this population varies among studies, patients with UC and PSC have consistently demonstrated a markedly increased risk for the development of both dysplasia and colon cancer compared to patients with UC without PSC (5, 16-20). The overall incidence of CRC in patients with UC and PSC was between 16% and 25% in a Swedish population-based study after 10 years of disease duration (17). This risk of neoplastic changes in UC patients with PSC has also been noted to occur earlier in the disease course than UC patients without PSC.

4. Definition of dysplasia

In UC, the term dysplasia is defined as neoplastic changes confined to the colonic epithelium. Tissue that is positive for dysplasia is most commonly identified as either low grade (LGD) or high grade (HGD) (21). Dysplasia is also characterized based on its endoscopic appearance, and outcomes of progression to cancer are associated with this endoscopic classification. Historically, flat dysplasia has been defined as dysplasia identified only by histological and not endoscopic features. However, recent studies have demonstrated that most lesions classified as flat dysplasia were obtained from targeted biopsies of visible lesions (22, 23). Raised lesions that are not endoscopically resectable are termed dysplasia associated mass or lesion or DALMs. The term ALM (adenoma-like mass) refers to a raised, endoscopically resectable lesion that resembles a sporadic adenoma by endoscopic and histological characteristics.

5. Biology of IBD-associated cancer

Although initiating mechanisms of carcinogenesis in IBD remain unknown, neoplastic lesions likely result from a combination of genetic alterations and inflammatory mediators that activate cell-signaling pathways. These pathways in turn promote deregulations in growth and apoptosis. Several molecular changes occurring in IBD-CRC are similar to those seen in sporadic CRC. In contrast to solitary lesions in sporadic colon cancer, however, neoplastic lesions in IBD are often multifocal. This finding likely reflects the widespread field defects throughout the UC involved mucosa that increase the risk for neoplastic changes. Moreover, expression changes in coding and non-coding (microRNA) genes that are seen in malignant transformation, also occur in chronic UC, further supporting this hypothesis (24-26).

Genomic instability characterized by either chromosomal instability or microsatellite instability occurs in both sporadic and IBD-associated CRC. In fact, frequencies of these genetic abnormalities (chromosomal instability – 85%, microsatellite instability – 15%) are similar in IBD-CRC and sporadic CRC (27-30).

Genetic changes in the tumor suppressor, p53, are believed to play an important role in the development of IBD-associated neoplasia. Loss of heterozygosity and p53 mutations have both been reported in colons with IBD-associated neoplasia (31-33). It is believed that changes in p53 may occur prior to the development of dysplastic lesions in 'at risk' mucosa (32). Moreover, reactivity of p53 antibodies increase with histologic progression from UC patients without dysplasia to those with dysplasia and CRC (34). Positive p53 immunostaining can also occur prior to the development of dysplasia in chronic UC mucosa (35, 36).

The WNT pathway is deregulated in IBD-associated cancer development as occurs in sporadic colorectal carcinogenesis. Similar to genetic changes in p53, it appears that up-regulation of WNT signaling occurs early in UC-associated neoplastic progression (37). In addition to overexpression of proteins in the WNT signaling cascade, hypermethylation of WNT-suppressor genes in this pathway occur during neoplastic development in IBD (38). Such methylations could lead to silencing of tumor suppressor genes. In contrast to sporadic colon cancer, however, it appears that APC loss of function mutations play a less significant role in initiating WNT signaling (39-41). Increased mutations in the oncogene, K-ras, have also been described in IBD-associated colon cancer (31). However, the timing of K-ras mutations in neoplastic progression needs to be clarified in larger studies.

In addition to genetic changes, previous studies in animal models of ulcerative colitis and colitis-associated colon cancer have demonstrated involvement of other key signaling pathways including the vitamin D receptor, NFκB, transforming growth factor beta (TGFβ), cyclooxygenase-2 (COX2), toll-like receptor-4 (TLR4), and the epidermal growth factor receptor (EGFR). Several mouse studies have shown that active vitamin D or its analogues inhibit progression in murine models of inflammation-associated colitis (42, 43) Furthermore, one retrospective analysis identified decreased expression of VDR in IBD-associated dysplastic lesions (44). NFκB controls a vast array of functions and is a master regulator of many pro-inflammatory cytokines including TNF-α and IL-1β. NFκB overexpression is known to contribute to both inflammation and malignant transformation in several cancers (45). NFκB has also been demonstrated to contribute to malignant transformation in a mouse model of inflammation-associated cancer (46). In the study by Greten et al, NFκB in epithelial cells was essential for survival signals, allowing mutant clones to expand, whereas NFκB in stromal cells increased cytokines and growth factors required for tumor growth (46). Furthermore, NFκB mediates TNF-α activation of cytidine deaminase in human colonic epithelial cells and colitis-associated cancers. Activation induced cytidine deaminase plays a critical role in physiological antibody diversification, but also contributes to malignant lymphocytic transformation (47). In addition to NFκB up-regulation, TLR4 overexpression occurs in colitis-associated colon cancer that enhances Cox-2 expression via an EGFR-dependent mechanism (48). Recent studies from our laboratory have demonstrated that EGFR signals were required for Cox-2 up-regulation in this model (49).

6. Surveillance for IBD-associated neoplasia

There are no randomized controlled trials investigating the mortality benefit of surveillance colonoscopy in patients with UC. The best evidence to support routine endoscopic surveillance comes from retrospective case-controlled studies. In a retrospective analysis of patients with CRC, Choi et al. reported that patients who underwent surveillance had a carcinoma detected at an earlier Dukes stage and improved 5-year survival rate (50). A second analysis by Lashner and colleagues found that in 186 patients with extensive UC who underwent surveillance, patients had an improved survival and delayed time to colectomy, although the decrease in mortality was not related to cancer free survival (51). A Swedish population-based nested case-control study examining patients who died from CRC reported that two of 40 patients with UC who had died from colon cancer had undergone at least one screening exam, compared to 18 of 102 controls with UC who did not die from colon cancer (52). Similar protective effects of surveillance were seen in a second retrospective cohort (13). In a Cochrane database analysis of these studies published in 2006, the authors concluded that there was indirect evidence that surveillance is likely to show a cost benefit and be effective in reducing the risk of death from IBD-associated CRC (53).

The current standard of care recommended for the prevention of cancer in IBD is regular surveillance colonoscopy. The ability to prevent cancer with this strategy relies on the early detection of precancerous lesions. Most strategies for early detection involve both random biopsies and targeted biopsies of suspicious lesions. The major challenge with this strategy is sampling error. With random biopsies, it has been estimated 33 biopsies are needed to exclude dysplasia with 90% certainty and 64 biopsies are need for a 95% certainty. Most gastroenterologists do not approach such numbers of biopsies during surveillance exams (54, 55). Several recent studies, however, indicate that the yield of targeted biopsies is much greater than random biopsies of the colon. One possible explanation for these findings was suggested by three recent retrospective analyses. These studies concluded that most dysplastic lesions can be visualized with white light colonoscopy (22, 23, 56).

Recent experience with chromoendoscopy, however, has consistently shown superior detection of dysplastic lesions with super vital staining compared to uncontrasted white light examinations (57-61). Chromoendoscopy is typically done with either indigo carmine or methylene blue dye. In a recent meta-analysis of six studies, the difference in proportion of lesions detected by chromoendoscopy vs. white light only was 44% (62). Autofluorescence with narrow band imaging (NBI) has been suggested to improve detection of dysplastic lesions in UC as well, although studies testing the benefit of NBI compared to high definition colonoscopy have been inconclusive (63-65).

Several recommendations have been published to guide surveillance strategies in patients with UC (66-69). The most recent consensus statement was released by the American Gastroenterological Association (AGA) and recommended initiating surveillance no later than 8 years of disease duration for patients with left-sided or pancolitis (69). During surveillance examinations, multiple biopsies should be obtained from each anatomic location in the colon. This statement included chromoendoscopy as a recommended alternative to random biopsies by endoscopists who have expertise with the technique. The AGA recommended repeat examinations every 1-3 years and to decrease the interval to every 1-2 years after 20 years of disease duration. For patients with PSC, surveillance exams should be performed at the time of diagnosis and then yearly thereafter, because of an increased risk earlier in the disease course.

7. Outcome after a diagnosis of dysplasia

After a diagnosis of flat HGD, colectomy has been universally recommended because there is a significant risk of harboring a synchronous CRC. One systematic review calculated this risk as 42% (70). A subsequent prospective analysis from St. Marks Hospital reported a 45% incidence of synchronous carcinomas in patients undergoing immediate colectomy after diagnosis of HGD (9). In this analysis, eight patients underwent surveillance. Of these eight, one developed CRC and seven developed further dysplasia (6 HGD, 1 LGD) (9). There appears to be a similar risk of development of cancer in patients with endoscopically unresectable DALMs (70, 71). Because of the high risk of CRC development, colectomy is warranted for any patient with a DALM or flat HGD.

In contrast to HGD, the management of patients with IBD-associated indeterminate dysplasia (IND) or LGD remains controversial. Previous studies have varied in their reported rates of progression from low-grade lesions to advanced neoplasia from 16% to 54% (9, 70, 72-76). The discrepancy in reported rates of progression to advanced neoplasia is likely secondary to the population heterogeneity of these studies. Within the classification of LGD, outcomes are different for flat dysplastic lesions and adenoma-like dysplastic lesions (ALMs). For patients who have an ALM in the absence of surrounding dysplasia, the risk of development of cancer appears to be minimal (77-79). For this reason, patients with polypoid lesions that resemble a sporadic adenoma without surrounding flat dysplasia can be managed with endoscopic resection and surveillance. Conversely, flat dysplastic lesions carry a higher risk of malignant progression and of harboring a synchronous CRC at the time of diagnosis (72, 74, 78). Total abdominal colectomy should be discussed with patients following a diagnosis of flat LGD. For patients with controlled disease who elect to undergo surveillance of flat LGD lesions, close follow up with endoscopic evaluations, initially at 3 to 6 month intervals is warranted.

Although neoplastic changes may develop in the pouch or in the anal transition zone, the risk of dysplasia appears to be low for patients with UC who undergo a restorative proctocolectomy with ileoanal anastomosis. One large analysis of 23 observational studies and over 2000 patients estimated that only slightly more than 1% of patients have confirmed dysplasia in the pouch or anal transition zone at follow up (80). A more recent analysis of over 3000 patients from the Cleveland Clinic reported the incidence of neoplasia to be 0.9%, 1.3%, 1.9%, 4.2%, and 5.1% at 5, 10, 15, 20, and 25 years after surgery, respectively (81). In both these studies, the risk of neoplastic transformation was significantly higher in patients who had dysplasia or cancer as their indication for initial colectomy. Although there are no published guidelines for surveillance after restorative proctocolectomy, many clinicians recommend a surveillance program because there remains a risk of neoplastic transformation, albeit low. It is postulated that performing a hand-sewn ileoanal anastomosis may decrease the risk of neoplasia. However, published studies have reported no difference between a stapled technique and hand-sewn anastomosis with mucosectomy (81, 82).

8. Chemoprevention

The primary goal of chemoprevention is to decrease the incidence of neoplastic lesions in those at increased risk. An effective chemopreventive agent offers the theoretical advantage over surveillance endoscopy alone by deceasing the frequency, cost, and risk of colonoscopy, as well as reducing need for colectomy.

The majority of studies examining chemopreventive agents in IBD have focused on the use of 5-aminosalicylates (5-ASA). There are several postulated mechanisms by which 5-ASA inhibits malignant transformation. These include inhibition of NFκB, increased apoptosis of mutant clones, decreased proliferation, and prevention of oxygen-radical induced DNA damage (83-85). A meta-analysis of nine case control studies examining the efficacy of 5-ASA in preventing dysplasia or cancer revealed a pooled odds ratio of 0.51 (95% CI, 0.38-0.69) (86). However, several studies that have been published subsequent to this meta-analysis have not found a protective effect of 5-ASA therapy (87-90). Taken together, data to support 5-ASA chemoprevention in IBD is inconclusive, likely due to the heterogeneity of individuals in these studies. Furthermore, it is not known what effect 5-ASA has on CRC risk in patients who have achieved mucosal healing with other therapies.

The bile acid, ursodeoxycholic acid, has been used as a chemopreventive agent in UC patients with PSC. In animal models, UDCA is protective against the development of colon cancer (91-94). The mechanism of UDCA's chemopreventive activity remains uncertain, although it is likely multifactorial (92, 94) There have been two retrospective analyses of UDCA in patients with UC and PSC with conflicting results (93, 95-97). In a randomized placebo-controlled trial of UDCA at the dose of 13-15mg/kg-body wt/day, the relative risk for dysplasia or cancer in the group receiving UDCA was 0.26 (95% CI, 0.06-0.92). However, a more recent randomized placebo-controlled trial examining high dose UDCA (28-30 mg/kg-body wt/day) in UC patients with PSC found that patients taking UDCA had a higher risk of developing colorectal neoplasia (98). Currently, the American Association for the Study of Liver Diseases (AASLD) does not recommend UDCA for chemoprevention in patients with UC and PSC as larger prospective studies of low dose UDCA are needed to further evaluate this potential chemopreventive agent (99).

Other chemopreventive agents that have been studied in IBD-associated colitis include folic acid, immunomodulators, and vitamin D. Although a recent analysis of thiopurines in IBD found their use to be protective, the majority of studies investigating the chemopreventive efficacy of immunomodulators have not shown a benefit (10, 75, 100, 101). While folic acid deficiency is associated with decreased risk of sporadic CRC in epidemiological studies and folic acid is protective of other malignancies, the studies examining folic acid in the chemoprevention of CRC in patients with IBD have not demonstrated a benefit (102-104). The data on chemoprevention with folic acid in IBD comes from small retrospective analyses that have failed to show a statistical difference in the risk of dysplasia (105, 106). Finally, vitamin D has shown chemopreventive efficacy in murine models of sporadic and inflammation-associated colon cancer (42, 43, 107). Although vitamin D supplementation has not been examined in humans with UC, decreased vitamin D receptor expression is seen in cancers of patients with IBD and vitamin D appears to be chemopreventive of human CRC in epidemiological studies (44, 108). For this reason, vitamin D might offer a potential benefit to patients with chronic UC, although there have been no controlled studies in an IBD population.

9. Conclusion

Patients with chronic ulcerative colitis are at increased risk for the development of colon cancer. Because of this risk, colonoscopic surveillance is recommended for early detection of precancerous lesions. Successful implementation of surveillance programs has likely limited the mortality from CRC in this high-risk population. The outcome after detection of dysplastic lesions needs to be better defined in future studies as endoscopic imaging techniques improve our ability to detect early neoplastic changes. Identification of effective chemopreventive agents against CRC development in UC could decrease the incidence and morbidity of colitis-associated neoplasia. To date, however, there is a lack of data to recommend the use of any specific chemopreventive agents in UC. Because of the cost and morbidity in the detection and treatment of neoplastic lesions in chronic UC, future research is urgently needed to identify efficacious, safe, and cost-effective chemopreventive agents and to establish clinical and biological predictors of dysplasia in order to tailor personalized surveillance strategies.

10. References

[1] Prior P, Gyde SN, Macartney JC, Thompson H, Waterhouse JA, Allan RN. Cancer morbidity in ulcerative colitis. Gut. 1982;23(6):490-7.

[2] Ekbom A, Helmick C, Zack M, Adami HO. Ulcerative colitis and colorectal cancer. A population-based study. N Engl J Med. 1990;323(18):1228-33.

[3] Winther KV, Jess T, Langholz E, Munkholm P, Binder V. Long-term risk of cancer in ulcerative colitis: a population-based cohort study from Copenhagen County. Clin Gastroenterol Hepatol. 2004;2(12):1088-95.

[4] Gyde SN, Prior P, Allan RN, Stevens A, Jewell DP, Truelove SC, Lofberg R, Brostrom O, Hellers G. Colorectal cancer in ulcerative colitis: a cohort study of primary referrals from three centres. Gut. 1988;29(2):206-17.

[5] Bergeron V, Vienne A, Sokol H, Seksik P, Nion-Larmurier I, Ruskone-Fourmestraux A, Svrcek M, Beaugerie L, Cosnes J. Risk factors for neoplasia in inflammatory bowel disease patients with pancolitis. Am J Gastroenterol. 2010;105(11):2405-11.

[6] Devroede GJ, Taylor WF, Sauer WG, Jackman RJ, Stickler GB. Cancer risk and life expectancy of children with ulcerative colitis. N Engl J Med. 1971;285(1):17-21.

[7] Eaden JA, Abrams KR, Mayberry JF. The risk of colorectal cancer in ulcerative colitis: a meta-analysis. Gut. 2001;48(4):526-35.

[8] Jess T, Loftus EV, Jr., Velayos FS, Harmsen WS, Zinsmeister AR, Smyrk TC, Schleck CD, Tremaine WJ, Melton LJ, 3rd, Munkholm P, Sandborn WJ. Risk of intestinal cancer in inflammatory bowel disease: a population-based study from olmsted county, Minnesota. Gastroenterology. 2006;130(4):1039-46.

[9] Rutter MD, Saunders BP, Wilkinson KH, Rumbles S, Schofield G, Kamm MA, Williams CB, Price AB, Talbot IC, Forbes A. Thirty-year analysis of a colonoscopic surveillance program for neoplasia in ulcerative colitis. Gastroenterology. 2006;130(4):1030-8.

[10] Rutter M, Saunders B, Wilkinson K, Rumbles S, Schofield G, Kamm M, Williams C, Price A, Talbot I, Forbes A. Severity of inflammation is a risk factor for colorectal neoplasia in ulcerative colitis. Gastroenterology. 2004;126(2):451-9.

[11] Gupta RB, Harpaz N, Itzkowitz S, Hossain S, Matula S, Kornbluth A, Bodian C, Ullman T. Histologic inflammation is a risk factor for progression to colorectal neoplasia in ulcerative colitis: a cohort study. Gastroenterology. 2007;133(4):1099-105; quiz 340-1.

[12] Velayos FS, Loftus EV, Jr., Jess T, Harmsen WS, Bida J, Zinsmeister AR, Tremaine WJ, Sandborn WJ. Predictive and protective factors associated with colorectal cancer in ulcerative colitis: A case-control study. Gastroenterology. 2006;130(7):1941-9.

[13] Eaden J, Abrams K, Ekbom A, Jackson E, Mayberry J. Colorectal cancer prevention in ulcerative colitis: a case-control study. Aliment Pharmacol Ther. 2000;14(2):145-53.

[14] Nuako KW, Ahlquist DA, Mahoney DW, Schaid DJ, Siems DM, Lindor NM. Familial predisposition for colorectal cancer in chronic ulcerative colitis: a case-control study. Gastroenterology. 1998;115(5):1079-83.

[15] Askling J, Dickman PW, Karlen P, Brostrom O, Lapidus A, Lofberg R, Ekbom A. Family history as a risk factor for colorectal cancer in inflammatory bowel disease. Gastroenterology. 2001;120(6):1356-62.

[16] Shetty K, Rybicki L, Brzezinski A, Carey WD, Lashner BA. The risk for cancer or dysplasia in ulcerative colitis patients with primary sclerosing cholangitis. Am J Gastroenterol. 1999;94(6):1643-9.

[17] Kornfeld D, Ekbom A, Ihre T. Is there an excess risk for colorectal cancer in patients with ulcerative colitis and concomitant primary sclerosing cholangitis? A population based study. Gut. 1997;41(4):522-5.

[18] Marchesa P, Lashner BA, Lavery IC, Milsom J, Hull TL, Strong SA, Church JM, Navarro G, Fazio VW. The risk of cancer and dysplasia among ulcerative colitis patients with primary sclerosing cholangitis. Am J Gastroenterol. 1997;92(8):1285-8.

[19] Brentnall TA, Haggitt RC, Rabinovitch PS, Kimmey MB, Bronner MP, Levine DS, Kowdley KV, Stevens AC, Crispin DA, Emond M, Rubin CE. Risk and natural history of colonic neoplasia in patients with primary sclerosing cholangitis and ulcerative colitis. Gastroenterology. 1996;110(2):331-8.

[20] D'Haens GR, Lashner BA, Hanauer SB. Pericholangitis and sclerosing cholangitis are risk factors for dysplasia and cancer in ulcerative colitis. Am J Gastroenterol. 1993;88(8):1174-8.

[21] Riddell RH, Goldman H, Ransohoff DF, Appelman HD, Fenoglio CM, Haggitt RC, Ahren C, Correa P, Hamilton SR, Morson BC, et al. Dysplasia in inflammatory bowel disease: standardized classification with provisional clinical applications. Hum Pathol. 1983;14(11):931-68.

[22] Rubin DT, Rothe JA, Hetzel JT, Cohen RD, Hanauer SB. Are dysplasia and colorectal cancer endoscopically visible in patients with ulcerative colitis? Gastrointest Endosc. 2007;65(7):998-1004.

[23] Rutter MD, Saunders BP, Wilkinson KH, Kamm MA, Williams CB, Forbes A. Most dysplasia in ulcerative colitis is visible at colonoscopy. Gastrointest Endosc. 2004;60(3):334-9.

[24] Noble CL, Abbas AR, Cornelius J, Lees CW, Ho GT, Toy K, Modrusan Z, Pal N, Zhong F, Chalasani S, Clark H, Arnott ID, Penman ID, Satsangi J, Diehl L. Regional variation in gene expression in the healthy colon is dysregulated in ulcerative colitis. Gut. 2008;57(10):1398-405.

[25] Okahara S, Arimura Y, Yabana T, Kobayashi K, Gotoh A, Motoya S, Imamura A, Endo T, Imai K. Inflammatory gene signature in ulcerative colitis with cDNA macroarray analysis. Aliment Pharmacol Ther. 2005;21(9):1091-7.

[26] Pekow JR, Dougherty U, Mustafi R, Zhu H, Kocherginsky M, Rubin DT, Hanauer SB, Hart J, Chang EB, Fichera A, Joseph LJ, Bissonnette M. miR-143 and miR-145 are downregulated in ulcerative colitis: Putative regulators of inflammation and protooncogenes. Inflamm Bowel Dis. 2011. epub ahead of print.

[27] Tahara T, Inoue N, Hisamatsu T, Kashiwagi K, Takaishi H, Kanai T, Watanabe M, Ishii H, Hibi T. Clinical significance of microsatellite instability in the inflamed mucosa

for the prediction of colonic neoplasms in patients with ulcerative colitis. J Gastroenterol Hepatol. 2005;20(5):710-5.

[28] Umetani N, Sasaki S, Watanabe T, Shinozaki M, Matsuda K, Ishigami H, Ueda E, Muto T. Genetic alterations in ulcerative colitis-associated neoplasia focusing on APC, K-ras gene and microsatellite instability. Jpn J Cancer Res. 1999;90(10):1081-7.

[29] Xie J, Itzkowitz SH. Cancer in inflammatory bowel disease. World J Gastroenterol. 2008;14(3):378-89.

[30] Goel GA, Kandiel A, Achkar JP, Lashner B. Molecular pathways underlying IBD-associated colorectal neoplasia: therapeutic implications. Am J Gastroenterol. 2011;106(4):719-30.

[31] Leedham SJ, Graham TA, Oukrif D, McDonald SA, Rodriguez-Justo M, Harrison RF, Shepherd NA, Novelli MR, Jankowski JA, Wright NA. Clonality, founder mutations, and field cancerization in human ulcerative colitis-associated neoplasia. Gastroenterology. 2009;136(2):542-50 e6.

[32] Brentnall TA, Crispin DA, Rabinovitch PS, Haggitt RC, Rubin CE, Stevens AC, Burmer GC. Mutations in the p53 gene: an early marker of neoplastic progression in ulcerative colitis. Gastroenterology. 1994;107(2):369-78.

[33] Burmer GC, Rabinovitch PS, Haggitt RC, Crispin DA, Brentnall TA, Kolli VR, Stevens AC, Rubin CE. Neoplastic progression in ulcerative colitis: histology, DNA content, and loss of a p53 allele. Gastroenterology. 1992;103(5):1602-10.

[34] Yoshizawa S, Matsuoka K, Inoue N, Takaishi H, Ogata H, Iwao Y, Mukai M, Fujita T, Kawakami Y, Hibi T. Clinical significance of serum p53 antibodies in patients with ulcerative colitis and its carcinogenesis. Inflamm Bowel Dis. 2007;13(7):865-73.

[35] Gerrits MM, Chen M, Theeuwes M, van Dekken H, Sikkema M, Steyerberg EW, Lingsma HF, Siersema PD, Xia B, Kusters JG, van der Woude CJ, Kuipers EJ. Biomarker-based prediction of inflammatory bowel disease-related colorectal cancer: a case-control study. Cell Oncol (Dordr). 2011;34(2):107-17.

[36] van Schaik FD, Oldenburg B, Offerhaus GJ, Schipper ME, Vleggaar FP, Siersema PD, van Oijen MG, Ten Kate FJ. Role of immunohistochemical markers in predicting progression of dysplasia to advanced neoplasia in patients with ulcerative colitis. Inflamm Bowel Dis. 2011. epub ahead of print.

[37] Claessen MM, Schipper ME, Oldenburg B, Siersema PD, Offerhaus GJ, Vleggaar FP. WNT-pathway activation in IBD-associated colorectal carcinogenesis: potential biomarkers for colonic surveillance. Cell Oncol. 2010;32(4):303-10.

[38] Dhir M, Montgomery EA, Glockner SC, Schuebel KE, Hooker CM, Herman JG, Baylin SB, Gearhart SL, Ahuja N. Epigenetic regulation of WNT signaling pathway genes in inflammatory bowel disease (IBD) associated neoplasia. J Gastrointest Surg. 2008;12(10):1745-53.

[39] You XJ, Bryant PJ, Jurnak F, Holcombe RF. Expression of Wnt pathway components frizzled and disheveled in colon cancer arising in patients with inflammatory bowel disease. Oncol Rep. 2007;18(3):691-4.

[40] Kukitsu T, Takayama T, Miyanishi K, Nobuoka A, Katsuki S, Sato Y, Takimoto R, Matsunaga T, Kato J, Sonoda T, Sakamaki S, Niitsu Y. Aberrant crypt foci as precursors of the dysplasia-carcinoma sequence in patients with ulcerative colitis. Clin Cancer Res. 2008;14(1):48-54.

[41] Aust DE, Terdiman JP, Willenbucher RF, Chang CG, Molinaro-Clark A, Baretton GB, Loehrs U, Waldman FM. The APC/beta-catenin pathway in ulcerative colitis-related colorectal carcinomas: a mutational analysis. Cancer. 2002;94(5):1421-7.

[42] Fichera A, Little N, Dougherty U, Mustafi R, Cerda S, Li YC, Delgado J, Arora A, Campbell LK, Joseph L, Hart J, Noffsinger A, Bissonnette M. A vitamin D analogue inhibits colonic carcinogenesis in the AOM/DSS model. J Surg Res. 2007;142(2):239-45.

[43] Kikuchi H, Murakami S, Suzuki S, Kudo H, Sassa S, Sakamoto S. Chemopreventive effect of a vitamin D(3) analog, alfacalcidol, on colorectal carcinogenesis in mice with ulcerative colitis. Anticancer Drugs. 2007;18(10):1183-7.

[44] Wada K, Tanaka H, Maeda K, Inoue T, Noda E, Amano R, Kubo N, Muguruma K, Yamada N, Yashiro M, Sawada T, Nakata B, Ohira M, Hirakawa K. Vitamin D receptor expression is associated with colon cancer in ulcerative colitis. Oncol Rep. 2009;22(5):1021-5.

[45] Mantovani A. Molecular pathways linking inflammation and cancer. Curr Mol Med. 2010;10(4):369-73.

[46] Greten FR, Eckmann L, Greten TF, Park JM, Li ZW, Egan LJ, Kagnoff MF, Karin M. IKKbeta links inflammation and tumorigenesis in a mouse model of colitis-associated cancer. Cell. 2004;118(3):285-96.

[47] Clevers H. At the crossroads of inflammation and cancer. Cell. 2004;118(6):671-4.

[48] Fukata M, Chen A, Vamadevan AS, Cohen J, Breglio K, Krishnareddy S, Hsu D, Xu R, Harpaz N, Dannenberg AJ, Subbaramaiah K, Cooper HS, Itzkowitz SH, Abreu MT. Toll-like receptor-4 promotes the development of colitis-associated colorectal tumors. Gastroenterology. 2007;133(6):1869-81.

[49] Dougherty U, Cerasi D, Taylor I, Kocherginsky M, Tekin U, Badal S, Aluri L, Sehdev A, Cerda S, Mustafi R, Delgado J, Joseph L, Zhu H, Hart J, Threadgill D, Fichera A, Bissonnette M. Epidermal growth factor receptor is required for colonic tumor promotion by dietary fat in the azoxymethane/dextran sulfate sodium model: roles of transforming growth factor-{alpha} and PTGS2. Clin Cancer Res. 2009;15(22):6780-9.

[50] Choi PM, Nugent FW, Schoetz DJ, Jr., Silverman ML, Haggitt RC. Colonoscopic surveillance reduces mortality from colorectal cancer in ulcerative colitis. Gastroenterology. 1993;105(2):418-24.

[51] Lashner BA, Kane SV, Hanauer SB. Colon cancer surveillance in chronic ulcerative colitis: historical cohort study. Am J Gastroenterol. 1990;85(9):1083-7.

[52] Karlen P, Kornfeld D, Brostrom O, Lofberg R, Persson PG, Ekbom A. Is colonoscopic surveillance reducing colorectal cancer mortality in ulcerative colitis? A population based case control study. Gut. 1998;42(5):711-4.

[53] Collins PD, Mpofu C, Watson AJ, Rhodes JM. Strategies for detecting colon cancer and/or dysplasia in patients with inflammatory bowel disease. Cochrane Database Syst Rev. 2006(2):CD000279.

[54] Rubin CE, Haggitt RC, Burmer GC, Brentnall TA, Stevens AC, Levine DS, Dean PJ, Kimmey M, Perera DR, Rabinovitch PS. DNA aneuploidy in colonic biopsies predicts future development of dysplasia in ulcerative colitis. Gastroenterology. 1992;103(5):1611-20.

[55] Bernstein CN, Weinstein WM, Levine DS, Shanahan F. Physicians' perceptions of dysplasia and approaches to surveillance colonoscopy in ulcerative colitis. Am J Gastroenterol. 1995;90(12):2106-14.

[56] Blonski W, Kundu R, Lewis J, Aberra F, Osterman M, Lichtenstein GR. Is dysplasia visible during surveillance colonoscopy in patients with ulcerative colitis? Scand J Gastroenterol. 2008;43(6):698-703.

[57] Kiesslich R, Fritsch J, Holtmann M, Koehler HH, Stolte M, Kanzler S, Nafe B, Jung M, Galle PR, Neurath MF. Methylene blue-aided chromoendoscopy for the detection of intraepithelial neoplasia and colon cancer in ulcerative colitis. Gastroenterology. 2003;124(4):880-8.

[58] Kiesslich R, Goetz M, Lammersdorf K, Schneider C, Burg J, Stolte M, Vieth M, Nafe B, Galle PR, Neurath MF. Chromoscopy-guided endomicroscopy increases the diagnostic yield of intraepithelial neoplasia in ulcerative colitis. Gastroenterology. 2007;132(3):874-82.

[59] Marion JF, Waye JD, Present DH, Israel Y, Bodian C, Harpaz N, Chapman M, Itzkowitz S, Steinlauf AF, Abreu MT, Ullman TA, Aisenberg J, Mayer L, Chromoendoscopy Study Group at Mount Sinai School of M. Chromoendoscopy-targeted biopsies are superior to standard colonoscopic surveillance for detecting dysplasia in inflammatory bowel disease patients: a prospective endoscopic trial. Am J Gastroenterol. 2008;103(9):2342-9.

[60] Hurlstone DP, Sanders DS, Lobo AJ, McAlindon ME, Cross SS. Indigo carmine-assisted high-magnification chromoscopic colonoscopy for the detection and characterisation of intraepithelial neoplasia in ulcerative colitis: a prospective evaluation. Endoscopy. 2005;37(12):1186-92.

[61] Rutter MD, Saunders BP, Schofield G, Forbes A, Price AB, Talbot IC. Pancolonic indigo carmine dye spraying for the detection of dysplasia in ulcerative colitis. Gut. 2004;53(2):256-60.

[62] Subramanian V, Mannath J, Ragunath K, Hawkey CJ. Meta-analysis: the diagnostic yield of chromoendoscopy for detecting dysplasia in patients with colonic inflammatory bowel disease. Aliment Pharmacol Ther.33(3):304-12.

[63] van den Broek FJ, Fockens P, van Eeden S, Reitsma JB, Hardwick JC, Stokkers PC, Dekker E. Endoscopic tri-modal imaging for surveillance in ulcerative colitis: randomised comparison of high-resolution endoscopy and autofluorescence imaging for neoplasia detection; and evaluation of narrow-band imaging for classification of lesions. Gut. 2008;57(8):1083-9.

[64] Dekker E, van den Broek FJ, Reitsma JB, Hardwick JC, Offerhaus GJ, van Deventer SJ, Hommes DW, Fockens P. Narrow-band imaging compared with conventional colonoscopy for the detection of dysplasia in patients with longstanding ulcerative colitis. Endoscopy. 2007;39(3):216-21.

[65] van den Broek FJ, Fockens P, van Eeden S, Stokkers PC, Ponsioen CY, Reitsma JB, Dekker E. Narrow-band imaging versus high-definition endoscopy for the diagnosis of neoplasia in ulcerative colitis. Endoscopy. 2011;43(2):108-15.

[66] Carter MJ, Lobo AJ, Travis SP, Ibd Section BSoG. Guidelines for the management of inflammatory bowel disease in adults. Gut. 2004;53 Suppl 5:V1-16.

[67] Kornbluth A, Sachar DB. Ulcerative colitis practice guidelines in adults (update): American College of Gastroenterology, Practice Parameters Committee. Am J Gastroenterol. 2004;99(7):1371-85.

[68] Itzkowitz SH, Present DH, Crohn's, Colitis Foundation of America Colon Cancer in IBDSG. Consensus conference: Colorectal cancer screening and surveillance in inflammatory bowel disease. Inflamm Bowel Dis. 2005;11(3):314-21.

[69] Farraye FA, Odze RD, Eaden J, Itzkowitz SH, McCabe RP, Dassopoulos T, Lewis JD, Ullman TA, James T, 3rd, McLeod R, Burgart LJ, Allen J, Brill JV, Diagnosis AGAIMPPo, Management of Colorectal Neoplasia in Inflammatory Bowel D. AGA medical position statement on the diagnosis and management of colorectal neoplasia in inflammatory bowel disease. Gastroenterology. 2010;138(2):738-45.

[70] Bernstein CN, Shanahan F, Weinstein WM. Are we telling patients the truth about surveillance colonoscopy in ulcerative colitis? Lancet. 1994;343(8889):71-4.

[71] Blackstone MO, Riddell RH, Rogers BH, Levin B. Dysplasia-associated lesion or mass (DALM) detected by colonoscopy in long-standing ulcerative colitis: an indication for colectomy. Gastroenterology. 1981;80(2):366-74.

[72] Ullman T, Croog V, Harpaz N, Sachar D, Itzkowitz S. Progression of flat low-grade dysplasia to advanced neoplasia in patients with ulcerative colitis. Gastroenterology. 2003;125(5):1311-9.

[73] Jess T, Loftus EV, Jr., Velayos FS, Harmsen WS, Zinsmeister AR, Smyrk TC, Tremaine WJ, Melton LJ, 3rd, Munkholm P, Sandborn WJ. Incidence and prognosis of colorectal dysplasia in inflammatory bowel disease: a population-based study from Olmsted County, Minnesota. Inflamm Bowel Dis. 2006;12(8):669-76.

[74] Ullman TA, Loftus EV, Jr., Kakar S, Burgart LJ, Sandborn WJ, Tremaine WJ. The fate of low grade dysplasia in ulcerative colitis. Am J Gastroenterol. 2002;97(4):922-7.

[75] Connell WR, Lennard-Jones JE, Williams CB, Talbot IC, Price AB, Wilkinson KH. Factors affecting the outcome of endoscopic surveillance for cancer in ulcerative colitis. Gastroenterology. 1994;107(4):934-44.

[76] Lim CH, Dixon MF, Vail A, Forman D, Lynch DA, Axon AT. Ten year follow up of ulcerative colitis patients with and without low grade dysplasia. Gut. 2003;52(8):1127-32.

[77] Odze RD, Farraye FA, Hecht JL, Hornick JL. Long-term follow-up after polypectomy treatment for adenoma-like dysplastic lesions in ulcerative colitis. Clin Gastroenterol Hepatol. 2004;2(7):534-41.

[78] Pekow JR, Hetzel JT, Rothe JA, Hanauer SB, Turner JR, Hart J, Noffsinger A, Huo D, Rubin DT. Outcome after surveillance of low-grade and indefinite dysplasia in patients with ulcerative colitis. Inflamm Bowel Dis.16(8):1352-6.

[79] Engelsgjerd M, Farraye FA, Odze RD. Polypectomy may be adequate treatment for adenoma-like dysplastic lesions in chronic ulcerative colitis. Gastroenterology. 1999;117(6):1288-94; discussion 488-91.

[80] Scarpa M, van Koperen PJ, Ubbink DT, Hommes DW, Ten Kate FJ, Bemelman WA. Systematic review of dysplasia after restorative proctocolectomy for ulcerative colitis. Br J Surg. 2007;94(5):534-45.

[81] Kariv R, Remzi FH, Lian L, Bennett AE, Kiran RP, Kariv Y, Fazio VW, Lavery IC, Shen B. Preoperative colorectal neoplasia increases risk for pouch neoplasia in patients with restorative proctocolectomy. Gastroenterology. 2010;139(3):806-12, 12 e1-2.

[82] Al-Sukhni W, McLeod RS, MacRae H, O'Connor B, Huang H, Cohen Z. Oncologic outcome in patients with ulcerative colitis associated with dysplasia or cancer who underwent stapled or handsewn ileal pouch-anal anastomosis. Dis Colon Rectum.53(11):1495-500.

[83] Kaiser GC, Yan F, Polk DB. Mesalamine blocks tumor necrosis factor growth inhibition and nuclear factor kappaB activation in mouse colonocytes. Gastroenterology. 1999;116(3):602-9.

[84] Reinacher-Schick A, Seidensticker F, Petrasch S, Reiser M, Philippou S, Theegarten D, Freitag G, Schmiegel W. Mesalazine changes apoptosis and proliferation in normal mucosa of patients with sporadic polyps of the large bowel. Endoscopy. 2000;32(3):245-54.

[85] Allgayer H, Kolb M, Stuber V, Kruis W. Modulation of base hydroxylation by bile acids and salicylates in a model of human colonic mucosal DNA: putative implications in colonic cancer. Dig Dis Sci. 1999;44(4):761-7.

[86] Velayos FS, Terdiman JP, Walsh JM. Effect of 5-aminosalicylate use on colorectal cancer and dysplasia risk: a systematic review and metaanalysis of observational studies. Am J Gastroenterol. 2005;100(6):1345-53.

[87] Terdiman JP, Steinbuch M, Blumentals WA, Ullman TA, Rubin DT. 5-Aminosalicylic acid therapy and the risk of colorectal cancer among patients with inflammatory bowel disease. Inflamm Bowel Dis. 2007;13(4):367-71.

[88] Jess T, Loftus EV, Jr., Velayos FS, Winther KV, Tremaine WJ, Zinsmeister AR, Scott Harmsen W, Langholz E, Binder V, Munkholm P, Sandborn WJ. Risk factors for colorectal neoplasia in inflammatory bowel disease: a nested case-control study from Copenhagen county, Denmark and Olmsted county, Minnesota. Am J Gastroenterol. 2007;102(4):829-36.

[89] Bernstein CN, Nugent Z, Blanchard JF. 5-aminosalicylate is not chemoprophylactic for colorectal cancer in IBD: a population based study. Am J Gastroenterol. 2011;106(4):731-6.

[90] Ullman T, Croog V, Harpaz N, Hossain S, Kornbluth A, Bodian C, Itzkowitz S. Progression to colorectal neoplasia in ulcerative colitis: effect of mesalamine. Clin Gastroenterol Hepatol. 2008;6(11):1225-30; quiz 177.

[91] Earnest DL, Holubec H, Wali RK, Jolley CS, Bissonette M, Bhattacharyya AK, Roy H, Khare S, Brasitus TA. Chemoprevention of azoxymethane-induced colonic carcinogenesis by supplemental dietary ursodeoxycholic acid. Cancer Res. 1994;54(19):5071-4.

[92] Wali RK, Frawley BP, Jr., Hartmann S, Roy HK, Khare S, Scaglione-Sewell BA, Earnest DL, Sitrin MD, Brasitus TA, Bissonnette M. Mechanism of action of chemoprotective ursodeoxycholate in the azoxymethane model of rat colonic carcinogenesis: potential roles of protein kinase C-alpha, -beta II, and -zeta. Cancer Res. 1995;55(22):5257-64.

[93] Khare S, Mustafi R, Cerda S, Yuan W, Jagadeeswaran S, Dougherty U, Tretiakova M, Samarel A, Cohen G, Wang J, Moore C, Wali R, Holgren C, Joseph L, Fichera A, Li YC, Bissonnette M. Ursodeoxycholic acid suppresses Cox-2 expression in colon cancer: roles of Ras, p38, and CCAAT/enhancer-binding protein. Nutr Cancer. 2008;60(3):389-400.

[94] Batta AK, Salen G, Holubec H, Brasitus TA, Alberts D, Earnest DL. Enrichment of the more hydrophilic bile acid ursodeoxycholic acid in the fecal water-soluble fraction after feeding to rats with colon polyps. Cancer Res. 1998;58(8):1684-7.

[95] Tung BY, Emond MJ, Haggitt RC, Bronner MP, Kimmey MB, Kowdley KV, Brentnall TA. Ursodiol use is associated with lower prevalence of colonic neoplasia in

patients with ulcerative colitis and primary sclerosing cholangitis. Ann Intern Med. 2001;134(2):89-95.

[96] Wolf JM, Rybicki LA, Lashner BA. The impact of ursodeoxycholic acid on cancer, dysplasia and mortality in ulcerative colitis patients with primary sclerosing cholangitis. Aliment Pharmacol Ther. 2005;22(9):783-8.

[97] Khare S, Cerda S, Wali RK, von Lintig FC, Tretiakova M, Joseph L, Stoiber D, Cohen G, Nimmagadda K, Hart J, Sitrin MD, Boss GR, Bissonnette M. Ursodeoxycholic acid inhibits Ras mutations, wild-type Ras activation, and cyclooxygenase-2 expression in colon cancer. Cancer Res. 2003;63(13):3517-23.

[98] Eaton JE, Silveira MG, Pardi DS, Sinakos E, Kowdley KV, Luketic VA, Harrison ME, McCashland T, Befeler AS, Harnois D, Jorgensen R, Petz J, Lindor KD. High-Dose Ursodeoxycholic Acid Is Associated With the Development of Colorectal Neoplasia in Patients With Ulcerative Colitis and Primary Sclerosing Cholangitis. Am J Gastroenterol. 2011. epub ahead of print.

[99] Chapman R, Fevery J, Kalloo A, Nagorney DM, Boberg KM, Shneider B, Gores GJ, American Association for the Study of Liver D. Diagnosis and management of primary sclerosing cholangitis. Hepatology.51(2):660-78.

[100] van Schaik FD, van Oijen MG, Smeets HM, van der Heijden GJ, Siersema PD, Oldenburg B. Thiopurines prevent advanced colorectal neoplasia in patients with inflammatory bowel disease. Gut. 2011.epub ahead of print.

[101] Matula S, Croog V, Itzkowitz S, Harpaz N, Bodian C, Hossain S, Ullman T. Chemoprevention of colorectal neoplasia in ulcerative colitis: the effect of 6-mercaptopurine. Clin Gastroenterol Hepatol. 2005;3(10):1015-21.

[102] Heimburger DC, Alexander CB, Birch R, Butterworth CE, Jr., Bailey WC, Krumdieck CL. Improvement in bronchial squamous metaplasia in smokers treated with folate and vitamin B12. Report of a preliminary randomized, double-blind intervention trial. JAMA. 1988;259(10):1525-30.

[103] Freudenheim JL, Graham S, Marshall JR, Haughey BP, Cholewinski S, Wilkinson G. Folate intake and carcinogenesis of the colon and rectum. Int J Epidemiol. 1991;20(2):368-74.

[104] Butterworth CE, Jr., Hatch KD, Gore H, Mueller H, Krumdieck CL. Improvement in cervical dysplasia associated with folic acid therapy in users of oral contraceptives. Am J Clin Nutr. 1982;35(1):73-82.

[105] Lashner BA, Heidenreich PA, Su GL, Kane SV, Hanauer SB. Effect of folate supplementation on the incidence of dysplasia and cancer in chronic ulcerative colitis. A case-control study. Gastroenterology. 1989;97(2):255-9.

[106] Lashner BA, Provencher KS, Seidner DL, Knesebeck A, Brzezinski A. The effect of folic acid supplementation on the risk for cancer or dysplasia in ulcerative colitis. Gastroenterology. 1997;112(1):29-32.

[107] Wali RK, Bissonnette M, Khare S, Hart J, Sitrin MD, Brasitus TA. 1 alpha,25-Dihydroxy-16-ene-23-yne-26,27-hexafluorocholecalciferol, a noncalcemic analogue of 1 alpha,25-dihydroxyvitamin D3, inhibits azoxymethane-induced colonic tumorigenesis. Cancer Res. 1995;55(14):3050-4.

[108] Gorham ED, Garland CF, Garland FC, Grant WB, Mohr SB, Lipkin M, Newmark HL, Giovannucci E, Wei M, Holick MF. Optimal vitamin D status for colorectal cancer prevention: a quantitative meta analysis. Am J Prev Med. 2007;32(3):210-6.

14

Ulcerative Colitis and Lung

Nilgün Yılmaz Demirci

Ataturk Chest Disease and Chest Surgery Training and Research Hospital,
Pulmonary Medicine Department, Ankara
Turkey

1. Introduction

Inflammatory bowel disease (IBD) refers to a group of conditions characterised by inflammation in the intestinal tract. Crohn disease (CD) and ulcerative colitis (UC) account for the majority of these conditions. Since these disorders have both distinct and overlapping pathologic and clinical characteristics in this part both diseases are discussed together.

Multiple studies have evaluated the epidemiology of IBD in various geographic regions. In North America, incidence rates range from 2.2 to 14.3 cases per 100,000 person-years for UC and 3.1 to 14.6 cases per 100,000 person-year for CD ([1]). Prevalence rates range from 37 to 246 per 100,000 persons for UC and from 26 to 201 cases per 100,000 for CD. The incidence and prevalence of CD and UC appear to be lower in Asia, Japan, and South America ([2]). IBD can present at any age, although the peak incidence occurs between the ages of 15 and 30 years. A second peak in the incidence of CD occurs between the ages of 50 to 80. There is no gender specificity ([3, 4]).

While numerous environmental factors have been hypothesized to affect risk of a phenotype of IBD, only a few associations have been reproducible and implicated in the pathogenesis of IBD. These factors as smoking, appendectomy, infection, oral contraceptives, isotretinoin are more likely to contribute to disease in susceptible subjects ([2]).

The strongest evidence for an environmental factor has been the association between cigarette smoking and IBD. Several studies have demonstrated a negative correlation between smoking and UC, but a positive correlation between smoking and CD recurrence ([5, 6, 7, 8, 9, 10]).

A variety of conditions arise outside of the gastrointestinal tract that are associated with IBD; these are termed extraintestinal manifestations of IBD which are very common: dermatological manifestations, erythema nodosum and pyoderma gangrenosum; ocular manifestations, uveitis and episcleritis; hepatobiliary manifestations, primary sclerosing cholangitis and autoimmune hepatitis; musculoskeletal manifestations, peripheral arthritis and axial arthropathy. In contrast, pulmonary involvement is rare ([11]).

Involvement of the respiratory tract, although relatively rare, is increasingly recognized in patients with IBD since the original report in 1976 of six patients with unexplained chronic purulent sputum production ([12]). These abnormalities are generally related to the underlying bowel disease, although interstitial lung disease can also be induced by administration of certain drugs, including sulfasalazine, 5-aminosalicylic acid, methotrexate, azathioprine and infliximab ([13, 14, 15, 16, 17]).

2. Demographic considerations

Respiratory complications have been more commonly described with ulcerative colitis than with Crohn's disease. In one study of 33 patients, for example, 27 had ulcerative colitis and six had Crohn's disease. The three patterns of presentation (airway disease, parenchymal disease, and serositis) had somewhat different characteristics in terms of sex preponderance and activity of the bowel disease ([12]). There was a female preponderance of almost 2:1 for all bronchopulmonary complications as a whole and 3 to 4:1 for bronchial complications. In contrast, serositis occurred with roughly equal frequency in men and women.

Bronchopulmonary complications followed the onset of inflammatory bowel disease in 80 to 85 percent of patients, preceded bowel disease in 10 to 15 percent, and developed concomitantly in 5 to 10 percent ([12]).

Respiratory involvement in IBD is disclosed with some pathophysiological mechanisms: both the colonic and respiratory epithelia share embryonic origin from the primitive foregut, and both types of epithelial cells include goblet cells and submucosal glands; and the lungs and gastrointestinal tract contain submucosal lymphoid tissue and play crucial roles in host mucosal defense. The similarity in the mucosal immune system causes the same pathogenetic changes. The aberrations in both innate and acquired immunity that are involved in the pathogenesis of IBD are complex and still incompletely understood ([11, 17]). In this context it has been speculated that colonic surgery may promote the onset of respirtory, as suggested by case histories ([12]).

The patterns of involvement in IBD are ([11, 17]):
- Upper airway: glottic/subglottic stenosis, tracheal inflammation and stenosis;
- Bronchi: chronic bronchitis, bronchiectasis, and chronic bronchial suppuration;
- Small airways: bronchiolitis obliterans, bronchiolitis, and diffuse pan-bronchiolitis;
- Lung parenchyma: bronchiolitis obliterans-organizing pneumonia, nonspecific interstitial pneumonia, granulomatous interstitial lung disease, desquamative interstitial pneumonitis, pulmonary infiltrates and eosinophilia, and sterile necrobiotic nodules;
- Sarcoidosis, α1 antitrypsin deficiency;
- Pulmonary vascular disease; Wegener's granulomatosis, Churg-Strauss syndrome, microscopic polyangiitis, and pulmonary vasculitis, venous thromboembolism; and - Serositis: pleural and pericardial manifestations.

3. Respiratory symptoms

The prevalence of respiratory symptoms in IBD patients without pulmonary pathology has been examined in a number of small studies. Among 44 randomly selected IBD patients, Douglas et al ([18]) found that 48% had unspecified respiratory symptoms. Songur et al ([19]) found that 16 of 36 IBD patients (44%) in a gastroenterology clinic had symptoms of wheeze, cough, sputum production, or breathlessness. Finally, Ceyhan and others ([20]) found 15 of 30 consecutively surveyed IBD patients had symptoms of dyspnea, cough, sputum, or wheeze for > 1 month. These investigations, while limited in scope, suggest that patients with IBD have pulmonary symptoms with greater frequency than the general population.

4. Radiologic findings

Chest radiography is often normal in patients with respiratory symptoms and IBD. Bronchiectasis is the classic pulmonary manifestation of IBD, and is noted in 66% of cases of IBD that involve the large airways (Figure 1)([17]).

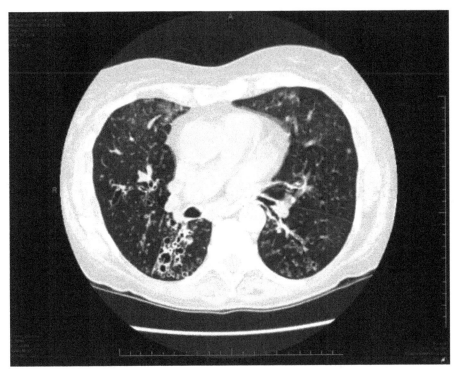

Fig. 1. CT showing bronchiectasis and inflammatory nodules in a 72-year-old woman with UC ([17])

Mahadeva et al ([21]) have found bronchiectasis in 13 of 17 patients with IBD, in whom sputum production was present in 10. In contrast, bronchiectasis was identified in only two patients in the present study. In the study of Yilmaz et al, the most frequent finding on HRCT was peribronchial thickness. The most common respiratory association of IBD is inflammation of the airways. Biopsy shows either severe nonspecific chronic inflammation or non-caseating tuberculoid granulomas. They concluded that these appearances have been associated with those in the bowel, and it is possible that the gut and the lung are both affected because they share common antigens. This inflammation is perceived on HRCT as an increase in bronchial wall thickness or an increase in diameter of pulmonary artery branches. In these patients, bronchial dilatation is commonly present and results from traction by fibrous tissue on the bronchial walls and results in bronchiectasis. Consequently, they suggested that peribronchial thickness might reflect inflammation, which usually responds well to steroids. They concluded that in this way, bronchiectasis can be prevented. And so this finding suggests a direct pathogenic link to IBD as well ([11]).

5. Pulmonary function

A number of investigations have focused on results of pulmonary function testing (PFT) among patients with IBD. Case-control studies designed to investigate the hypothesis that IBD is associated with abnormal pulmonary function have been limited by low numbers of patients and poor choice of control subjects. A number of reports have demonstrated a decrease in diffusion capacity of the lung for carbon monoxide (DLco). Two studies by Tzanakis et al ([22, 23]) have shown that DLco was significantly lower among IBD patients with active GI disease than those in remission. In the same study an increased prevalence of small airway dysfunction among IBD patients have shown. Marvisi et al ([24]) reported a similar finding in a smaller cohort with UC. This suggests that degree of GI inflammation may correlate with the severity of lung disease in these patients.

Other reports have employed less conventional measures of airflow obstruction to identify subclinical pulmonary disease. Patients with active UC had increased airway obstruction compared with patients with inactive UC. Pasquis et al ([25]) found an increase in functional residual capacity among a small number of patients with CD. Two groups, Mansi and colleagues ([26]) and Louis et al ([27, 28]) have documented increased bronchial response to methacholine, a measure of airway hyperactivity, among patients with both UC and CD, but this was not confirmed in another study. Ceyhan et al revealed that the prevalence of allergic symptoms, positive skin tests, and functional abnormalities was significantly higher in patients with IBD. ([20]).

Nitric oxide (NO) is a mediator of inflammation in a number of pathological processes. It is elevated in exhaled air (eNO) from asthmatic patients compared with healthy volunteers, and also in aspirated colonic gas from patients with Crohn's disease. Koek et al studied 31 patients with Crohn's disease and 24 with ulcerative colitis. The authors found that eNO was elevated in active IBD, and in addition, observed a negative correlation between spirometry values and disease activity in patients with Crohn's disease ([29]). Ozyilmaz et al evaluated the value of fractional concentration of exhaled NO (FeNO) level for the diagnosis of pulmonary involvement due to IBD and to investigate any correlation between FeNO level and disease activity. They concluded that an increased FeNO level may be used for identifying patients with IBD who need further pulmonary evaluation ([30]) .

6. Patterns of involvement

Upper airway: Glottic/subglottic stenosis, tracheal inflammation and stenosis; are associated with inflammation, friability, and pseudotumors in the trachea which results in airway narrowing. The primary symptoms are cough and hoarseness, although some patients develop upper airway obstruction with resulting stridor and severe dyspnea ([20]). In endoscopic examination glottic/subglottic oedema, inflammation can be seen.

Airway inflammation: Chronic bronchitis, bronchiectasis, and chronic bronchial suppuration; inflammation of the trachea, bronchi, and bronchioles can occur in inflammatory bowel disease, with bronchial involvement being most common, accounting for 39% of all cases reviewed ([12, 31, 32, 33]). Patients with large airways disease may also have coincident nonthoracic extraintestinal manifestations, including microangiopathic hemolytic anemia, pyoderma gangrenosum, primary sclerosing cholangitis, episcleritis, and peripheral and axial arthritis. Bronchial involvement may be manifested as unexplained chronic bronchitis or as bronchiectasis. Bronchiectasis is the classic pulmonary manifestation of IBD, noted in 66% of instances of IBD involving the large airways ([17]). Patients can be asymptomatic or present with cough and variable amounts of mucopurulent sputum production. Cultures of bronchial secretions are typically unrevealing, and the symptoms are generally not responsive to antibiotics. Chest radiographs are frequently normal or show nonspecific changes resulting from bronchial wall thickening or bronchiectasis. High resolution chest CT scanning is more sensitive than plain chest radiographs, often demonstrating findings of bronchial wall thickening, dilated airways with thickened walls, or branched opacities suggestive of mucoid impaction ([34, 35]).

Interestingly, nine patients, mostly with UC, presented with or had a recrudescence of bronchiectasis within 1 year of colectomy. In one case, bronchiectasis presented within weeks of colectomy. This temporal link between colonic resection and onset or worsening of pulmonary disease has fueled speculation that colectomy may actually induce pulmonary disease in these patients ([12]). Alternatively, this phenomenon may be related to the discontinuation of immunosuppressive therapies after presumed surgical cure of the disease ([17]).

Small airway involvement: Bronchiolitis obliterans, bronchiolitis, and diffuse pan-bronchiolitis; can cause cough, variable sputum production, wheezing, and airflow obstruction. Small airway involvement in IBD tends to present at a younger age and at an earlier point in the disease course than abnormalities of the large airways. In contrast to other airway manifestations, diseases of the small airways more commonly occur before symptomatic GI disease (29% of surveyed cases) ([17]). Pathologic findings include nonspecific inflammation, narrowing, and fibrosis of small airways; granulomatous bronchiolitis (58.8%) has also been reported ([15, 36]). Small airway involvement can cause abnormalities in pulmonary function in patients with normal chest radiographs. In one series of 82 patients with IBD and normal plain chest radiographs, 47 (57 percent) had abnormal findings on complete pulmonary function tests ([16]). Most of these patients had findings consistent with restrictive lung disease. High resolution chest CT can demonstrate mosaic perfusion or tree-in-bud ([12]).

Pulmonary parenchymal disease: Bronchiolitis obliterans-organizing pneumonia(BOOP), nonspecific interstitial pneumonia, granulomatous interstitial lung disease, desquamative interstitial pneumonitis, pulmonary infiltrates and eosinophilia, and sterile necrobiotic nodules.

Several patterns of lung parenchymal involvement have now been described in inflammatory bowel disease, with bronchiolitis obliterans with organizing pneumonia and interstitial lung disease being most common ([12, 13]). UC is the underlying form of IBD in the majority of reported cases of IBD-associated parenchymal lung disease. Age of onset varies, and there is a slight female predominance. One study of 85 patients with ulcerative colitis and 47 patients with Crohn's disease found that diffusing capacity was significantly lower during exacerbations of bowel disease than when gastrointestinal disease was quiescent ([22]). No pulmonary symptoms were associated with these transient physiologic derangements. These results have been confirmed in other reports, suggesting that pulmonary inflammation commonly accompanies inflammation of the bowel ([24]).

BOOP presents in an acute or subacute fashion with variable combinations of fever, dyspnea, cough, and pleuritic chest pain ([12]). Chest radiographic findings range from patchy focal opacities to diffuse infiltrates, while CT scanning often demonstrates the opacities to be pleural-based and sometimes associated with air bronchograms (Figure 2) ([21]).

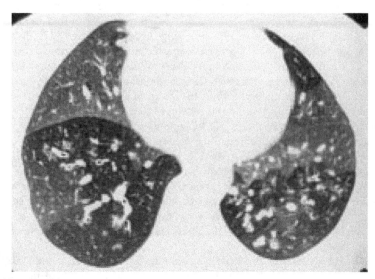

Fig. 2. High resolution computed tomography. On expiration, there is evidence of extensive air trapping in keeping with obliterative bronchiolitis ([21])

Sarcoidosis: IBD and sarcoidosis are usually considered to be distinct entities. However, the cumulative volume of case reports documenting coexistence of these two entities suggests a link between them. Fifty-three cases of IBD and concomitant sarcoidosis have been reported in the literature ([17]). The pathophysiologic basis of a relationship between IBD and sarcoidosis is unclear. Genetic susceptibility and derangements of cellular immunity play important roles in the development of both. Barr et al reported that human leukocyte antigen (HLA)-B8 and HLA-DR3 haplotypes were present in three of eight patients with UC and sarcoidosis, a higher proportion than expected ([37]). Papadopoulos et al reported a greater incidence of a variety of autoimmune diseases in patients with sarcoidosis, and suggested that HLA-linked genetic susceptibility (HLA-B8/DR3) predisposes sarcoidosis patients to a variety of autoimmune diseases ([38]). Finally, IBD and sarcoidosis share comparable dermatologic, ocular, and joint manifestations, further suggesting a pathogenic link. Nontuberculous Mycobacterium species have been postulated as an infectious cause of, and have been detected in tissues from patients with, both IBD and sarcoid ([39]). Elevated CD4:CD8 ratios on BAL, a characteristic but not diagnostic finding in sarcoidosis, have also been documented in patients with CD ([40, 41]).

α_1 - **antitrypsin deficiency:** α_1 - antitrypsin deficiency can lead to the development of pulmonary emphysema and hepatic dysfunction. In a study 10 patients, 7 with emphysema, who had concomitant α_1- antitrypsin deficiency and IBD have identified. Combined with the complex effects of smoking on the prevalence and course of UC and CD, this observation has lead the authors to propose that, as in the lung, imbalances in neutrophil elastase regulation exhibited in α_1-antitrypsin deficiency may enhance potential local tissue damage in the gastroenterological tract from smoking ([42]).

Intestinal manifestations of a pulmonary vasculitis such asWegener granulomatosis, Churg-Strauss syndrome, microscopic polyangiitis, and pulmonary vasculitis have been reported. Bloody diarrhea, abdominal pain, and intestinal perforation have been described in these patients. The symptoms can mimic IBD and make diagnosis difficult without biopsy ([15]).

Pulmonary infiltrates with eosinophilia (PIE syndrome); is a recognized complication of sulfasalazine, which is commonly used in the therapy of ulcerative colitis. There are also case reports of eosinophilic pneumonia in association with mesalamine therapy. However, this syndrome can occur in patients with inflammatory bowel disease who have no history of sulfasalazine use. Eosinophilia is frequently present in the peripheral blood, and chest radiographs often show peripheral infiltrates typical of chronic eosinophilic pneumonia ([2]).

Necrobiotic nodules resemble radiographically the cavitating nodules that can be seen with either septic pulmonary emboli or Wegener's granulomatosis . Histologically, the nodules are composed of sterile aggregates of neutrophils with necrosis, findings that are similar to those of pyoderma gangrenosum, a cutaneous complication of inflammatory bowel disease ([43]).

Serositis: As a complication of inflammatory bowel disease, serositis involving intrathoracic structures has occurred in the form of pleural effusions, pericarditis, pleuropericarditis, and myopericarditis ([12]). The serosal fluid is exudative, with a cellular content generally composed primarily of neutrophils. In a single case in which pleural biopsy was reported, nonspecific inflammation without granulomas was found. The pericardium is uniquely involved in 45% of cases ([44]).

Pulmonary embolism: Venous thromboembolism (VTE) represents a relevant cause of morbidity and mortality among patients with IBD. Compared to non-IBD subjects, patients with IBD are at a 3- to 4-fold increased risk of VTE and are affected by VTE at a younger age ([45, 46, 47]). The majority of thromboembolic events among IBD patients are VTE, manifested as either deep venous thrombosis or pulmonary embolism, but arterial thromboembolism and venous thrombosis at unusual sites have also been reported ([48]). The pathogenesis of increased thrombotic risk among patients with IBD is unclear. The prevalence of inherited prothrombotic disorders is no higher among patients with IBD than in the general population. While laboratory markers of activation of the coagulation system have been found in some patients with IBD, the significance of this finding is unclear. IBD patients often have acquired thrombosis risk factors in conjunction with their disease or its treatment, including immobility, surgery, and central venous catheters. However, up to one third of thrombotic events among IBD patients occur while their disease is quiescent, suggesting ongoing thrombotic risk unrelated to disease activity or therapy ([49, 50, 51]). Active disease, fistulas, and abscesses are present in the majority of IBD patients at the time of the thromboembolic event. Furthermore, IBD patients are more often exposed to disease-related risk factors that may provoke VTE, including surgery, immobilization, dehydration, and central venous catheters ([47, 48, 52]). Patients who present with the acute development of unexplained pulmonary symptoms, tachycardia, lower extremity swelling, and/or hypoxemia should be assessed for possible pulmonary embolism ([17]).

Drug-induced Complications: Patients with inflammatory bowel disease are often treated with sulfasalazine and 5-aminosalicylic acid (5-ASA), both of which can cause pulmonary disease ([14, 53, 54]). Methotrexate, infliximab, and azathioprine / 6-mercaptopurine are also used in selected patients, and can induce pulmonary toxicity.

Sulfasalazine: Pneumonitis, commonly seen in conjunction with fever and rash, is a recognized complication of sulfasalazine therapy. Nearly one-half of affected patients present with the clinical syndrome of pulmonary infiltrates with eosinophilia. The infiltrates are commonly in upper lobe (Figure 3) ([53]).

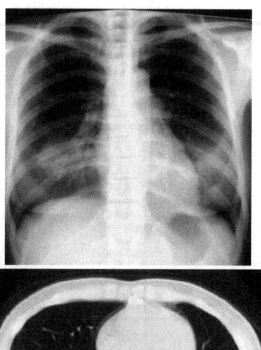

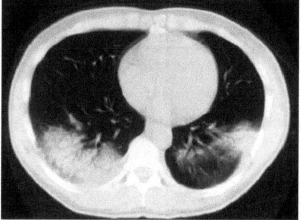

Fig. 3. Chest radiograph and computed tomography of the patient showing bilaterally interstitial infiltrates with air-bronchogram in both lower lung fields ([53])

Other pulmonary disorders have also been associated with sulphasalazine, including interstitial lung disease, bronchiolitis obliterans with organizing pneumonia, granulomatous lung disease, and rarely pleural effusion ([12, 55]).

Most reactions related to sulfasalazine or mesalamine are seen between 2-6 months of drug administration. The most common symptoms are dyspnea (76%), fever (68%), chest pain (65%) and cough (22%). Peripheral eosinophilia is found in almost half of the reported cases, diffusion capacity was decreased in a large percentage of patients and most had bilateral infiltrates or opacities on chest radiograph ([15]). A pulmonary picture consistent with Wegener's granulomatosis has also been attributed to sulfasalazine ([56]).

In general, patients with sulphasalazine-induced pulmonary disease improve with drug-withdrawal; in one analysis, two of three patients who continued on the drug died ([52]).

5-aminosalicylic acid: Pulmonary toxicity attributable to 5-aminosalicylic acid (5-ASA or mesalamine) is less common than with sulfasalazine. Some affected patients have diffuse or basilar infiltrates, sometimes with eosinophilia or may develop bronchiolitis obliterans ([53]).

Methotrexate: Methotrexate is an analogue of the vitamin folic acid and inhibits cellular proliferation by inducing an acute intracellular deficiency of certain folate coenzymes. Serious toxicity may affect the lungs, liver, and bone marrow. Methotrexate can cause pneumonitis that can become life threatening. Symptoms typically include progressive shortness of breath, cough, and fever. Hypoxemia and tachypnea are always present, and chest radiograph often reveals a diffuse interstitial or mixed interstitial and alveolar infiltrate, commonly in the lower lung fields. Pulmonary function tests show a restrictive pattern with diffusion abnormalities ([15]).

Azathioprine and 6-mercaptopurine: Immunomodulatory drugs, such as azathioprine (AZA) and 6-mercaptopurine (6-MP) can potentiate the therapeutic effect of glucocorticoids and exert a glucocorticoid-sparing effect in patients with glucocorticoid-dependent ulcerative colitis. Drug-induced hypersensitivity pneumonitis is a rare but potentially serious complication of therapy with these agents. Other pathologic patterns, such as usual interstitial pneumonia and bronchiolitis obliterans with organizing pneumonia, have rarely been reported in patients with inflammatory bowel disease treated with AZA or 6-MP ([57]).

Infliximab: Infliximab, an inhibitor of tumor necrosis factor-alpha, is used in selected patients with Crohn's disease, particularly those with fistulizing disease. Infectious complications from use of infliximab are well-described, most notably in the development of tuberculosis ([58]). There are also case reports of interstitial pneumonitis developing in patients with rheumatoid arthritis and Crohn's disease treated with infliximab (Figure 4) ([59]).

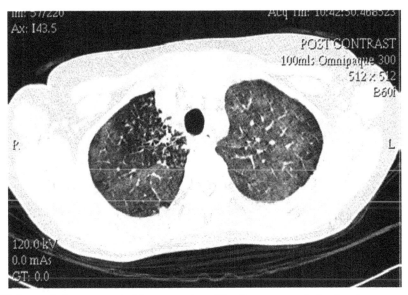

Fig. 4. High-resolution computed tomography of the thorax revealed extensive ground glass shadowing with right apical peribronchial consolidation ([59])

7. Diagnosis and treatment

The first step in determining appropriate therapy is to consider the possible role of drug-induced disease and the possibility of superimposed bacterial infection. When patients with inflammatory bowel disease who are treated with sulfasalazine or 5-ASA develop pulmonary infiltrates with eosinophilia, it is reasonable to assume initially that drug-induced disease is present and to discontinue the drug ([12]). The possible role of drug toxicity is less clear with other clinical presentations of parenchymal lung disease, such as interstitial disease or bronchiolitis obliterans with organizing pneumonia. In this setting, any decision concerning cessation of drug therapy should consider the relative severity of the pulmonary disease and the inflammatory bowel disease, which could flare if the drug is withdrawn. Possible superimposed bacterial or mycobacterial infection should be excluded in patients with fever, cough, or purulent sputum production. Appropriate antimicrobial therapy should be given if infection is found. Prophylaxis against venous thromboembolism (VTE) should be considered in hospitalized patients without evidence of gastrointestinal bleeding or other contraindications, since the risk of VTE may be increased in patients with inflammatory bowel disease ([47, 49, 52,60, 61]).

Antiinflammatory drugs: For those patients in whom neither drug therapy nor infection seems to be playing a role, inhaled or systemic glucocorticoids may be effective, depending upon the type of pulmonary complication. Inhaled glucocorticoid therapy, often in relatively high doses (eg, beclomethasone 1500-2000 mcg/day), is frequently effective in the various forms of airway inflammation. Large airway inflammation tends to be more responsive than bronchiolitis, presumably due to relatively poor delivery of the inhaled medication to the affected small airways. Patients with copious sputum production (greater than 50 mL/day) and those with bronchiectasis are also less likely to respond to inhaled glucocorticoids and may require oral glucocorticoids. Potentially life-threatening airway inflammation, as with subglottic involvement causing upper airway obstruction, may require intravenous glucocorticoids. The pulmonary parenchymal complications of inflammatory bowel disease require oral glucocorticoid therapy; we usually use prednisone at an initial dose of 0.5 to 1.0 mg/kg per day. Most patients have a good response to glucocorticoid therapy. The duration of treatment has not been well established, but is likely to be a number of months ([2]).

Serositis in the form of pleural effusions may need therapy if the effusions produce symptoms. Nonsteroidal antiinflammatory therapy should be tried initially, but glucocorticoids may be necessary if the patient does not respond. A single case of cardiac tamponade requiring pericardial drainage has been reported ([17]). There is insufficient evidence to support the use of infliximab or other agents directed against tumor necrosis factor in the management of pulmonary disease associated with IBD.

In conclusion, although most patients have subclinical disease, the pulmonologist must be aware of the multiple potential pulmonary manifestations that can occur in a patient with IBD. To get over this problem a complex work-up is needed (Table 1. Based on Storch Et al. [15]). Otherwise, they tend to generate persistent and annoying symptoms, and can lead to destructive and irreversible changes in the airway wall, or the "end-stage lung" ([12]).

Blood work
  Complete blood count with differential
  Comprehensive metabolic panel
  Antineutrophil cytoplasmic antibodies
  Angiotensin converting enzyme level
  Erythrocyte sedimentation rate
Radiographic
  Chest x-ray
  Computed tomography
Other
  Sputum culture/acid fast stain
  Purified Protein Derivative
  Kveim test
Advanced
  Pulmonary function testing
  Bronchoscopy with alveolar lavage
  Pulmonary biopsy
  Lower extremity Doppler
  Ventilation/perfusion scan
  Computed tomography — angiogram
  Hypercoagulability work-up

Table 1. Work-up of pulmonary disease in IBD

8. References

[1] Loftus EV Jr. Clinical epidemiology of inflammatory bowel disease: Incidence, prevalence, and environmental influences. Gastroenterology 2004; 126:1504.

[2] http://www.uptodate.com/contents/pulmonary-complications-of-inflammatory-bowel-disease (accessed June 2, 2011).

[3] Shivananda S, Lennard-Jones J, Logan R, et al. Incidence of inflammatory bowel disease across Europe: is there a difference between north and south? Results of the European Collaborative Study on Inflammatory Bowel Disease (EC-IBD). Gut 1996; 39:690.

[4] Trallori G, Palli D, Saieva C, et al. A population-based study of inflammatory bowel disease in Florence over 15 years (1978-92). Scand J Gastroenterol 1996; 31:892.

[5] Boyko EJ, Koepsell TD, Perera DR, Inui TS. Risk of ulcerative colitis among former and current cigarette smokers. N Engl J Med 1987; 316:707.

[6] Logan RF, Edmond M, Somerville KW, Langman MJ. Smoking and ulcerative colitis. Br Med J (Clin Res Ed) 1984; 288:751.

[7] Harries AD, Baird A, Rhodes J. Non-smoking: a feature of ulcerative colitis. Br Med J (Clin Res Ed) 1982; 284:706.

[8] Tobin MV, Logan RF, Langman MJ, et al. Cigarette smoking and inflammatory bowel disease. Gastroenterology 1987; 93:316.

[9] Vessey M, Jewell D, Smith A, et al. Chronic inflammatory bowel disease, cigarette smoking, and use of oral contraceptives: findings in a large cohort study of women of childbearing age. Br Med J (Clin Res Ed) 1986; 292:1101.

[10] Mahid SS, Minor KS, Soto RE, et al. Smoking and inflammatory bowel disease: a meta-analysis. Mayo Clin Proc 2006; 81:1462.

[11] Yilmaz A, Yilmaz Demirci N, Hoşgün D, Uner E, Erdoğan Y, Gökçek A, Cağlar A. Pulmonary involvement in inflammatory bowel disease. World J Gastroenterol. 2010 Oct 21; 16(39):4952-7.

[12] Camus P, Piard F, Ashcroft T, et al. The lung in inflammatory bowel disease. Medicine (Baltimore) 1993; 72:151.

[13] Casey MB, Tazelaar HD, Myers JL, et al. Noninfectious lung pathology in patients with Crohn's disease. Am J Surg Pathol 2003; 27: 213.

[14] Parry SD, Barbatzas C, Peel ET, Barton JR. Sulphasalazine and lung toxicity. Eur Respir J 2002; 19:756.

[15] Storch I, Sachar D, Katz S. Pulmonary manifestations of inflammatory bowel disease. Inflamm Bowel Dis 2003; 9:104-115.

[16] Kuzela L, Vavrecka A, Prikazska M, et al. Pulmonary complications in patients with inflammatory bowel disease. Hepatogastroenterology 1999; 46:1714.

[17] Black H, Mendoza M, Murin S. Thoracic manifestations of inflammatory bowel disease. Chest 2007; 131:524.

[18] Douglas JG, McDonald CF, Leslie MJ, et al. Respiratory impairment in inflammatory bowel disease: does it vary with disease activity? Respir Med 1989; 83:389-394.

[19] Songur N, Songur Y, Tuzun M, et al. Pulmonary function tests and high-resolution CT in the detection of pulmonary involvement in inflammatory bowel disease. J Clin Gastroenterol 2003; 37:292-298.

[20] Ceyhan BB, Karakurt S, Cevik H, et al. Bronchial hyperreactivity and allergic status in inflammatory bowel disease. Respiration 2003; 70:60-66.

[21] Mahadeva R, Walsh G, Flower CD, Shneerson JM. Clinical and radiological characteristics of lung disease in inflammatory bowel disease. Eur Respir J 2000; 15: 41-48.

[22] Tzanakis N, Bouros D, Samiou M, et al. Lung function in patients with inflammatory bowel disease. Respir Med 1998; 92: 516-522.

[23] Tzanakis N, Samiou M, Bouros D, et al. Small airways function in patients with inflammatory bowel disease. Am J Respir Crit Care Med 1998; 157:382-386.

[24] Marvisi M, Borrello PD, Brianti M, et al. Changes in the carbon monoxide diffusing capacity of the lung in ulcerative colitis. Eur Respir J 2000; 16:965-968.

[25] Pasquis P, Colin R, Denis P, et al. Transient pulmonary impairment during attacks of Crohn's disease. Respiration 1981; 41:56-59.

[26] Mansi A, Cucchiara S, Greco L, et al. Bronchial hyperresponsiveness in children and adolescents with Crohn's disease. Am J Respir Crit Care Med 2000; 161:1051-1054.

[27] Louis E, Louis R, Drion V, et al. Increased frequency of bronchial hyperresponsiveness in patients with inflammatory bowel disease. Allergy 1995; 50:729-733.

[28] Louis E, Louis R, Shute J, et al. Bronchial eosinophilic infiltration in Crohn's disease in the absence of pulmonary disease. Clin Exp Allergy 1999; 29:660-666.

[29] Koek GH, Verleden GM, Evenepoel P, Rutgeerts P. Activity related increase of exhaled nitric oxide in Crohn's disease and ulcerative colitis: a manifestation of systemic involvement? Respir Med. 2002; 96: 530-5.

[30] Ozyilmaz E, Yildirim B, Erbas G, Akten S, Oguzulgen IK, Tunc B, Tuncer C, Turktas H. Value of fractional exhaled nitric oxide (FE NO) for the diagnosis of pulmonary involvement due to inflammatory bowel disease. Inflamm Bowel Dis. 2010 Apr;16(4):670-6.

[31] Higenbottam T, Cochrane GM, Clark TJ, et al. Bronchial disease in ulcerative colitis . Thorax 1980; 35:581.

[32] Kuźniar T, Sleiman C, Brugière O, et al. Severe tracheobronchial stenosis in a patient with Crohn's disease. Eur Respir J 2000; 15:209.

[33] Mansi A, Cucchiara S, Greco L, et al. Bronchial hyperresponsiveness in children and adolescents with Crohn's disease. Am J Respir Crit Care Med 2000; 161:1051.

[34] Garg K, Lynch DA, Newell JD. Inflammatory airways disease in ulcerative colitis: CT and high-resolution CT features. J Thorac Imaging 1993; 8:159.

[35] Spira A, Grossman R, Balter M. Large airway disease associated with inflammatory bowel disease. Chest 1998; 113:1723.

[36] Vandenplas O, Casel S, Delos M, et al. Granulomatous bronchiolitis associated with Crohn's disease. Am J Respir Crit Care Med 1998; 158:1676.

[37] Barr GD, Shale DJ, Jewell DP. Ulcerative colitis and sarcoidosis. Postgrad Med J 1986; 62: 341–345.

[38] Papadopoulos KI, Hornblad Y, Liljebladh H, et al. High frequency of endocrine autoimmunity in patients with sarcoidosis. Eur J Endocrinol 1996; 134:331–336.

[39] Storch I, Rosoff L, Katz S. Sarcoidosis and inflammatory bowel disease. J Clin Gastroenterol 2001; 33:345.

[40] Smiejan JM, Cosnes J, Chollet-Martin S, et al. Sarcoid-likelymphocytosis of the lower respiratory tract in patients with active Crohn's disease. Ann Intern Med 1986; 104:17–21.

[41] Bernstein CN, Wajda A, Blanchard JF. The clustering of other chronic inflammatory diseases in inflammatory bowel disease: a population-based study. Gastroenterology 2005; 129:827–836.

[42] Yang P, Tremaine WJ, Meyer RL, et al. α_1 -Antitrypsin deficiency and inflammatory bowel diseases. Mayo Clin Proc 2000; 75: 450–455.

[43] Kasuga I, Yanagisawa N, Takeo C, et al. Multiple pulmonary nodules in association with pyoderma gangrenosum. Respir Med 1997; 91: 493.

[44] Swinburn CR, Jackson GJ, Cobden I, et al. Bronchiolitis obliterans organising pneumonia in a patient with ulcerative colitis. Thorax 1988; 43:735–736.

[45] W. Sloan, A. Bargen and R. Gage, Life histories of patients with chronic ulcerative colitis: a review of 2000 cases, Gastroenterology (1950), pp. 25–38.

[46] C.N. Bernstein, J.F. Blanchard and D.S. Houston et al., The incidence of deep venous thrombosis and pulmonary embolism among patients with inflammatory bowel disease: a population-based cohort study, Thromb Haemost (2001), pp. 430–434.

[47] W. Miehsler, W. Reinisch and E. Valic et al., Is inflammatory bowel disease an independent and disease specific risk factor for thromboembolism?, Gut (2004), pp. 542–548.

[48] Talbot RW, Heppell J, Dozois RR, et al. Vascular complications of inflammatory bowel disease. Mayo Clin Proc 1986; 61:140 –145.

[49] Quera R, Shanahan F. Thromboembolism: an important manifestation of inflammatory bowel disease. Am J Gastroenterol 2004; 99:1971–1973.

[50] Papa A, Danese S, Grillo A, et al. Review article: inherited thrombophilia in inflammatory bowel disease. Am J Gastroenterol2003; 98:1247–1251.

[51] Oldenburg B, Fijnheer R, van der Griend R, et al. Homocysteine in inflammatory bowel disease: a risk factor for thromboembolic complications? Am J Gastroenterol 2000; 95:2825–2830.

[52] C.A. Solem, E.V. Loftus and W.J. Tremaine *et al.*, Venous thromboembolism in inflammatory bowel disease, *Am J Gastroenterol* (2004), pp. 97–101.

[53] Tanigawa K, Sugiyama K, Matsuyama H, et al. Mesalazine-induced eosinophilic pneumonia. Respiration 1999; 66:69.

[54] Bitton A, Peppercorn MA, Hanrahan JP, Upton MP. Mesalamine-induced lung toxicity. Am J Gastroenterol 1996; 91:1039.

[55] Hamadeh MA, Atkinson J, Smith LJ. Sulfasalazine-induced pulmonary disease. Chest 1992; 101:1033.

[56] Salerno SM, Ormseth EJ, Roth BJ, et al. Sulfasalazine pulmonary toxicity in ulcerative colitis mimicking clinical features of Wegener's granulomatosis. Chest 1996; 110:556.

[57] Ananthakrishnan AN, Attila T, Otterson MF, et al. Severe pulmonary toxicity after azathioprine/6-mercaptopurine initiation for the treatment of inflammatory bowel disease. J Clin Gastroenterol 2007; 41:682.

[58] Keane J, Gershon S, Wise RP, et al. Tuberculosis associated with infliximab, a tumor necrosis factor alpha-neutralizing agent. N Engl J Med 2001; 345:1098.

[59] Weatherhead M, Masson S, Bourke SJ, et al. Interstitial pneumonitis after infliximab therapy for Crohn's disease. Inflamm Bowel Dis 2006; 12:427.

[60] Bonderman D, Jakowitsch J, Adlbrecht C, et al. Medical conditions increasing the risk of chronic thromboembolic pulmonary hypertension. Thromb Haemost 2005; 93:512.

[61] Sonoda K, Ikeda S, Mizuta Y, et al. Evaluation of venous thromboembolism and coagulation-fibrinolysis markers in Japanese patients with inflammatory bowel disease. J Gastroenterol 2004; 39:948.

15

Mucosal Remodeling and Alteration of Stromal Microenvironment in Ulcerative Colitis as Related to Colorectal Tumorigenesis

Isao Okayasu, Tsutomu Yoshida, Tetuo Mikami, Jun Mitsuhashi,
Masaaki Ichinoe, Nobuyuki Yanagisawa, Wataru Tokuyama,
Kiyomi Hana and Yuichi Ishibashi
Department of Pathology,
Kitasato University School of Medicine, Sagamihara, Kanagawa,
Japan

1. Introduction

As an organ-specific, chronic inflammation-carcinoma sequence, it is well known that colorectal neoplasia is prone to appear in long-standing ulcerative colitis (UC) (Lennard-Jones et al., 1983). It has been shown that the tumor suppressor gene, *p53* mutation, which results from chromosomal instability due to inflammation-driven DNA damage plays an important role in the early stage of tumorigenesis (Hussain et al., 2000; Yoshida et al., 2003; 2006). However, the incidence of *p53* mutation is approximately up to 50% in dysplasia and carcinoma lesions in UC, according to our examination with our novel combined method of microdissection and polymerase chain reaction (PCR)-direct sequencing of the full-length *p53* gene from single crypts in long-standing UC (Yoshida et al., 2004). Instead, we have shown that mucosal remodeling and stromal genomic instability can be raised as another factor for carcinoma development. In this chapter, we describe the mucosal remodeling and genomic instability of stromal cells as well as epithelial cells, suggesting insufficient cross-talk between epithelium and stroma in long-standing UC.

2. Mucosal remodeling, correlative to the duration of ulcerative colitis (UC)

2.1 Colorectal mucosal remodeling in long-standing UC

Regarding the structural alterations of colorectal mucosa formerly, there were no systemic analyses but there were sporadic descriptions such as distortion and atrophy of crypts, and Paneth cell metaplasia in UC (Floren et al., 1987; Day et al., 2003). For a general image of mucosal remodeling in long-standing UC, we reconstituted 3-dimensional features after taking serial histological sections of UC cases. Representative three-dimensional reconstructed images are shown in Fig. 1.

In order to find risk factors for cancer development in long-standing UC, according to these general features, we tried to assess mucosal remodeling of rectal mucosa, including decreased number (/cm), height (µm) and angle (degree) of crypts and increased fused crypts (/100 crypts), metaplastic Paneth cells (/100 crypts) and thickening of muscularis mucosa (µm) quantitatively, and found most of items correlated significantly with the duration of illness in UC (Fig. 2).

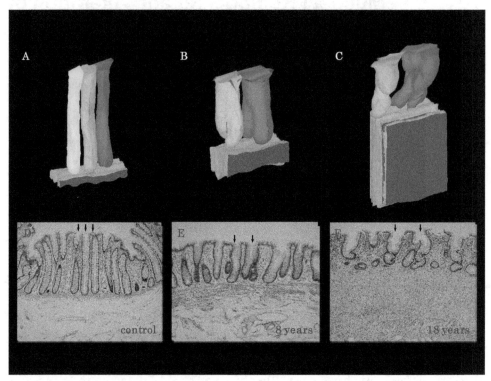

Fig. 1. A three-dimensional, reconstructed figure of rectal mucosa in UC (Control and UC cases for 8 and 18 years) (Mitsuhashi et al., *Pathol Int*, 2005)

However, there were no significant differences of increased or decreased correlation lines of each marker between the two groups, UC, inactive, without neoplasia and with neoplasia, or between the two groups, UC, active without neoplasia and with neoplasia. For immunohistochemical markers, Ki-67 (for cellular proliferative activity), p53, p21 and ssDNA (for apoptosis) labeling indices (LI) (%) were significantly correlated with the duration of illness (Fig. 3). The period-dependent increase of epithelial p53 and p21 LI is clearly shown. Furthermore, epithelial p53 and p21 LI were significantly higher in the non-neoplastic rectal mucosa of long-standing UC patients with colorectal neoplasia compared with those without neoplasia (Mitsuhashi et al., 2005).

Epithelial p53 and p21 overexpression means acceleration of G1 check point due to inflammatory oxidative stress, indicating accumulation of DNA damage in line with pathway for tumorigenesis (Yoshida et al., 2003; 2006). Canonical discriminative analysis using duration of UC illness, number of crypts, angles of crypts and thickness of muscularis mucosa gave no clear difference between UC with neoplasia and without neoplasia (Fig. 4-

Mucosal Remodeling and Alteration of Stromal Microenvironment in Ulcerative Colitis as Related to
Colorectal Tumorigenesis

257

1). However, in particular, Ki-67LI, p53LI and p21LI can give reliable canonical discriminative values to estimate the risk of cancer development as compared with UC without neoplasia (Fig. 4-2).

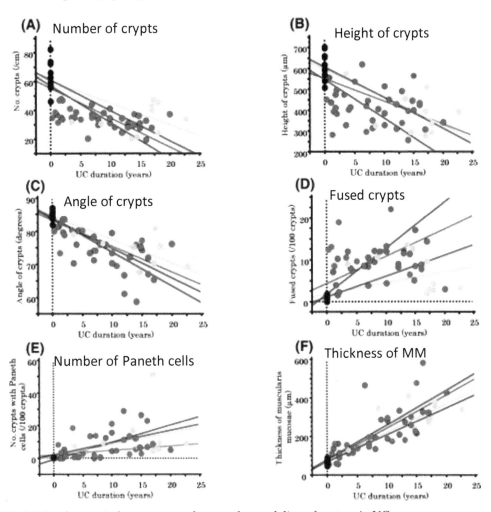

Fig. 2. Morphometrical assessment of mucosal remodeling of rectum in UC
(A) Number, (B) height and (C) angle of crypts, (D) fused crypts , (E) crypts with Paneth cells and (F) thickness of muscularis mucosa (MM) with relation to the duration of UC illness and cancer development (○ UC, active with neoplasia; UC, active without neoplasia; UC, inactive with neoplasia; ○ UC, inactive without neoplasia) (Mitsuhashi et al., *Pathol Int*, 2005)

Thus, the above described markers in rectal biopsy specimens can be useful to predict the risk of colorectal tumor development in long-standing UC, using canonical discriminative analysis.

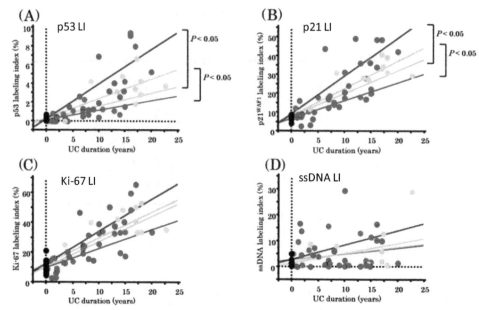

Fig. 3. (A) p53, (B) p21, (C) Ki-67 and (D) ssDNA labeling indices (LI) with relation to the duration of UC illness and cancer development (○ UC, active with neoplasia; ○ UC, active without neoplasia; ○ UC, inactive with neoplasia; ○ UC, inactive without neoplasia) (Mitsuhashi et al., *Pathol Int*, 2005)

2.2 The increase of stem-cell mutated crypts as related to the duration of UC illness

O-acetylation of epithelial sialoglycoprotein identified by mild PAS staining can show N-acetyl neuraminic acid phenotypes (Fig. 5). Mutated crypts in UC patients of heterozygous O-acetylation (oat^a/oat^b), which show a positive reaction with mild periodic acid-Schiff (PAS) staining in negative background mucosa (Fig. 5), were counted per 10,000 crypts. With this method, mutated crypts increased correlatively with the UC duration. Furthermore, clusters of crypts, positive with mild PAS staining, indicating regenerated crypts covered by a single tissue stem cell after erosion, also increased correlatively with the duration of the UC illness (Fig. 6). Moreover, non-neoplastic mucosal crypts in cases of sporadic colorectal carcinoma also showed significant increase of mutated crypts with mild PAS staining, although angles of their correlation lines were extremely low compared with those in UC cases. Elongated lines of the correlation between two factors showed 0 crypts at 0 years old, indicating gradual appearance of mutated crypts after birth. Thus, mutated crypts appear extremely higher in UC patients than non-UC patients (Fig. 6).

These results indicate the base of a chronic inflammation- carcinoma sequence (Okayasu et al., 2002; 2006).

2.3 Shortening of telomere length of colonic epithelial cells in UC

In addition to chromosomal alterations due to chronic inflammation-driven DNA damage through the generation and effects of reactive oxygen species, telomere shortening in mucosal epithelia is an important factor in tumorigenesis. The telomere shortening in colonic

Canonical discriminative   Can 1
analysis 1

Can 1 = 0.061 X (Duration)
     − 0.014 X (Number of crypts)
     − 0.102 X (Angle of crypts)
     + 0.006 X (Thickness of MM)

Can 2= 0.244 X (Duration)
     + 0.015 X (Number of crypts)
     + 0.162 X (Angle of crypts)
     - 0.005 X (Thickness of MM)

UC+Cancer active

UC+Cancer inactive

UC active

UC inactive

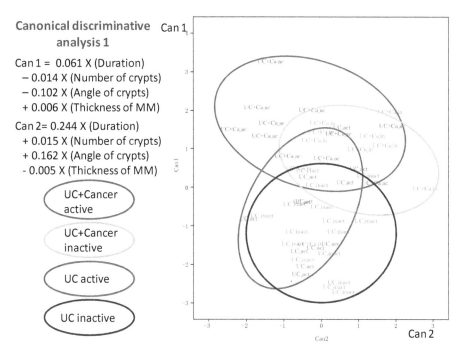

Fig. 4-1. Canonical discriminative analysis with number and angle of crypts and thickness of
muscularis mucosa (MM) among UC active or inactive and with or without neoplasia

epithelia is reported in long-standing UC, particularly in patients with colorectal cancers,
suggesting an unstable state of chromosomes in which cells can easily mutate (Risques et al.,
2008; 2011, Bronner et al., 2008). In addition to UC, telomere shortening is detected in
esophageal Barrett's mucosa-Barrett's adenocarcinoma sequence by our group (Shiraishi et
al., 2009). This phenomenon suggests an accelerated aging in inflamed lesions (Risques et
al., 2008; 2011).

3. Alteration of subepithelial (pericryptal) myofibroblasts and interstitial fibrosis in UC

We have clearly shown that subepithelial myofibroblasts forming crypt niches have various
phenotypic expressions of α-smooth muscle actin (αSMA), NCAM, PGP9.5, HSP47 and
cytoglobin (Cygb) by immunohistochemistry (Fig. 7) or immunofluorescence (Fig. 8) and
immunoelectron microscope (Fig.9). Therefore, we first identified these subepithelial
myofibroblasts as colonic stellate cells (also known as perisinusoidal cells or Ito cells, fat
storing cells in perisinusoidal spaces of the liver). Subepithelial myofibroblasts are localized
between mucosal epithelia and capillaries, similar to hepatic stellate cells between liver cells
and sinusoids. Further, subepithelial myofibroblasts occasionally have small lipid droplets
indicating vitamin A storage. Subepithelial myofibroblasts are localized more at the crypt
base than they are at the crypt surface, similar to the dense localization of hepatic stellate
cells at the periportal area in hepatic lobules. These features indicate that subepithelial
myofibroblasts correspond to colonic stellate cells (Okayasu et al., 2009; 2011).

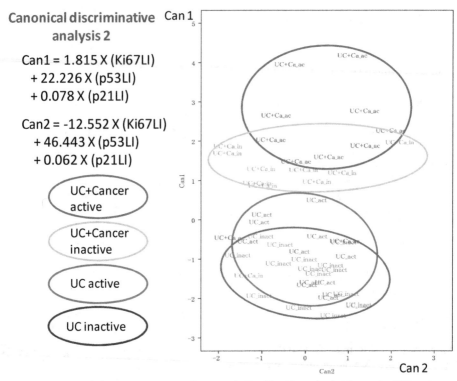

Fig. 4-2. Canonical discriminative analysis with Ki-67, p53 and p21LI among UC active or inactive and with or without neoplasia. There is no overlap between UC+Cancer and UC groups.

It is known that subepithelial myofibroblasts secrete pericryptin, a specific extracellular matrix protein, which recruits activated fibroblasts and forms collagen fibrils, supporting the growth of epithelial components after mechanical stress in tissue repair processes (Shimazaki et al., 2008).

Cytoglobin (Cygb), a novel member of the globin family is also expressed in splanchnic fibroblasts-like cells, including hepatic stellate cells and colonic subepithelial myofibroblasts. A recent study demonstrated that Cygb served as a defensive mechanism against oxidative stress under hypoxic conditions in a kidney ischemia-reperfusion experimental system (Nishi et al., 2011). Thus, subepithelial myofibroblasts at the crypt base play important roles to protect and support crypt stem cells and their differentiation and maturation as stem cell niches.

Furthermore, we reported the decrease of subepithelial myofibroblasts, along with the inversely correlated increase of interstitial myofibroblasts and fibrosis, in relation to the duration of UC illness (Okayasu et al., 2009) (Table 1). Loss of subepithelial myofibroblasts means dysregulation of colonic crypt stem cell protection and differentiation. Interstitial fibrosis with the increase of stromal myofibroblasts in colonic mucosa, may also accelerate erroneous interactions between epithelial and stromal cells. These alterations might be major components of a microenvironment conductive to tumorigenesis (Fig. 11).

Mucosal Remodeling and Alteration of Stromal Microenvironment in Ulcerative Colitis as Related to
Colorectal Tumorigenesis

261

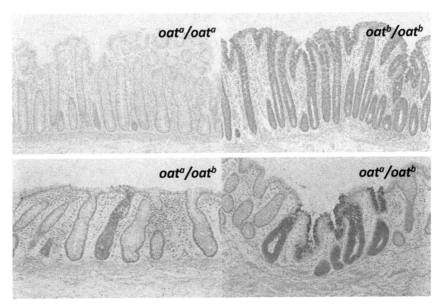

Fig. 5. *O*-acetylation phenotypes (*o*-acetyl transferase) in colonic mucosa with mild PAS
staining. Single mutated crypt and a cluster of mutated crypts in UC patients of
heterozyogous *O*-acetylation (*oat^a/oat^b*) are shown in the lower left and right figures,
respectively. (Okayasu et al., *Cancer Res*, 2002)

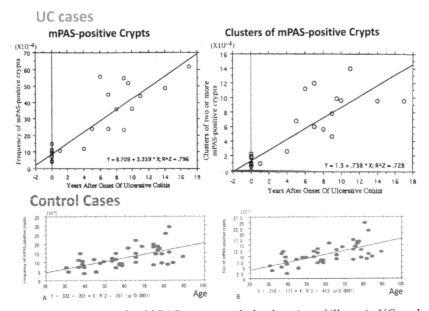

Fig. 6. Correlative increase of mild PAS+ crypts with the duration of illness in UC, and with
the age in control cases (/1x10^5 crypts) (Okayasu et al., *Cancer Res*, 2002; *Cancer Sci*, 2006)

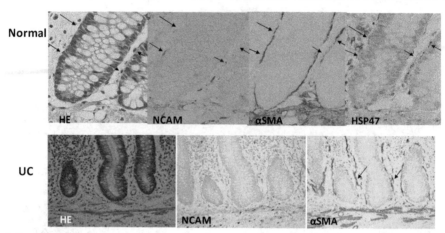

Fig. 7. Immunohistochemical phenotypes of subepithelial myofibroblasts (arrows) in UC.
Subepithelial myofibroblasts (arrows) are located around the crypts. Identification of
subepithelial myofibroblasts as colonic stellate cells (Ito cells, fat-storing cells) by findings of
αSMA+, NCAM+, HSP47+, Cytoglobin+ and lipid droplets. (Okayasu et al., *Pathol Int*, 2009;
Histol Histopathol, 2011)

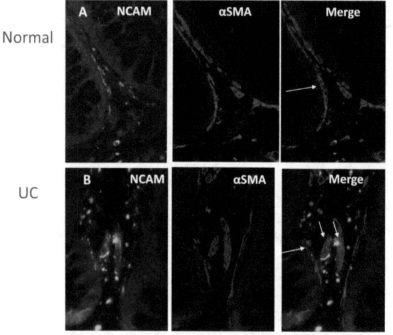

Fig. 8. Double immunofluorescences of subepithelial myofibroblasts (arrows) in UC. Double
positive reactions are shown in subepithelial myofibroblasts (large arrows) of normal
mucosa and in both subepithelial myofibroblasts (large arrow) and interstitial
myofibroblasts (small arrows) of UC-mucosa. (Okayasu et al., *Pathol Int*, 2009)

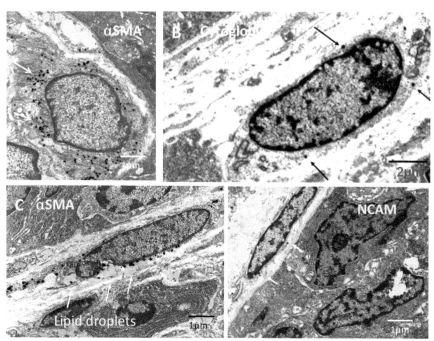

Fig. 9. Immunoelectron microscopic features of subepithelial myofibroblasts (arrows,
immunogold deposits). A, Smooth muscle actin (αSMA); B, Cytoglobin; C, αSMA. Lipid
droplets (arrows) in a subepithelial myofibroblast, indicating a vitamin A storage cell; D,
NCAM. (Okayasu et al., *Pathol Int*, 2009; *Histol Histopathol*, 2011)

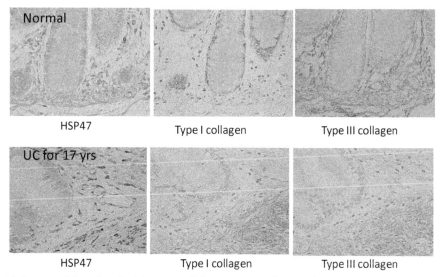

Fig. 10. Immunohistochemical features of the stroma in the rectal mucosa in UC for 17 years
and control. (Okayasu et al., *Pathol Int*, 2009)

4. Epithelial and stromal genomic instability in UC and its relation to tumorigenesis

We have analyzed genomic instability, microsatellite instability (MSI) and loss of heterozygosity (LOH) in stromal cells, as well as epithelial cells, in order to see the role of stromal cell alterations in UC-associated tumorigenesis, using a combination of laser-captured microdissection and the Gene-scan approach (Fig. 12). Stromal genomic instability kept the same incidences in dysplasia and invasive carcinoma lesions as those of regenerative mucosa. The frequency of LOH or MSI for 5 tumor suppressor gene (TSG) markers, D9S161 (close to p16[INK4A]), D7S486 (close to ST-7), D13S268 (close to Rb), D18S474 (close to Smad 4 and DCC) and D3S1300 (close to the FHIT [fragile histidine triad]) was almost constantly found to be increased in stromal components of all lesion types (regenerative mucosa, dysplasia and carcinoma). In contrast, the epithelial cells showed a step-up increase of MSI in tumor progression and a constant increase of LOH for TSG markers. In epithelium, LOH for 4 chromosome17 markers, D17S796 (17p13 close to the *p53* gene, TP53 (17p13, the *p53* gene locus), D17S786 (17p13, close to the *p53* gene) and D17S579 (p17q21, close to *BRCA1*) increased along with histological progression. In stroma, LOH was relatively low, but there was a constant incidence in all types of lesions. When data were combined for TSG and chromosome 17 markers, the tendency was prominent that stromal cells showed a constantly increased incidence of both MSI and LOH in all types of lesions, including regenerative mucosa, dysplasia and carcinoma, compared with the step-up increase in epithelium along with histological progression (Matsumoto et al., 2003a; 2003b; Yagishita et al., 2008). On the other hand, genomic instability for NCI-recommended standard microsatellite markers for colorectal cancers, BAT25, BAT26, D2S123, D3S346 and D17S250 (Boland et al., 1998) was not remarkable, indicating that chromosome 17 and tumor suppressor gene markers are more sensitive in UC-associated mucosal lesions (Matsumoto et al., 2003a).

	Mucosa propria			Muscularis mucosae		
	Without neoplasia		With neoplasia	Without neoplasia		With neoplasia
Total duration	<5 years	≥5 years	≥5 years	<5 years	≥5 years	≥5 years
Thickness†	↓	↓▽	↓▽	↑	↑△	↑▲▲
Subepithelial myofibroblasts						
α-SMA+ cells	↓	↓▽	↓▽			
NCAM+ cells	↓	↓	↓▽ ▼			
HSP47+ cells	↑	↑	↓▽ ▼			
Interstitium in lamina propria						
NCAM+ interstitial cells	→	→	↓▼			
α-SMA+ interstitial cells	↑	↑	↑△ ▲			
CD68+ macrophages	↑	→	▲			
Collagen type I	↑	↑	↑	↑	↑△	↑△
Collagen type III	↑	↑	↑	↑	↑△	↑△

‡Inactive phase according to the Seo clinical activity index at surgical operation. †Partly from Ref 19.

↓or ↑ significantly decreased or increased, compared to the normal control group.

▽ or △ significantly decreased or increased, compared to the group (<5 years).

▼ or ▲ significantly decreased or increased, compared to the group (≥5 years, without neoplasia).

→ not significant, compared to the normal control group.

Table 1. Summary of stromal cell alterations in the rectal mucosa in UC (Okayasu et al., *Pathol Int*, 2009)

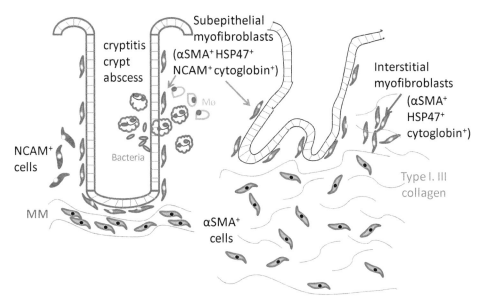

Fig. 11. Schema of mucosal remodeling in UC (Lt, early active lesion; Rt, long-standing UC)
MM, muscularis mucosa

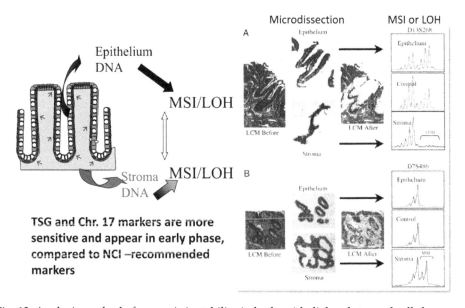

Fig. 12. Analysis method of genomic instability in both epithelial and stromal cells by a
combination of microdissection and PCR-gene scan
MSI, microsatellite instability; LOH, loss of heterozygosity; LCM, laser-captured
microdissection (Yagishita et al, *Scand J Gastroenterol*, 2008)

Tumor Suppressor
Gene markers
(TSG, 6 markers):
Smad 4, p16,Rb,
WT1, ST-7, FHIT

Chromosome 17
markers (Chr.17, 4
markers): D17S796,
TP53, D17S786,
D17S579 (close to
BRCA1)

TSG and Chr. 17
markers
(10 markers)

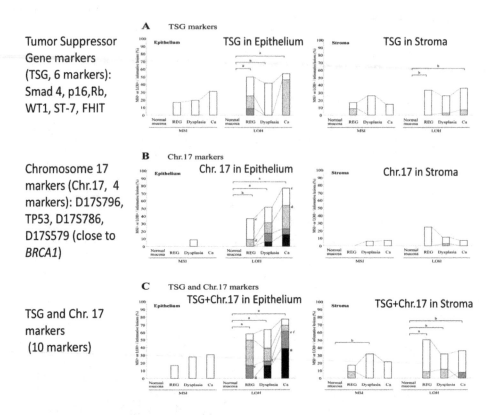

Fig. 13. MSI and LOH incidences in mucosal epithelial and stromal cells in UC
MSI, microsatellite instability; LOH, loss of heterozygosity. Bars on horizontal axis show
normal mucosa, regenerative mucosa, dysplasia and carcinoma, respectively. Open bars,
positive for 1 marker; dotted bars, for 2 markers; gray bars, for 3 markers; black bars for 4 or
more markers. Horizontal lines indicate significant difference (p<0.05~0.01) between two
bars (lesion groups). Left part shows MSI, and right part shows LOH in each figure.
(Yagishita et al., *Scand J Gastroenterol*, 2008)

Genomic instability in sporadic colorectal tumorigenesis, including *de novo* carcinogenesis
and the adenoma-carcinoma sequence, was prominent in epithelium compared with a low
incidence in stroma (Ishiguro et al., 2006; Ogawa et al., 2006). We also demonstrated that
genomic instability was accelerated in stromal cells in Barrett's mucosa and Barrett's
adenocarcinoma sequence in the esophagus similarly to UC tumorigenesis (Shiraishi et al.,
2006).
Contribution of genomic instability in stromal cells to carcinogenesis is variable in the
tumorigenesis of various organs. It has been demonstrated that stromal genomic instability
due to hormonal dysfunction precedes in tumorigenesis of the breast (Moinfar et al., 2000;
Shekhar et al., 2001). Thus, enhanced genomic instability in stromal cells is important in the
chronic inflammation-carcinoma sequence.

Mucosal Remodeling and Alteration of Stromal Microenvironment in Ulcerative Colitis as Related to
Colorectal Tumorigenesis

267

5. Stochastic pathways in a chronic inflammation-carcinoma sequence

Various kinds of inflammatory cytokines, cell cycle regulators and other cell signal molecules
are repeatedly cycle regulators are repeatedly or continuously activated in chronic

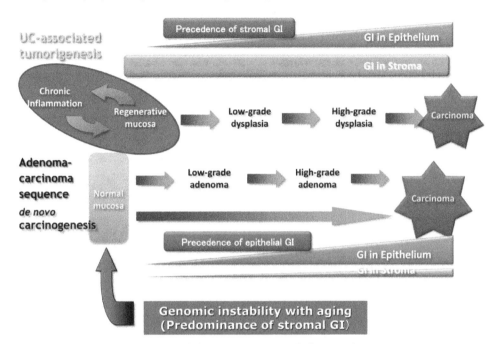

Fig. 14. Summary of genomic instability patterns in epithelium and stroma in various
carcinogenesis of the colorectum. GI, genomic instability

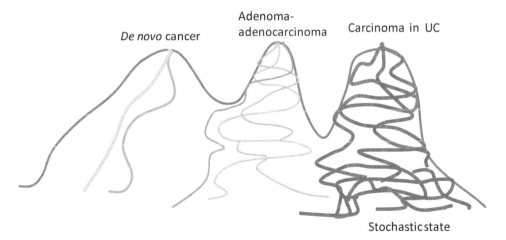

Fig. 15. Schema of tumorigenesis in colorectal cancers

inflammation, such as TNF-α, IL-8, IL-6, toll-like receptors, cell cycle G1-check point and NF-kB (Yoshida et al., 2003, 2004; Ohkusa et al., 2009). Compared to de novo cancer development and the adenoma-carcinoma sequence, stochastic pathways to tumor development can be proposed in a chronic inflammation-carcinoma sequence. In a mountain climbing analogy, it is obvious that various climbing pathways connecting with that various climbing pathways connecting with each other showing stochasticity at the mountain-base are reduced to several paths and then even fewer paths as one approaches closer to the top of the mountain. The analogy in the body is that stochastic (probabilistic) pathways to tumor development over time gain commonalty through chronic inflammatory stimulation (Kobayashi and Inoue, 2008; Inoue and Kobayashi, 2011).

6. Conclusions

Not only chromosomal instability, telomere shortening and genomic instability of epithelial cells due to chronic inflammation-driven DNA damage, we also stressed the important role of mucosal remodeling, including morphological alterations and genomic instability of stromal cells, suggesting insufficient crosstalk between epithelial and stromal cells, as it relates to UC-associated tumorigenesis.

7. References

Boland CR, Thibodeau SN, Hamilton SR, Sidransky D, Eshleman JR, Burt RW, Meltzer SJ, Rodriguez-Bigas MA, Fodde R, Ranzani GN & Srivastava S (1998). A National Cancer Institute Workshop on Microsatellite Instability for cancer detection and familial predisposition: development of international criteria for the determination of microsatellite instability in colorectal cancer. Cancer Res, 58, 5248-5257.

Bronner MP, O'Sullivan JN, Rabinovitch PS, Crispin DA, Chen L, Emond MJ, Rubin CE & Brentnall TA (2008). Genomic biomarkers to improve ulcerative colitis neoplasia surveillance. Am J Pathol, 173, 1853-1860.

Day DW, Jass JR, Price AB, Shepherd NA, Sloan JS, Talbot IC, Warren BF & Williams GT (2003). Morson Dawson's Gastrointestinal Pathology, 4th ed, 496-497, Blackwell Science Ltd, Oxford, UK.

Floren CH, Benoni C & Willen R (1987). Histologic and colonoscopic assessment of disease extension in ulcerative colitis. Scand J Gastroenterol, 22, 459-462.

Hom YK, Young P, Wiesen JF, Miettinen PJ, Derynck R, Werb Z & Cunha GR (1998). Uterine and vaginal organ growth requires epidermal growth factor receptor signaling from stroma. Endocrinology, 139, 913-921.

Hussain SP, Amstad P, Raja K, Ambs S, Nagashima M, Bennett WP, Shields, PG, Ham AJ, Swenberg JA, Marrogi AJ & Harris CC (2000). Increased p53 mutation load in noncancerous colon tissue from ulcerative colitis: a cancer-prone chronic inflammatory disease. Cancer Res, 60, 3333-3337.

Inoue T & Kobayashi Y (2011). Commonalty and stochasticity in gene expression profiles during aging process. SOT 50th Annual Meeting & ToxExpoTM, Washington DC, Morning Sessions on March 7.

Ishiguro K, Yoshida T, Yagishita H, Numata Y & Okayasu I (2006). Epithelial and stromal genetic instability contributes to genesis of colorectal adenoma. Gut, 55, 695-702.

Kobayashi Y & Inoue T (2008). Principles of data mining in toxicogenomics, In: *Toxicogenomics: A Powerful Tool for Toxicity Assessment*, Sahu SC, 57-84, John Wiley &Sons Ltd, Chichester, West Sussex, UK.

Lennard-Jones JE, Morson BC, Ritchie JK & Williams CB (1983). Cancer surveillance in ulcerative colitis. Experience over 15 years. *Lancet*, 2 (8342), 149-152.

Matsumoto N, Yoshida T & Okayasu I (2003). High epithelial and stromal genetic instability of chromosome 17 in ulcerative colitis-associated carcinogenesis. *Cancer Res*, 63, 6158-6161.

Matsumoto N, Yoshida T, Yamashita K, Numata Y & Okayasu I (2003). Possible alternative carcinogenesis pathway featuring microsatellite instability in colorectal cancer stroma. *Br J Cancer*, 89, 707-712.

Mitsuhashi J, Mikami T, Saigenji K & Okayasu I (2005). Significant correlation of morphological remodeling in ulcerative colitis with disease duration and between elevated p53 and p21 expression in rectal mucosa and neoplastic development. *Pathol Int*, 55, 113-121.

Moinfar F, Man YG, Arnould L, Bratthauer GL, Ratschek M & Tavassoli FA (2000). Concurrent and independent genetic alterations in the stroma and epithelial cells of mammary carcinoma: implications for tumorigenesis. *Cancer Res*, 60, 2562-2566.

Nishi H, Inagi R, Kawada N, Yishizato K, Mimura I, Fujita T& Nangaku M (2011). Cytoglobin, a novel member of the globin family, protects kidney fibroblasts against oxidative stress under ischemic conditions. *Am J Pathol*, 178, 128-139.

Ogawa T, Yoshida T, Tsuruta T, Saigenji K & Okayasu I (2006). Tumor budding is predictive of lymphatic involvement and lymph node metastases in submucosal invasive colorectal adenocarcinomas and in non-polypoid compared with polypoid growths. *Cancer Sci*, 97, 1335-1342.

Ohkusa T, Yoshida T, Sato N, Watanabe S, Tajiri H & Okayasu I (2009). Commensal bacteria can enter colonic epithelial cells and induce proinflammatory cytokine secretion: a possible pathogenic mechanism of ulcerative colitis. *J Med Microbiol*, 58, 535-545.

Okayasu I., Hana K, Yoshida T, Mikami T, Kanno J & Fujiwara M (2002). Significant increase of colonic mutated crypts in ulcerative colitis correlatively with duration of illness. *Cancer Res*, 62, 2236-2238.

Okayasu I, Hana K, Tsuruta T, Okamura T, Tokuyama W, Kajita S, Yoshida T & Mikami T (2006). Significant increase of colonic mutated crypts correlates with age in sporadic cancer and diverticulosis cases, with higher frequency in the left- than right-side colorectum. *Cancer Sci*, 97, 362-367.

Okayasu I. Yoshida T, Mikami T, Hana K, Yokozawa M, Araki K, Mitsuhashi J, Kikuchi M, Adachi E & Sada M (2009). Mucosal remodeling in long-standing ulcerative colitis with colorectal neoplasia: significant alterations of NCAM+ or alpha-SMA+ subepitheial myofibroblasts and interstitial cells. *Pathol Int*, 59, 701-711.

Okayasu I. Mikami T, Yoshida T, Hana K, Yokozawa M, Sada M, Fujiwara M & Kawada N (2011). Cytoglobin expression of rectal subepithelial myofibroblasts: Significant alterations of cytoglobin+ stromal cells in long-standing ulcerative colitis. *Histol Histopathol*, 26, 679-688.

Risques RA, Lai LA, Brentnall TA, Li L, Feng Z, Gallaher J, Mandelson MT, Potter JD, Bronner MP & Rabinovitch PS (2008). Ulcerative colitis is a disease of accelerated colon aging: evidence from telomere attrition and DNA damage. *Gastroenterology*, 135, 410-418.

Risques RA, Lai LA, Himmetoglu C, Ebaee A, Li L, Feng Z, Bronner MP, Al-Lahham B, Kowdley KV, Lindor KD, Rabinovitch PS & Brentnall TA (2011). Ulcerative colitis-associated colorectal cancer arises in a field of short telomeres, senescence, and inflammation. *Cancer Res*, 71, 1669-1679.

Shekhar MP, Werdell J, Santner SJ, Pauley RJ & Tait L (2001). Breast stroma plays a dominant regulatory role in breast epithelial growth and differentiation: implications for tumor development and progression. *Cancer Res*, 61, 1320-1326.

Shimazaki M, Nakamura K, Kii I, Kashima T, Amizuka N, Li M, Saito M, Fukuda K, Nishiyama T, Kitajima S, Saga Y, Fukayama M, Sato M & Kudo A (2008). Periostin is essential for cardiac healing after acute myocardial infarction. *J Exp Med*, 205, 295-303.

Shiraishi H, Miakami T, Yoshida T, Tanabe S, Kobayashi N, Watanabe M & Okayasu I (2006). Early genetic instability of both epithelial and stromal cells in esophageal squamous cell carcinomas, contrasted with Barrett's adenocarcinomas. *J Gastroenterol*, 41, 1186-1196.

Shiraishi H, Mikami T, Aida J, Nakamura K, Izumiyama-Shimomura N, Arai T, Watanabe M, Okayasu I & Takubo K (2009). Telomere shortening in Barrett's mucosa and esophageal adenocarcinoma and its association with loss of hetgerozygosity. *Scand J Gastroenterol*, 44, 538-544.

Yagishita H, Yoshida T, Ishiguro K, Numata Y & Okayasu I (2008). Epithelial and stromal genetic instability linked to tumor suppressor genes in ulcerative colitis-associated tumorigenesis. *Scand J Gastroenterol*, 43, 559-566.

Yoshida T, Miami T, Mitomi H & Okayasu I (2003). Diverse p53 alterations in ulcerative colitis-associated low-grade dysplasia: full-length gene sequencing in microdissected single crypts. *J Pathol*, 199, 166-175.

Yoshida T, Matsumoto N, Mikami T & Okayasu I (2004). Upregulation of p16[INK4A] and Bax in *p53* wild/p53-overexpressing crypts in ulcerative colitis-associated tumours. *Br J Cancer*, 91, 1081-1088.

Yoshida T, Haga S, Numata Y, Yamashita K, Mikami T, Ogawa T, Ohkusa T & Okayasu I (2006). Disruption of the p53-p53r2 DNA repair system in ulcerative colitis contributes to colon tumorigenesis. *Int J Cancer*, 118, 1395-1403.

16

Nephritis Associated with Ulcerative Colitis

Hirobumi Tokuyama, Shu Wakino, Koichi Hayashi and Hiroshi Itoh

Department of Internal Medicine, School of Medicine, Keio University, Tokyo, Japan

1. Introduction

Ulcerative colitis (UC) is an idiopathic chronic inflammatory disease of the colon and rectum, characterized by mucosal inflammation and typically presenting with bloody diarrhea. Crohn's disease is characterized by transmural inflammation of the gut wall and can affect any part of the tubular gastrointestinal tract. Although the underlying etiology and exact pathogenesis remain fully unclarified, current hypothesis favors dysregulation of gastrointestinal immune system in genetically predisposed individuals [1]. Extra-intestinal manifestations of inflammatory bowel disease (IBD) are common, ensuing in approximately 40% of patients [2], many of which are postulated to be associated with autoimmune mechanisms [3]. Renal manifestations associated with IBD, however, have rarely been reported. Sulfasalazine reaches the colon intact, where it is metabolized to 5-aminosalicylic acid (5-ASA, mesalazine, mesalamine) and a sulfapyridine moiety. It is therefore used for colonic disease, either as initial therapy or to maintain remission. Adverse effects are mainly caused by the sulfapyridine moiety and include headache, vomiting, and abdominal pain. A reduction in dose is usually beneficial. Newer 5-ASA preparations lack the sulfa moiety of sulfasalazine and are associated with fewer side effects. Mesalamines are slow-release formulae of 5-ASA and are effective as a primary tool for initial and maintenance therapy of IBD. Rare hypertensitivity reactions occur and include pneumonitis, pancreatitis, and hepatitis. Recently, several case reports have been published suggesting an association between the use of 5-ASA and the development of chronic tubulointerstitial nephritis in patients with IBD [4, 5]. Because of adverse effects of these agents, differentiation of renal complications subtending these therapies from the true extraintestinal manifestations of IBD involves much difficulty.

In this review, we note the drugs including 5-ASA associated nephrotoxicity and also show case reports of UC related nephritis.

2. Drugs of the treatment for IBD associated nephrotoxicity

2.1 Epidemiology of nephrotoxicity in IBD

Sulfasalazine has been used in the treatment of IBD, both for UC and for Crohn's disease. Newer 5-ASA preparations lack the sulfa moiety of sulfasalazine and are associated with fewer side effects. Mesalamines are slow-release formulae of 5-ASA and are effective as a primary tool for initial and maintenance therapy of IBD. Azad Khan et al. studied the therapeutic activity of the component parts of sulfasalazine and found that 5-ASA was the therapeutically active component of the drug [6]. In moderate active UC, both sulfasalazine and 5-ASA have proven to be effective in inducing and maintaining clinical remission. However, a number of cases have shown the 5-ASA related toxicity [7, 8]. In particular, nephrotoxicity has been described in some patients with IBD treated with 5-ASA [7, 8]. In this respect, both acetylsalicylic acid and phenacetin, which have been implicated in the occurrence of nonsteroidal antiinflammatory drug-induced nephropathy, share structural similarities with 5-ASA [9, 10]. Furthermore, previous studies reported that 5-ASA may cause injuries to tubular epithelial cells in animals when fed in high doses [9, 10]. The actual incidence of nephrotoxicity in IBD patients with 5-ASA therapy has not been determined, but it has been suggested that renal impairment may occur in up to 1% of patients treated with 5-ASA. A recent prospective study revealed that renal impairment was observed in 2-3% of IBD patients with and without concomitant 5-ASA treatment [11]. More recently, a case-control analysis found that IBD patients treated with 5-ASA had an increased risk of renal disease [12]. However, after adjustment for several factors and variables, the risk of 5-ASA users was comparable to controls. This study found that IBD patients without 5-ASA also had increased risk of renal disease. Taken together, although users of 5-ASA may have an increased risk of renal disease, it may be partly attributable to the underlying disease [12].

2.2 Monitoring markers in IBD
Microalbuminuria has been demonstrated to be present in the majority of IBD patients, and it seems to be related to disease activity. However, other studies have shown that microalbuminuria is not present in patients with IBD [13]. Some authors have concluded that an increased prevalence of tubular proteinuria may be attributed to high doses of 5-ASA [14]. Nevertheless, differences among these studies may be related to differences in disease activity of IBD. Taken together, it is important to conduct a systematic evaluation of the effect of 5-ASA treatment on renal function in patients with IBD.
5-ASA treatment-related nephrotoxicity is reported most often within the first 12 months, but also delayed presentation after several years has been observed. Thus, regular monitoring of renal function should be performed during the therapy.
Several attempts have been made to measure early signs of renal impairment in patients with IBD treated with 5-ASA using sensitive markers of glomerular and tubular dysfunction. Riley et al. found that the incidence of elevated urinary markers such as N-acetyl-D-glucosamidase is low in patients with quiescent UC, which is independent of the dose and duration of 5-ASA treatment [15]. When renal damage occurs, its presence is unlikely to be detected by urinalysis in its early remediable stages. Although tubular enzymuria may be a more sensitive and specific marker of renal damage, it is not yet available as a screening method and the correlation between the several urinary markers of renal damage and 5-ASA treatment remains unproven. These limitations emphasize the importance of monitoring serum creatinine in patients with IBD treated with 5-ASA.

2.3 The incidence of renal disease in IBD
It has been suggested that mesalazine may induce renal impairment more frequently than sulfasalazine [16]. In an analysis of spontaneous reports of adverse events in the UK, 5-ASA-related nephrotoxicity seemed more frequent in mesalazine-treated patients compared with

sulfasalazine-treated patients [17]. Recently, data from the UK General Practice Research Database were used to estimate the incidence of renal disease in adult patients with IBD, and mesalazine and sulfasalazine users had comparable risks of nephrotoxicity (0.17 versus 0.29 cases per 100 person-years, respectively) [12]. It can be conluded that the nephrotoxicity potential of mesalazine and sulfasalazine seems to be similar, and,even if differences exist, they are probably small. Mesalazine should be withdrawn when renal impairment manifests in a patient with IBD in whom no other cause can be readily identified. If withdrawal of 5-ASA treatment does not result in a fall in serum creatinine, then the patient should be referred for consideration of renal biopsy to make sure whether interstitial nephritis or glomerulonephritis associated with IBD is the cause of the persistent impaired renal function.

2.4 Treatment for renal impairment in IBD

Steroids and azathioprine have been used in patients with renal impairment due to mesalazine-associated interstitial nephritis, but the evidence for beneficial roles is anecdotal and uncontrolled. Partial improvement or even complete recovery of renal function after steroid therapy has been reported by several authors. However, other studies have been unable to demonstrate a beneficial effect of these immunosuppressive drugs. Nevertheless, it has been suggested that a trial of high-dose steroid (60 mg/day or 1 mg day/kg for up to 3 months) may be recommended in patients whose renal function does not respond to drug withdrawal alone [7]. Although most case reports indicate reversibility after cessation of the drug, in some cases permanent clinical kidney dysfunction has been observed. Thus, it has been calculated that 10% of the patients with 5-ASA nephrotoxicity will develop end-stage renal disease [5].

3. Case reports of UC related nephritis

3.1 ANCA related nephritis

UC is typically associated with antineutrophil cytoplasmic antibodies of perinuclear type (p-ANCA). These antibodies are not usually considered to carry potential for the development of systemic vasculitis as they lack specificity for proteinase 3 (PR3) or myeloperoxidase (MPO). ANCA can be detected in sera from patients with a wide variety of inflammatory diseases including UC. In one study of 50 patients with UC, 54% were shown to be either p-ANCA or c-ANCA positive but none of these antibodies reacted with PR3 or MPO [18]. In another study, ANCA-positive patients with UC were followed for a year during which no evidence of glomerulonephritis was found [19].

3.2 IgA nephropathy

UC may be associated with a number of extraintestinal complications, involving almost any organ system. The organs most commonly involved include the skin, joints, biliary tract and eyes [3, 20]. However, renal and genitourinary tract manifestations are quite rare, particularly glomerulonephritis. They reported that a patient of IgA nephropathy with UC and chronic intermittent episodes of indolent macrohematuria [21]. IgA nephropathy can be primary in most cases or secondary but is rarely associated with UC [22, 23]. Altered T-helper cells' function might be the initial common derangement of both UC and IgA nephropathy [24, 25]. In IgA nephropathy such alteration in CD4-positive T cells causes a nonspecific stimulus on plasma cells in the bone marrow to secrete polymeric IgA1 into the circulation [26, 27] and of IgG1 and IgG3 in UC [28, 29] culminating in both cases with a common state of local cytokine secretion and tissue inflammation.

3.3 UC related interstitial nephritis

Lately, we reported a patient with UC who has developed acute interstitial nephritis and the subsequent renal failure following a long pause of the treatment with mesalazine [30]. In this case, we observed progressive decline in renal function in a patient with UC. Although the patient exhibited stable levels of serum Cr during the 3 year period after the treatment with mesalazine and sulfapyridine was discontinued, he developed severe interstitial nephritis associated with moderately active UC (Figure 1). His renal biopsy samples showed evidence of severe active tubulointerstitial nephritis along with intense renal interstitial infiltration of CD3-positive T cells (Figure 2). Colonic fiberscopic examination also revealed moderate UC activity and the mucosal infiltration of CD3-positive cells, thus suggesting the common immune mechanism possibly mediated by T-cell dysregulation. Since the patient had not used any nephrotoxic agent for at least three years, it was reasonable to conclude

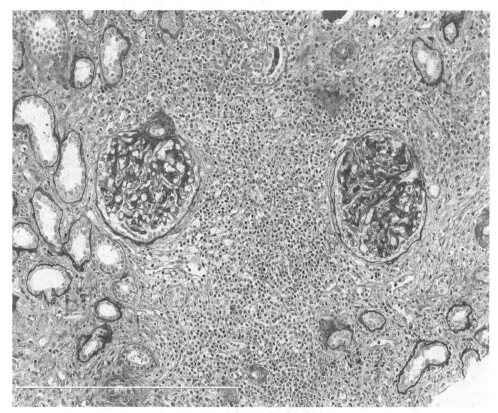

Fig. 1. UC related interstitial nephritis (PAS staining)

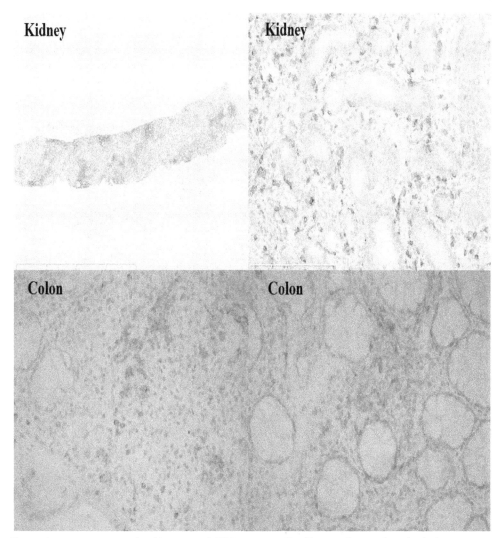

Fig. 2. Intense interstitial infiltration of CD3-positive T cells was detected in the kidney (Upper). The infiltration of CD3-positive cells into the intestinal mucosa was also observed (Lower)

that the main precipitating cause of the progression of renal injury during the medication-free period is attributable to the disease activity of UC *per se*, rather than the flare-up of the reminiscence of mesalazine effect.

Drug-induced nephropathy constitutes a critical problem that precludes the continued use of the agent. Nephrotoxicity has been described in patients with IBD treated with 5-ASA [4, 5]. In the literature survey, 5-ASA-associated nephrotoxicity is reported most often within the first 12 months from the initiation of the drug [31], but delayed presentation has also been shown rarely, with the onset of the renal manifestation after several years of the treatment [32, 33]. In most of their reports, however, 5-ASA was given continuously during the latent period. In our case, by contrast, nephrotoxic agents, including mesalazine or sulfapyridine, were discontinued for at least three years, during which renal function remained relatively stable. Collectively, it appears unlikely that the aggravating process after the cessation of the drugs is associated with the direct nephrotoxic effect of these agents.

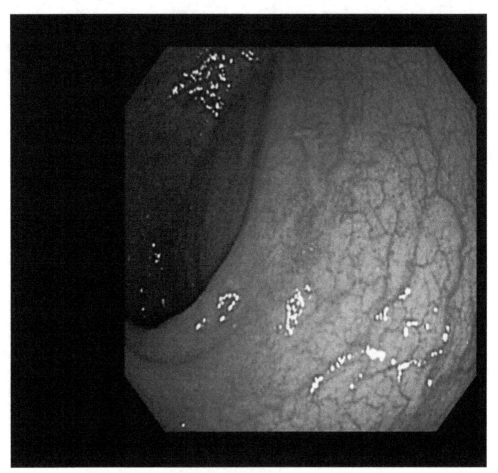

Fig. 3. Colonic fiberscopic findings unveiled moderate UC activity

Since IBD is acknowledged as autoimmune disease affecting multiple extraintestinal organs, it is possible that the kidney is a target organ for the UC-associated systemic injury. Indeed, several types of kidney disease have been documented, including glomerulonephritis, membranous nephropathy and nephrotic syndrome as rare extra-intestinal manifestations of IBD [34-35]. In contrast to glomerular disease, tubulointerstitial nephritis unrelated to nephrotoxic agents has rarely been reported hitherto [36]. Of note, it has been shown that a substantial number of patients manifest pathological enzymuria [37]. Furthermore, a strong correlation between disease activity and tubular proteinuria has been reported in IBD [38]. In our recent case report, the patient shows moderate UC activity (Figure 3) and progressive course of interstitial nephritis with no nephrotoxic agent given during the antecedent 3-year period. Although there reported one case showing that the renal injury does not parallel the activity of IBD [33], the absence of other aggravating factors rather favors the recognition of the UC activity as a precipitating mechanism in this case.

Link between IBD and kidney disease merits comment. As shown in the present case, the kidney constitutes a target organ involved in the UC-induced systemic disorders. Furthermore, the kidney, where various drugs and their metabolites are condensed *in situ* and excreted in the urine, is susceptible to the nephrotoxicity of these agents. Of more clinical importance, the present case sheds light on the kidney as an organ affected in IBD albeit low incidence reported so far. To the extent that the kidney disease contributes substantially to the development of cardiovascular events, our observation would emphasize the need for increasing awareness of the kidney in the management of IBD.

4. Conclusion

A large number of biological agents as well as many biochemical substances and molecules specifically for the medical treatment of patients with IBD, have been developed. Sulfasalazine has been used in the treatment of IBD, both for UC and for Crohn's disease. Mesalamines are slow-release formulae of 5-ASA and are effective as a primary tool for initial and maintenance therapy of IBD. Recently, several case reports have been published suggesting an association between the use of 5-ASA and the development of chronic tubulointerstitial nephritis in patients with IBD. Because of adverse effects of these agents, differentiation of renal complications subtending these therapies from the true extraintestinal manifestations of IBD involves much difficulty. Since IBD is acknowledged as autoimmune disease affecting multiple extraintestinal organs, it is possible that the kidney is a target organ for the UC-associated systemic injury. Indeed, several types of kidney disease have been documented, including glomerulonephritis, membranous nephropathy and nephrotic syndrome as rare extra-intestinal manifestations of IBD. We also reported the case of acute interstitial nephritis associated with UC. As noted in our case report, we assume that the renal manifestation is attributed to intrinsic disease process of the UC-mediated immune dysregulation, and emphasize the need for the pathophysiological evaluation of the intestine and other organs in clinical situations.

5. References

[1] Podolsky DK. (2002). Inflammatory bowel disease. *N Engl J Med*, Vol 347, No. 6, (August 2002), pp. 417-429.
[2] Ricart E. (2004). Autoimmune disorders and extraintestinal manifestations in first-degree familial and sporadic inflammatory bowel disease: a case-control study. *Inflamm Bowel Dis*, Vol 10, No. 3, (May 2004), pp. 207-214.

[3] Das KM. (1999). Relationship of extraintestinal involvements in inflammatory bowel disease: new insights into autoimmune pathogenesis. *Dig Dis Sci.* Vol 44, pp. 1-13.

[4] Uslu N (2007). Acute tubular injury associated with mesalazine therapy in an adolescent girl with inflammatory bowel disease. *Dig Dis Sci.* Vol 52, pp. 2926-2929.

[5] Arend LJ (2004). Interstitial nephritis from mesalazine: case report and literature review. *Pediatr Nephrol.* Vol 19, No. 5, (May 2004), pp. :550-553.

[6] Azad Khan AK (1977). An experiment to determine the active therapeutic moiety of sulphasalazine. *Lancet.*Vol 29, No. 2, (October 1977), pp. 892-895.

[7] Corrigan G (2000). Review article: interstitial nephritis associated with the use of mesalazine in inflammatory bowel disease. *Aliment Pharmacol Ther.* Vol. 14, No. 1, (January 2000), pp. 1- 6.

[8] Loftus EV (2004). Systematic review: short-term adverse effects of 5-aminosalicylic acid agents in the treatment of ulcerative colitis. *Aliment Pharmacol Ther.* Vol.19, No. 2, (January 2004), pp. 179 -189.

[9] Calder IC (1972). Nephrotoxic lesions from 5-aminosalicylic acid. *BMJ.Vol. 15, No. 1,* (Jan 1972), pp. 52-54.

[10] Bilyard KG (1990). Mesalazine: an overview of key preclinical studies. *Scand J Gastroenterol Suppl.* Vol. 172, pp. 52-55.

[11] Elseviers MM (2004). Renal impairment in patients with inflammatory bowel disease: association with aminosalicylate therapy? *Clin Nephrol.* Vol. 61, No. 2, (February 2004), pp. 83- 89.

[12] Van Staa TP (2004). 5-Aminosalicylic acids and the risk of renal disease: a large British epidemiologic study.*Gastroenterology.* Vol. 126, No. 7, (June 2004), pp.1733-1739.

[13] Fraser JS (2001). Renal tubular injury is present in acute inflammatory bowel disease prior to the introduction of drug therapy. *Aliment Pharmacol Ther.* Vol.15, No. 8, (August 2001), pp. 1131-1137.

[14] Schreiber S (1997). Renal tubular dysfunction in patients with inflammatory bowel disease treated with aminosalicylate. *Gut.* Vol. 40, No. 6, (June 1997), pp. 761-766.

[15] Riley SA (1992). Tests of renal function in patients with quiescent colitis: effects of drug treatment. *Gut.* Vol. 33, No. 10, (October 1992), pp. 1348-1352.

[16] Birketvedt GS (2000). Glomerular and tubular renal functions after long-term medication of sulphasalazine, olsalazine, and mesalazine in patients with ulcerative colitis. *Inflamm Bowel Dis.* Vol. 6, No. 4, (November 2000), pp. 275-279.

[17] Ransford RA (2002). Sulphasalazine and mesalazine: serious adverse reactions re-evaluated on the basis of suspected adverse reaction reports to the Committee on Safety of Medicines. *Gut.* Vol. 51, No. 4, (October 2002), pp. 536-539.

[18] Cambridge G (1992). Antineutrophil antibodies in inflammatory bowel disease: prevalance and diagnostic role. *Gut.* Vol. 33, No. 5, (May 1992), pp. 668-674.

[19] Rosa M (1996). Does the presence of ANCA in patients with ulcerative colitis necessarily imply renal involvement? *Nephrol Dial Transplant.* Vol.11, No. 12, (December 1996), pp. 2426-2429.

[20] Monsen U (1990). Extracolonic diagnoses in ulcerative colitis: An epidemiological study. *Am J Gastroenterol.* Vol. 85, No. 6, (June 1990), pp. 711-716.

[21] Trimarchia HM (2001). Immunoglobulin A Nephropathy and Ulcerative Colitis. *Am J Nephrol*. Vol. 21, No. 5, (September 2001), pp. 400-405.

[22] Dard S (1983). A new association: Ankylosing spondylitis and Berger's disease. *Kidney Int*. Vol. 24, (August 1983), pp129.

[23] Bruneau C (1986). Seronegative spondyloarthropathies and IgA glomerulonephritis: A report of four cases and a review of the literature. *Semin Arthritis Rheum* Vol. 15, No. 3. (February 1986), pp. 179-184.

[24] Imasawa T (1999). Bone marrow transplantation attenuates murine IgA nephropathy: Role of a stem cell disorder. *Kidney Int*. Vol. 56, No. 5, (November 1999), pp. 1809-1817.

[25] Noris M (1999). IgA nephropathy: A stem cell disease? *Kidney Int*. Vol. 56, No. 5, (November 1999), pp. 1964-1966.

[26] Van den Wall Bake A (1989). Elevated production of polymeric and monomeric IgA1 by the bone marrow in IgA nephropathy. *Kidney Int* . Vol. 35, No. 6, (June 1989), pp. 1400-1404.

[27] Van Es L (1992). Pathogenesis of IgA nephropathy. *Kidney Int*. Vol. 41, No. 6, (June 1992), pp. 1720-1729.

[28] Scott M (1986). Spontaneous secretion of IgG subclasses by intestinal mononuclear cells: Differences between ulcerative colitis, Crohn's disease and control subjects. *Clin Exp Immunol*. Vol. 66, No. 1, (October 1986), pp. 209-216.

[29] Kett K (1987). Mucosal subclass distribution of immunoglobulin G-producing cells is different in ulcerative colitis and Crohn's disease of the colon. *Gastroenterology*. Vol. 93, pp. 919-924.

[30] Tokuyama H (2010). Acute interstitial nephritis associated with ulcerative colitis. *Clin Exp Nephrol*. Vol.14, No. 5, (October 2010), pp. 483-6.

[31] Popoola J (1998). Late onset interstitial nephritis associated with mesalazine treatment. *Brit Med J*. Vol. 317, (September 1998), pp. 795-797.

[32] Gisbert JP (2007). 5-Aminosalicylates and renal function in inflammatory bowel disease: a systematic review. *Inflamm Bowel Dis*. Vol. 13, No. 5, (May 2007), pp. 629-638.

[33] Wilcox GM (1990). Glomerulonephritis associated with inflammatory bowel disease. Report of a patient with chronic ulcerative colitis, sclerosing cholangitis, and acute glomerulonephritis. *Gastroenterology*. Vol. 98, No. 3, (March 1990), pp. 786-791.

[34] Ridder RM (2005). Membranous nephropathy associated with familial chronic ulcerative colitis in a 12-year-old girl. *Pediatr Nephrol*. Vol. 20, No. 9, (September 2005), pp. 1349-1351.

[35] Nand N (1991). Nephrotic syndrome in ulcerative colitis. *Nephrol Dial Transplant*. Vol.6, No. 3, pp.227.

[36] Khosroshahi HT (2006). Tubulointerstitial disease and ulcerative colitis. *Nephrol Dial Transplant*. Vol. 21, No. 8, (August 2006), pp. 2340.

[37] Kreisek W (1996). Renal tubular damage: an extraintestinal manifestation of chronic inflammatory bowel disease. *Eur J Gastroenterol Hepatol*. Vol. 8, No. 5, (May 1996), pp. 461-468.

[38] Herrlinger KR (2001). Minimal renal dysfunction in inflammatory bowel disease is related to disease activity but not to 5-ASA use. *Aliment Pharmacol Ther.* Vol.15, No. 3, (March 2001), pp.:363-369.

Permissions

The contributors of this book come from diverse backgrounds, making this book a truly international effort. This book will bring forth new frontiers with its revolutionizing research information and detailed analysis of the nascent developments around the world.

We would like to thank Mortimer B. O'Connor, for lending his expertise to make the book truly unique. He has played a crucial role in the development of this book. Without his invaluable contribution this book wouldn't have been possible. He has made vital efforts to compile up to date information on the varied aspects of this subject to make this book a valuable addition to the collection of many professionals and students.

This book was conceptualized with the vision of imparting up-to-date information and advanced data in this field. To ensure the same, a matchless editorial board was set up. Every individual on the board went through rigorous rounds of assessment to prove their worth. After which they invested a large part of their time researching and compiling the most relevant data for our readers. Conferences and sessions were held from time to time between the editorial board and the contributing authors to present the data in the most comprehensible form. The editorial team has worked tirelessly to provide valuable and valid information to help people across the globe.

Every chapter published in this book has been scrutinized by our experts. Their significance has been extensively debated. The topics covered herein carry significant findings which will fuel the growth of the discipline. They may even be implemented as practical applications or may be referred to as a beginning point for another development. Chapters in this book were first published by InTech; hereby published with permission under the Creative Commons Attribution License or equivalent.

The editorial board has been involved in producing this book since its inception. They have spent rigorous hours researching and exploring the diverse topics which have resulted in the successful publishing of this book. They have passed on their knowledge of decades through this book. To expedite this challenging task, the publisher supported the team at every step. A small team of assistant editors was also appointed to further simplify the editing procedure and attain best results for the readers.

Our editorial team has been hand-picked from every corner of the world. Their multi-ethnicity adds dynamic inputs to the discussions which result in innovative outcomes. These outcomes are then further discussed with the researchers and contributors who give their valuable feedback and opinion regarding the same. The feedback is then collaborated with the researches and they are edited in a comprehensive manner to aid the understanding of the subject.

Apart from the editorial board, the designing team has also invested a significant amount of their time in understanding the subject and creating the most relevant covers. They scrutinized every image to scout for the most suitable representation of the subject and create an appropriate cover for the book.

The publishing team has been involved in this book since its early stages. They were actively engaged in every process, be it collecting the data, connecting with the contributors or procuring relevant information. The team has been an ardent support to the editorial, designing and production team. Their endless efforts to recruit the best for this project, has resulted in the accomplishment of this book. They are a veteran in the field of academics and their pool of knowledge is as vast as their experience in printing. Their expertise and guidance has proved useful at every step. Their uncompromising quality standards have made this book an exceptional effort. Their encouragement from time to time has been an inspiration for everyone.

The publisher and the editorial board hope that this book will prove to be a valuable piece of knowledge for researchers, students, practitioners and scholars across the globe.

List of Contributors

Iftikhar Ahmed
Department of Gastroenterology, University of Bristol / North Bristol NHS Trust, Bristol, UK

Zafar Niaz
Mayo Hospital / King Edward Medical University Lahore, Pakistan

Manae S. Kurokawa, Takuya Yoshioka and Tomohiro Kato
Clinical Proteomics and Molecular Medicine, St. Marianna University Graduate School of Medicine, Japan

Moriaki Hatsugai, Yohei Noguchi and Hiroshi Yasuda
Division of Gastroenterology and Hepatology, Department of Internal Medicine, St. Marianna University School of Medicine, Japan

Hiroyuki Mitsui
Department of Orthopaedic Surgery, St. Marianna University School of Medicine, Kawasaki, Japan

Yutao Yan
Emory University, Atlanta, Georgia, USA

Zhanju Liu
Department of Gastroenterology, The Shanghai Tenth People's Hospital, Tongji University, Shanghai, China

Yurong Yang
College of Animal and Veterinary Engineering, Henan Agricultural University, Zhengzhou, China

Hiroshi Nakase, Minoru Matsuura, Sakae Mikami and Tsutomu Chiba
Department of Gastroenterology and Hepatology, Graduate School of Medicine, Kyoto University, Japan

Carla Cirillo, Giovanni Sarnelli and Rosario Cuomo
University of Naples "Federico II", Italy

Ramesh P. Arasaradnam and Chuka U. Nwokolo
Department of Gastroenterology, University Hospital Coventry & Warwickshire, Coventry, United Kingdom

Ramesh P. Arasaradnam
Clinical Sciences Research Institute, University of Warwick, Coventry, United Kingdom

Kenji Suzuki
Department of Medicine III, Niigata University Medical and Dental Hospital, Japan

Hiroyuki Yoneyama
Stelic Institute of Regenerative Medicine, Stelic Institute & Co., Japan

Hitoshi Asakura
The Koukann Clinics, Japan

Gino Caselli Morgado and George Pinedo Mancilla
Unit of Colorectal Surgery, Department of Digestive Surgery, Pontifical Catholic University of Chile, Santiago, Chile

Brian Huang, Lola Y. Kwan and David Q. Shih
Cedars Sinai Medical Center, Inflammatory Bowel and Immunobiology Institute (IB), USA

Antoni Stadnicki
Department of Basis Biomedical Sciences, Medical University of Silesia, Katowice, Poland
Section of Gastroenterology, District Hospital, Jaworzno, Poland

Gulbanu Erkan
Ufuk University Faculty of Medicine, Department of İnternal Medicine, Division of Gastroenterology, Turkey

Joel Pekow and Marc Bissonnette
Department of Medicine, Section of Gastroenterology, University of Chicago, USA

Nilgün Yılmaz Demirci
Ataturk Chest Disease and Chest Surgery Training and Research Hospital, Pulmonary Medicine Department, Ankara, Turkey

Isao Okayasu, Tsutomu Yoshida, Tetuo Mikami, Jun Mitsuhashi, Masaaki Ichinoe, Nobuyuki Yanagisawa, Wataru Tokuyama, Kiyomi Hana and Yuichi Ishibashi
Department of Pathology, Kitasato University School of Medicine, Sagamihara, Kanagawa, Japan

Hirobumi Tokuyama, Shu Wakino, Koichi Hayashi and Hiroshi Itoh
Department of Internal Medicine, School of Medicine, Keio University, Tokyo, Japan

Printed in the USA
CPSIA information can be obtained
at www.ICGtesting.com
JSHW011458221024
72173JS00005B/1119